Applying
Nursing Process

PROMOTING COLLABORATIVE CARE

Author Info

Rosalinda Alfaro-LeFevre, MSN, RN, is president of Teaching Smart/Learning Easy in Stuart, Florida. A recipient of a *1998–1999 Sigma Theta Tau Best Pick Award* for nursing books, she is an established and successful author who is known for making difficult topics easy to understand. Her work has been translated into five languages. She has over 20 years of clinical practice and teaching experience in both baccalaureate and associate degree nursing programs and has a wealth of nursing expertise to draw upon, whether writing, consulting, or leading seminars.

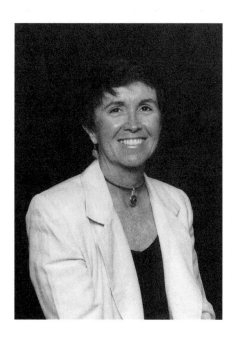

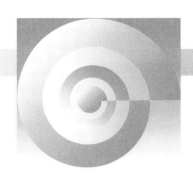

5TH EDITION

Applying
Nursing Process

PROMOTING COLLABORATIVE CARE

Rosalinda Alfaro-LeFevre, MSN, RN
President
Teaching Smart/Learning Easy
Stuart, Florida

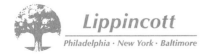
Lippincott
Philadelphia · New York · Baltimore

Acquisitions Editor: Ilze Rader
Managing Editor: Hilarie Surrena
Editorial Assistant: Jeanettie Hill
Production Editor: Debra Schiff
Senior Production Manager: Helen Ewan
Art Director: Carolyn O'Brien

Cover Design: Melissa Walters
Manufacturing Manager: William Alberti
Indexer: Lynne McCabe
Compositor: Peirce Graphic Services, Inc.
Printer: RR Donnelley

Edition 5

9 8 7 6 5 4 3 2

Library of Congress Cataloging-in-Publication Data
Alfaro-LeFevre, Rosalinda.
    Applying nursing process : promoting collaborative care / Rosalinda Alfaro-LeFevre. — 5th ed.
        p. ; cm.
    Includes bibliographical references and index.
    ISBN 0-7817-3140-2 (alk. paper)
    1. Nursing—Handbooks, manuals, etc. I. Title: Nursing process. II. Title.
    [DNLM: 1. Nursing Process. WY 100 A385a 2002]
RT51 .A6255 2002
610.73—dc21
                                                        2001037741

Care has been taken to confirm the accuracy of the information presented and to describe generally accepted practices. However, the authors, editors, and publisher are not responsible for errors or omissions or for any consequences from application of the information in this book and make no warranty, express or implied, with respect to the content of the publication.

The authors, editors, and publisher have exerted every effort to ensure that drug selection and dosage set forth in this text are in accordance with the current recommendations and practice at the time of publication. However, in view of ongoing research, changes in government regulations, and the constant flow of information relating to drug therapy and drug reactions, the reader is urged to check the package insert for each drug for any change in indications and dosage and for added warnings and precautions. This is particularly important when the recommended agent is a new or infrequently employed drug.

Some drugs and medical devices presented in this publication have Food and Drug Administration (FDA) clearance for limited use in restricted research settings. It is the responsibility of the health care provider to ascertain the FDA status of each drug or device planned for use in his or her clinical practice.

Dedication

To the nurses, physicians, staff, and patients of The Volunteers In Medicine Clinic, Stuart, FL. You inspire me in every way!

The Volunteers in Medicine Clinic is almost completely staffed by volunteer physicians, nurses, and helpers. The clinic's purpose is to meet the needs of people unable to afford basic health care services. A portion of the royalties from this book is donated to the clinic.

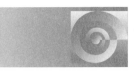# Advisors and Reviewers

A note of thanks: Without the timely and insightful reviews and advice of the experts listed on these pages, this book would not have been possible. The author wishes to also acknowledge the translators of previous editions: Aiko Emoto (Japanese), Maria Teresa Luis (Spanish), and Maria Augusta Soares, Miriam de Abreu Almeida, and Valéria Giordami Araújo (Portuguese).

USA

Elizabeth A. Ayello, PhD, RN, CS, CWOCN
Clinical Assistant Professor
New York University
New York, NY

Ledjie Ballard, CRNA, MSN
Affiliate Clinical Faculty
University of Washington
Seattle, WA

Joyce C. Begley, MSN, MA, RN
Assistant Professor of Nursing
Department of Baccalaureate and Graduate Nursing
Eastern Kentucky University
Richmond, KY

Suzanne C. Beyea, RN, PhD
Director of Research
Association of Operating Room Nurses
Denver, CO

Lynda Juall Carpenito, RN, MSN, FNPC
President
LJC Consultants
Mickleton, NJ
Family Nurse Practitioner
Ches-Penn Community Health Center
Chester, PA

Carol Ann Coltrin
Associate Professor
Ventura College
Ventura, CA

Judy Cummings, RNC, MS
Nursing Faculty
Yavapai College
Prescott, AZ

Jane Cunneen, MSN, RN, CCRN
Critical Care Clinical Nurse Specialist
Clarian Health, Methodist Hospital
Indianapolis, IN

Pam Di Vito-Thomas, RN, MS, PhD (c)
Nursing Faculty
Anna Vaughn School of Nursing
Oral Roberts University
Tulsa, OK

Bonnie Eyeler, MSN, RN, JD
Boca Raton, FL

Pauline McKinney Green, PhD, RN
Associate Professor
Howard University
College of Pharmacy, Nursing and Allied Health Sciences
Washington, DC

Elizabeth E. Hand, MS, BSN, RNII, CCRN
Adult Critical Care Clinical Instructor
St. John Medical Center
Adjunct Faculty
Oral Roberts University
Tulsa, OK

Ruth I. Hansten, FACHE, PhD (c), MBA, BSN
Principal, Hansten and Washburn
Bainbridge Island, WA

Esther Halvorson-Hill, RN, MN, MPA
Associate Professor
School of Nursing
Oregon Health Sciences University
Administrator
Halvorson-Hill Enterprises
Ashland, OR

Millie Hill, MSN, RN
Clinical Nurse Educator
Staff Development
Patient Education
Paoli Memorial Hospital
Paoli, PA

Carol Hutton, EdD, ARNP
President, Hutton Associates
Boca Raton, FL

Marilynn Jackson, PhD (c)
Principal, Hansten & Washburn
Tyler, TX

Sharon Johnson, MSN, RNC, CNA
Director
Jefferson Home Health/Main Line Hospitals
Bryn Mawr, PA

Ann E. J. Kobs
President/CEO
Type 1 Solutions, Inc
Cape Coral, FL

Debra Konicek, RN, BSN, BC
SNOMED Research Analyst
College of American Pathologists
Northfield, IL

Anita G. Kinser, MSN, RNC
Assistant Professor, Nursing
Riverside Community College
Riverside, CA

Heidi Pape Laird, BA, MLA, Cert Ed
Programmer
Highland Laboratories, Inc.
Ashland, MA

Karol Burkhart Lindow, RN, C, MSN
Associate Professor, Nursing
Kent State University, Tuscarawas Campus
New Philadelphia, OH

Cindy Ling, RN, MN, CCM
Case Manager
Santa Clara Valley Health and Hospital Systems
San Jose, CA

Linda McIntosh Liptok, RN, CS, BMus, MSN
Assistant Professor of Nursing
Kent State University, Tuscarawas Campus
New Philadelphia, OH

Jody M. Masterson, RN, MSN, CRRN
Adjunct Professor, College of Nursing
Villanova University
Villanova, PA

Carol R. Matz, MSN, RN
Retired Faculty
West Chester University
West Chester, PA

Barbara A. Musinski, RN, C, BS
Health Science Education Coordinator
Boca Raton Community High School
Boca Raton, FL

Terri Patterson, RN, MSN, CRRN
President
Nursing Consultation Services LTD and LifeTrak LTD
Norristown, PA

Josy Petr, MS, RN
Lecturer
Indiana University School of Nursing
Northwest Campus
Gary, IN

Joan P. Roache, MS, RN, CCRN
University of Massachusetts, Amherst
Amherst, MA

Mary Smathers-Himenez, RN, MSN
Assistant Professor of Nursing
Coastal Georgia Community College
Brunswick, GA

Terrie Snow, RN, MSN
Instructor, Nursing Department
Shasta College
Redding, CA

Melanie Sophocles
Nursing Student
Barry University
Miami, FL

Cindy Warren, MSN, RN
Kent State University, Tuscarawas Campus
College of Nursing
New Philadelphia, OH

Ervena Weingartner, MN, RN, CPNP
Professor
University of Cincinnati, Raymond Walters College
Cincinnati, OH

Mary Weisel
IVY Tech State College
South Bend, IN

Toni C. Wortham, RN, BSN, MSN
Professor
Madisonville Community College, Health Campus
Madisonville, KY

International

Cecile Boisvert, RN, MScN
Consultant–Educator in Nursing
Lecturer University of Paris (Bobigny)
International liaison on AFEDIR Board (Association Fran
cophone Europeenne des Diagnostics, Interventions et
Resultats des Soins Infirmiers)
St Aubin, France

Christian Bolan, Med, RN
Centre for Nursing Studies
Instructor II (Faculty)
St. John's, New Foundland, Canada

Veronica Broughton, RN, RM, MEdSt, FRCNA
Lecturer, School of Nursing and Midwifery
University of South Australia
Adelaide, South Australia, Australia

Emilia Campos de Carvalho, RN, PhD
Dean, University of São Paulo
Ribeirão College of Nursing
WHO Collaborating Centre for Nursing Research
Development
São Paulo, Brazil

Judy Boychuk Duchscher, RN, BScN, FCCM, MN
Faculty
Nursing Education Program of
Saskatchewan
SIAST Kelsey Campus
Saskatoon, Saskatchewan, Canada

Kaoru Fujisaki, RN
St.Luck's College of Nursing,
Doctoral (c)
Kobe, Japan

Maria Teresa Luis
Professora d'Infermeria Medicoquirúrgica
Campus de Bellvitge
Hospitalet del Llobregat
Barcelona, Spain

Judith Manning
Clinical Skills Coordinator
Clinical Education Development Unit
North Western Adelaide Health Service
Adelaide, South Australia, Australia

Jeanne Liliane Marlene Michel, RN, MSN
Assistant Professor, Department of Nursing
Technical-administrative Coordinator, Nursing
Universidade Federal de São Paulo
Direction, Hospital
São Paulo, Brazil

Nico Oud, RN, MNSc, Dipl.N.Adm
Consultant and Trainer of Aggression Management
Connecting
Amsterdam, The Netherlands

Ann Paterson, RN, BApp Sci, MA
Senior Lecturer in Nursing
Department of Nursing and Midwifery
RMIT University
Bundoora, VIC, Australia

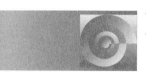

Preface

Nursing Process and Critical Thinking

In both practice and education, experts agree that applying the nursing process provides the foundation for the critical thinking skills required to function in a safe and effective way. Today's world of predetermined treatment plans doesn't replace the need for knowledge of nursing process. Rather, meeting standards and thinking independently and proactively to ensure competent, individualized care require thinking habits gained from application of principles and rules of nursing process.

In education, students have additional motivation for mastering the nursing process — state board exams are based on its use. To be able to think their way through the test that gives them the right to practice nursing, students must be thoroughly familiar with nursing process principles. For these reasons, this book aims to give a sound, reality-based guide that provides the basis for applying nursing process to think critically in today's fast-paced clinical setting.

What's New About This Edition

The title has been changed from the previous edition, which received a *1998–1999 Sigma Theta Tau Best Pick Award,* to reflect how the nursing process has changed to a more dynamic model that promotes collaborative approaches to improve outcomes.

New content and features include:

- A streamlined and revised description of the nursing process to reflect a more dynamic, less linear approach
- More on how the shift in thinking from *diagnose and treat* to *predict, prevent, and manage* requires nurses to be proactive, focusing on identifying risk factors, screening for common health problems, and predicting potential complications, as well as treating actual problems
- Detailed guidelines on how to develop (or adapt) specific outcomes and corresponding indicators to help you plan, give, and evaluate care
- Nurses' responsibilities related to preventing errors and improving consumer satisfaction by promoting empowered partnerships with patients and families
- Succinct, practical information on the use and misuse of standard nursing languages such as North American Nursing Diagnosis Association (NANDA), Nursing Intervention Classification (NIC), and Nursing Outcome Classification (NOC)

- More on such things as:
  - ○ Nurses' roles in homes, communities, and multidisciplinary practice
  - ○ The use of critical pathways and computers
  - ○ How nurses' roles as diagnosticians and case managers continue to evolve
  - ○ Cultural and spiritual aspects of nursing care
- *Voices* (quotes from nurses that are either inspirational or exemplary of current best practices) are placed throughout to illustrate key points. (*Think About It* displays, retained from the previous edition, provide "food for thought" from the author to stimulate thinking and reinforce content.)

What's the Same About This Edition

The overall goal continues to be to give a clear, concise presentation of the nursing process, using lots of examples to make content relevant and easy to understand. Great pains have been taken to make this a user-friendly book that helps you to move around the text as you please, reading what's most interesting first. Elements that promote critical thinking and enhance motivation to learn are integrated throughout (see page xiv).

Principles and rules that provide a basis for making decisions and adapting to the constant changes in health care are highlighted throughout. To help you master and apply content, you'll find critical thinking exercises placed at strategic places in the reading. Previously called *Practice Sessions,* they have been renamed *Critical Thinking Exercises* to reenforce that they are meant to stimulate thinking, rather than provide rote practice. Example responses for these exercises are found beginning on page 243.

The *Nursing Diagnosis Quick Reference Section* (beginning on page 203) provides easy access to information on diagnoses accepted for clinical testing by the NANDA. You can also find a comprehensive list of the latest terms from NIC and NOC on pages 255–262.

Key concepts include:

- The role of knowledge, skills, and caring in demonstrating nursing process expertise (see page 22)
- The importance of mastering communication, interpersonal, and critical thinking skills
- The importance of making changes early, based on assessment and reassessment, during *Implementation,* rather than waiting for a formal evaluation period
- The significance of ethical and legal implications
- The impact of cost-containment and insurance requirements

A Word About "Patient/Client" and "He/She"

Whenever possible, I've used a fictitious name, or "someone," "person," "consumer," or "individual" instead of "client" or "patient" to help us keep in mind that each client or patient is an individual who has unique needs, values, perceptions, and motivations. "He" and "she" are used interchangeably to avoid the awkwardness of using he/she over and over.

Comments and Suggestions Welcomed

I welcome and appreciate suggestions for improvement—often the most significant changes are made based on student and faculty suggestions.

Rosalinda Alfaro-LeFevre, MSN, RN
Email: *rozalfaro@aol.com*

Elements Used to Promote Critical Thinking and Enhance Motivation to Learn

1. Learning outcomes written at the cognitive level of analysis precede each chapter.
2. Advance organizers and chapter overviews precede content.
3. Relevant terms are defined in the glossary, and more difficult terms are clarified in the text by definition, discussion, and use within context.
4. Illustrations are placed throughout to establish relationships and clarify text.
5. Analogies, examples, and case studies are used to clarify information and demonstrate relevance of content.
6. Rationales are highlighted in guidelines and displays and integrated as needed in other parts of the text.
7. Questioning at the analysis level is used:
   - During content presentation to stimulate curiosity and give clues to what's important.
   - After the content (in Critical Thinking Exercises) to reinforce key points and provide the opportunity to test and refine knowledge.
8. Content is presented in such a way that those who need structure have it, without restricting those who require more creative freedom.
9. "Try This on Your Own" sessions are offered to allow for practice without concern about being evaluated by others.
10. Summaries are listed at the end of each chapter.

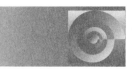# Acknowledgments

I want to thank my husband, Jim, for his love, support, and sense of humor and fun; and the rest of my family for being behind me all the way.

I also want to thank the following people for their belief in me and their contribution to my personal and professional growth: Louise and Nat Rochester, Heidi Laird, Ledjie Ballard, Annette Sophocles, Carol Taylor, Terry Valiga, Barbara Cohen, Lynda Carpenito, Mary Jo Boyer, John Payne, Charlie and Nancy Lindsay, Becky Resh, Diane Verity, Nancy Flynn, Carol Hutton, Bonnie Eyler, the Villanova University Nursing Faculty, Frank and Grace Nola, Chuck and Pat Morgan, and the past and present nurses at Paoli Memorial Hospital.

My special thanks go to the Nursing Editorial division of Lippincott Williams & Wilkins, especially to Ilze Rader, Senior Acquisitions Editor; Hilarie Surrena, Managing Editor; Jeanettie Hill, Editorial Assistant; Jane Velker, Manager of Development; and Debra Schiff, Production Editor, who stay focused on the details of this project, even when their desks are full of other priorities; and, of course, the sales and marketing department whose efforts have helped make this book a bestseller.

Contents

CHAPTER *3*

Diagnosis
78

CHAPTER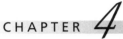

Planning
122

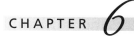

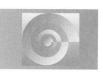

Critical Thinking Exercises

Nursing Process Overview

LEARNING OUTCOMES

After mastering the content in this chapter, you should be able to:

- Explain how the nursing process provides a dynamic way to promote critical thinking.
- Give three examples of how nurses can prove their value to consumers and employers.
- List four benefits of using the nursing process.
- Discuss how focusing on nursing process complements the focus of other health care professionals' treatment approaches.
- Describe three qualities required to be competent in using the nursing process.
- Name seven ethical principles and address how to apply them to advocating for client rights.
- Describe critical thinking in nursing using your own terms.
- Determine five critical thinking characteristics you want to acquire or improve.
- Identify behaviors that promote positive interpersonal relationships.
- Explain what it takes to be willing and able to care.

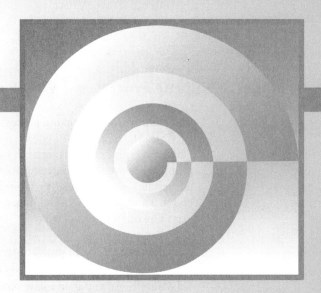

Critical Thinking Exercises

■ **Critical Thinking Exercise I:** Nursing Process in a Changing World

■ **Critical Thinking Exercise II:** Knowledge, Skills, and Willingness and Ability to Care

What's in this chapter?

This chapter defines nursing process and addresses the question, "Why learn about it?" It then presents a short overview of each step of the nursing process and explains how it provides a dynamic way to promote critical thinking in today's changing world. Recognizing the importance of protecting and advocating for client rights, it addresses seven major ethical principles that are central to giving humanistic care. Finally, it focuses on what it takes to be competent using the nursing process (knowledge, skills, and caring), and gives suggestions for how to develop critical thinking skills.

What Is the Nursing Process and Why Learn About It?

What is it? The nursing process—which consists of five interrelated steps, *Assessment, Diagnosis, Planning, Implementation, and Evaluation*—is a systematic, dynamic way of giving nursing care. Central to all nursing approaches, the nursing process promotes humanistic, outcome-focused (results-focused), cost-effective care. It also pushes nurses to continually examine what they're doing and to study how it can be done better. Think about the following, more detailed, description.

The nursing process is:

- **Systematic.** Like the problem-solving method, it consists of five steps during which you take deliberate steps to maximize efficiency and attain long-term beneficial results.
- **Dynamic.** As you gain more experience, you'll find yourself moving back and forth between the steps, sometimes combining activities, yet still getting the same end result. For example, new nurses often need to methodically assess a patient for quite some time before coming to a diagnosis, whereas experienced nurses often immediately suspect a diagnosis, then assess the patient more closely to see if they are correct.
- **Humanistic.** It's based on the belief that as we plan and deliver care, we must consider the unique interests, values, and desires of the consumer (person, family, and community). As nurses, we deal with the body, mind, and spirit. We strive to understand each individual's health problems and the corresponding impact on one's sense of well-being and ability to do daily activities.
- **Outcome-focused (results-oriented).** The steps of the nursing process are designed to keep the focus on determining whether people seeking health care are getting the best results in the most efficient way. The specific documentation requirements provide key data that can be studied to improve results for other patients in the similar situations.

Why Learn About it? Practice standards in both the United States and Canada mandate the use of the nursing process (see page 249 in the Appendix). The nursing process provides the basis for state board examinations—you need to be thoroughly familiar with it to think your way through the questions. We continue to become more dependent on computers and standard plans—to be able use the information they provide in a safe way, you *must* master the principles behind the nursing process. Only then can you become the thought-oriented, rather than task-oriented, nurse you must be in today's world. Only then will you be able to think critically about how to achieve the ultimate aims of nursing—to:

- Prevent illness and promote, maintain, or restore health (in terminal illness, to control symptoms and promote comfort and well-being until death)
- Maximize sense of well-being and ability to function in desired roles
- Provide cost-effective, efficient care that pays attention to individual wants and needs
- Find ways to improve consumer satisfaction with health care delivery

Steps of the Nursing Process[1]

Here's a brief description of what you do during each step of nursing process:

1. *Assessment.* You collect and examine information about health status, looking for evidence of abnormal function or risk factors that may contribute to health problems (eg, smoking). You also look for evidence of client strengths (eg, desire to learn).

2. *Diagnosis (Problem Identification).* You analyze the data and identify actual and potential problems, which are the basis for the plan of care. You also identify strengths, which are essential to developing an efficient plan.

3. *Planning.* Here, you do four key things:
   - **Determine immediate priorities:** Which problems need immediate attention? Which ones can wait? Which ones will nursing focus on? Which ones will you delegate or refer to someone else? Which ones require a multidisciplinary approach?
   - **Establish expected outcomes (expected results):** Exactly how will the person benefit from nursing care (what will the patient be able to do and in what time frame)?
   - **Determine interventions:** What interventions (nursing actions) will you prescribe to prevent or manage the problems and achieve the outcomes?
   - **Record or individualize the plan of care.** Will you write your own plan, or will you adapt a standard or computerized plan to meet your patient's specific situation?

4. *Implementation.* Put the plan into action—but don't just *act*. Think about it and reflect on what you're doing:
   - **Assess the person's current status before acting.** Are there any new problems? Has anything happened that requires an immediate change in the plan?
   - **Perform interventions and reassess to determine initial responses.** What's the response? Do you need to change something? Don't wait until the "formal" evaluation period to make changes if something needs changing today.
   - **Report and record.** Are there any signs you must report immediately? What are you going to chart and where and how are you going to chart it?

5. *Evaluation.* Has the person achieved the expected outcomes?
   - **How does the person's health status and ability to function compare with the expected outcomes?** Is he able to do what you expected? If not, why? Has something changed? Are you missing something? Are there new care priorities?
   - **If he achieved the outcomes, is the person ready to manage his care on his own?** Do you need to make referrals for health promotion or support? What made the plan work? What could have been done to make things easier?

---

[1]Throughout this book, *medical problem* refers to diseases or trauma diagnosed by primary care providers: physicians, physician's assistants, or advanced practice nurses (APNs). APNs have a wide scope of authority to act (may include treating some medical problems and prescribing some medications) by virtue of advanced credentials (usually completion of a master's program and certification). The term *medical order* refers to interventions prescribed by primary care providers to treat medical problems.

Keep in mind that the accuracy of all of these steps depends on factual, relevant, and comprehensive patient information. Study Table 1–1, which summarizes the steps of the nursing process and compares them with those of the familiar problem-solving method. Notice how the problem-solving method begins with *encountering a problem*, whereas the nursing process is more proactive, stressing *continuous assessment for risk factors* for problems.

Think About It

The Power of Partnerships. *Each patient and family holds the key to effective nursing care. When you establish partnerships through mutual trust and provide information and encourage people to take an active role in their plan of care, you empower them to maximize health and open the door to patient satisfaction and health care efficiency.*

Developing partnerships requires you to move from an I'll-take-care-of-you approach to one that asks, "How can I empower you to be independent?" Assume that patients know themselves well. Think about the power of statements like, "You know yourself best—tell me what you'd like to see happen," "What's most important to you?" and "I want you to be able to make informed choices—we share a common purpose and we're both responsible for what happens."

TABLE 1–1 Nursing Process Versus Problem-Solving Method	
Nursing Process	**Problem-Solving Method**
Assessment: Continuously collecting data about health status to monitor for evidence of health problems and risk factors that may contribute to health problems (eg, smoking).	**Encountering a problem:** Collecting data about the problem.
Diagnosis: Analyzing data to clearly identify actual and potential health problems and strengths.	**Analyzing data** to determine exactly what the problem is.
Planning: Determining desired outcomes (specific goals) and identifying interventions to achieve the outcomes.	**Making a plan** of action.
Implementation: Putting the plan into action and observing initial responses.	**Putting the plan into action.**
Evaluation: Determining how well the outcomes have been achieved and deciding whether changes need to be made.	**Evaluating the results.**

Relationships Among the Steps of the Nursing Process

To get a beginning idea of why we view the nursing process as being dynamic, it's important to remember that the steps are overlapping and interrelated, as described below.

Assessment and Diagnosis

Assessment and *Diagnosis* overlap significantly. As you gather information, you start to interpret what the information means, even though you haven't put the whole picture together yet. For example, you might be assessing someone and notice an irregular pulse, swollen ankles, and difficulty breathing. You may begin to make a tentative diagnosis (this patient may have a heart problem) as you continue with the assessment. **But remember:** If your assessment is incomplete or inaccurate, you're likely to make mistakes in diagnosing the problems. The following diagram illustrates the close relationship between *Assessment* and *Diagnosis.*

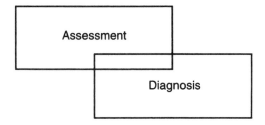

Diagnosis and Planning

Diagnosis and *Planning* are related for several reasons:

1. Accurate planning requires accurate diagnoses. If you miss problems or misunderstand them, you waste time developing a plan to solve the wrong problems. You also may allow key problems to persist or get worse because of neglect.
2. To achieve the overall desired outcome of care—that is, that the person is able to be as independent as possible—you must develop specific outcomes for each problem or diagnosis that *must* be managed to stay on track for expected discharge. Determining expected outcomes of care requires you to decide exactly what you expect to see when the diagnoses are corrected or improved. For example, if *Constipation* is major problem, an appropriate outcome might be *the person will have a soft bowel movement at least every other day.*
3. The interventions you identify during *Planning* must be designed to prevent, resolve, or control the problems identified during *Diagnosis.* For example, for *Constipation,* you'd plan interventions to promote bowel regularity (eg, teaching the need for adequate hydration, dietary roughage, and so forth).
4. There are times when you have to act quickly, implementing a mental plan of action, before identifying all the problems. For example, if you encounter a life-threatening

problem, take immediate action. Once the situation is under control, complete *Diagnosis* by analyzing all of the data in depth.

5. It's important to incorporate the strengths you identify during *Diagnosis* into the plan. For example, if you learn that someone is unable to plan meals but has relatives who are willing to help, you use the relatives as a resource (eg, teaching relatives how to include high-roughage foods in the diet).

The following diagram shows *Diagnosis* and *Planning* overlapping.

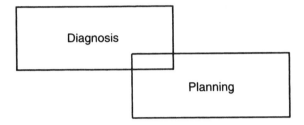

Think About It

Accurate Diagnosis Is Essential. *If you make a mistake in* Diagnosis—*if your diagnoses are inaccurate, incomplete, or vague—it's unlikely that your plan will be effective. It may even be dangerous.*

Planning and Implementation

Planning and *Implementation* are closely related and overlapping for two reasons.

1. The plan guides interventions performed during *Implementation*.

2. As you implement the plan, you may need to fine-tune the plan to get the results you want. Sometimes, you even have to go back and check whether your assessment and diagnosis information is correct. The following diagram shows *Planning and Implementation* overlapping.

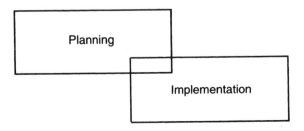

Implementation and Evaluation

Implementation and *Evaluation* overlap for an obvious reason. As the nurse, you can't be task-oriented—you must be thought-oriented, reflecting on initial responses to your actions, monitoring your patients carefully, and making changes early during *Implementation* as needed. The following diagram shows how *Implementation* and *Evaluation* overlap.

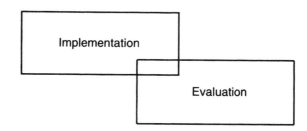

Evaluation and the Other Steps in the Nursing Process

Evaluation clearly is related to *Planning* because, assuming that your diagnoses are accurate and your outcomes are appropriate, the ultimate question to be answered during this phase is, "Have we achieved the outcomes determined during *Planning*?" However, because we can't assume that the diagnoses are accurate and outcomes are appropriate, and because we need to identify things that helped or hindered progress, *Evaluation* involves examining *all of the other steps,* as in the following illustration.

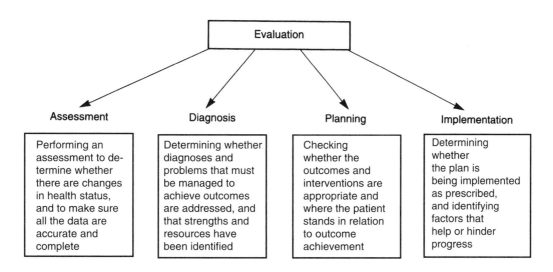

The following is a brief example of using the nursing process when caring for a specific person when the major concern is that of potential for injury.

- *Assessment:* Mr. Martin is 80 years old and lives alone. He wants to be independent and keeps an immaculate home. However, today he has a cold, is weak, and states that he is feeling very tired. Other than that, his health is unchanged.
- *Diagnosis:* You analyze the above data and realize that his fatigue puts him at risk for falls. You recognize his desire for independence is a strength, but you also know that it might be a weakness because he may not ask for help. You talk with Mr. Martin and tell him that you'd like him to have some extra help while he is ill because you're concerned that his weakness puts him at risk for simple falls, which can bring big injuries.
- *Planning:* Together with Mr. Martin, you agree on the following outcome: *Mr. Martin will be free of injury with reduced risk factors for falls.* You then develop a plan to prevent falls (eg, you arrange furniture so things are out of the way or easy to grasp for balance, you stress the importance of adequate nutrition and hydration with a cold, and you ask who might be able to come and help for a few days). You decide to monitor his blood pressure because you know that low blood pressure is a risk factor for falls.
- *Implementation:* You monitor him closely, checking vital signs, monitoring food and fluid intake, and finding out if he has help each day. Knowing of his desire for independence, you stress the importance of accepting help from others. You encourage him to keep up his strength by avoiding being in bed all day.
- *Evaluation:* You assess Mr. Martin and determine whether he is free from injury and whether the risk factors of weakness and fatigue still are present. If he has regained his strength, encourage him to continue his usual independent life style. If not, you reassess his health status and decide whether to make changes in the plan.

What Are the Benefits of Using the Nursing Process?

The nursing process complements other disciplines by focusing not only on medical problems, but also on the *human response*—how the person *responds to* medical problems, treatment plans, and changes in activities of daily life. For example, if someone has a broken leg, the physician focuses on treating the broken bones, and the physical therapist focuses on issues like promoting muscle strength and balance. You, as the nurse, focus on the whole person, for example, whether the person has pain, whether there's a risk for injury, how the person is doing with maintaining muscle strength and skin integrity, and what inconveniences are encountered by being incapacitated.

This holistic focus helps to ensure that interventions are tailored to the individual, not just the disease. Can you think what it would be like if you were hospitalized with a head laceration, a fractured arm, and a bruised kidney and everyone focused only on the medical problems? Can you imagine lying there with daily visits from a surgeon to check your head, an orthopedist to look at your arm, a urologist to check your kidney, and no one there to be concerned with how *you're* doing—to care about what *you* need and want?

Consider the following example of the difference between how a physician and nurse might analyze the same patient's data.

E X A M P L E

> **Physician's data (disease focus):** "Mrs. Garcia has pain and swelling in all joints. Diagnostic studies indicate that she has rheumatoid arthritis. We will start her on a course of anti-inflammatories to treat the rheumatoid arthritis." (*Focus is on treating the arthritis.*)
> **Nurse's data (holistic focus, considering both problems and their effect on the person's ability to function independently):** "Mrs. Garcia has pain and swelling in all joints, making it difficult to feed and dress herself. She has voiced that it's difficult to feel worthwhile when she can't even feed herself. She states that she is depressed because she misses seeing her two small grandchildren. We need to develop a plan to help her with her pain, to assist her with feeding and dressing, to work through feelings of low self-esteem, and for special visitations with the grandchildren." (*Focus is on Mrs. Garcia.*)

There are other real, tangible benefits of using the nursing process, and these are summarized in Display 1–1. Table 1–2 compares the nursing process and the medical process.

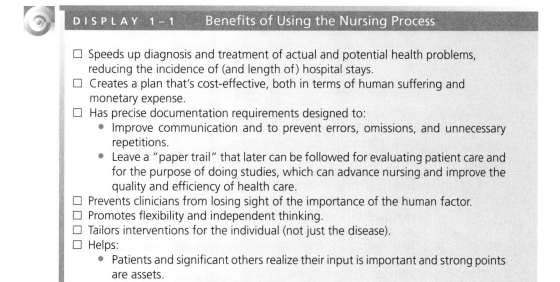

DISPLAY 1–1   Benefits of Using the Nursing Process

☐ Speeds up diagnosis and treatment of actual and potential health problems, reducing the incidence of (and length of) hospital stays.
☐ Creates a plan that's cost-effective, both in terms of human suffering and monetary expense.
☐ Has precise documentation requirements designed to:
  • Improve communication and to prevent errors, omissions, and unnecessary repetitions.
  • Leave a "paper trail" that later can be followed for evaluating patient care and for the purpose of doing studies, which can advance nursing and improve the quality and efficiency of health care.
☐ Prevents clinicians from losing sight of the importance of the human factor.
☐ Promotes flexibility and independent thinking.
☐ Tailors interventions for the individual (not just the disease).
☐ Helps:
  • Patients and significant others realize their input is important and strong points are assets.
  • Nurses have the satisfaction of getting results.

Nursing Process in Context of Today's Changing World

Understanding the nursing process requires you to think about its use in the context of today's changing world. For example, today nurses are increasingly accountable for showing how their care brings beneficial, cost-effective results (outcomes). We also have moved from a linear nursing process model—one in which we followed very specific steps to create plans "from scratch"—to a dynamic nursing process model,

TABLE 1–2 Comparison of Nursing Process and Medical Process	
Nursing Process	Medical Process
Broad, holistic approach that assesses body, mind, and spirit and aims to maximize people's ability to do activities that are important to them.	Comparatively narrow approach that assesses organs and systems and aims to keep them functioning normally.
Mainly considers how people are affected by problems with organ and system function (human responses).	Mainly considers problems with organ and system function.
Focuses on teaching how to maximize functioning and being independent.	Focuses on teaching about how diseases and trauma are treated.
Consults with medicine for treatment of diseases or trauma.	Consults with nursing for planning for activities of daily living.
Involved with individuals, their significant others, and with groups.	Mostly involved with individuals, sometimes with groups and families.

VOICES

People or Car Parts? "Never . . . has it been more important for nursing to take a holistic view of patient care than it is now . . . to maintain, in fact *insist* that the whole patient, not just bits and pieces like used-car parts, come under RNs' scientific and compassionate scrutiny and care."— *Harriet Forman, RN, EdD, CNAA*

(Forman, H. [2001]. Chop shop health care. *Nursing Spectrum, 10*[13FL], 3.)

where we adapt standard plans that already have been created for specific conditions. To reflect these changes, throughout this book, we'll approach using the nursing process from two perspectives:

1. How to create a comprehensive plan of care from beginning to finish using the five steps of *Assessment, Diagnosis, Planning, Implementation,* and *Evaluation.* Studying each of the steps in depth will help you gain the insights needed to be able to move on to using the nursing process in a more dynamic way. (The standards of the American Nurses Association [1995] address six steps, placing *Outcome Identification* between *Diagnosis* and *Planning.* For our purposes, *Outcome Identification* is addressed as a key component of Step 4, *Planning.*)

2. How to collect and analyze patient data and to adapt existing plans to make them appropriate for each unique individual.

   To give you a big picture of factors influencing the use of nursing process today, the next section gives some key points on health care delivery today.

Today's Health Care Reality

Expanding Nursing Roles. There's an increased demand for advanced practice nurses (APNs), who are prepared at the master's level and who have specialized skills to function in clinical, educational, research, and management roles. Nurse practitioners, who have advanced preparation in primary care, may function in collaboration with, or independent of, physicians, depending on state regulations. Studies demonstrate that APNs provide cost-effective outcomes, particularly for people with chronic illnesses such as diabetes and lung disease. APNs, who may be clinical nurse specialists or nurse practitioners, have advanced education in nursing science that prepares them to view patients holistically. They pay attention to the full range of human experiences, providing care beyond disease management to care of the whole person, talking to patients, spending time with them, and finding out what's important to them and gaining an understanding of the meaning of illness in their lives.

Diagnosis and Treatment: A Question of Competency and Authority. Nurses often diagnose and treat problems that once were in the medical domain, depending on competency (knowledge, skills, and credentials) and authority (what is allowed based on laws and facility policies). For example, in critical care units, nurses diagnose and treat hypertension, congestive heart failure, and numerous other problems using well-defined clinical protocols.

Highly Collaborative Practice. Patient acuity and pressure to address problems in a timely fashion require highly collaborative approaches. Some agencies require documentation of multidisciplinary team efforts in planning and giving care and in planning for discharge. Boundaries between health care professionals continue to be flexible and ever changing as nurses work together with other disciplines to improve outcomes.

Partnerships Nurtured. Professional, teacher–learner, and nurse–patient relationships are encouraged to be more equal, with an emphasis on developing partnerships that focus on common goals.

Monitoring Role Emphasized. The importance of having skilled nurses present to monitor signs and symptoms to detect, prevent, and treat potential complications early is stressed.

Diverse Responsibilities. Nurses at all levels in hospitals, homes, skilled nursing facilities, nursing homes, and communities are more accountable for diagnosis, prevention, and management of various health problems. Other responsibilities include primary health care, patient education, health promotion, rehabilitation, self-care, and alternative methods of healing. In many cases, nurses are responsible for overseeing care given by unlicensed assistive personnel. All of these factors require nurses to have diverse skills (Display 1–2, page 14).

Nurses Must Prove Value. Regulatory requirements stress that nurses must prove their value to both consumers and their employers, showing how they impact on patient outcomes (eg, how they promote health and independence; how they reduce health care costs). As health care facilities cut costs by hiring unlicensed workers, nurses are challenged to develop new frameworks for evaluating and showing their impact on patient care. For example, below are seven categories that nurses working in nonacute settings must consider to evaluate the impact of nursing care from a consumer perspective (Display 1–3).

DISPLAY 1–2   Diverse Skills Required to be a Nurse Today*

You must be able to

- ✓ Be flexible and adapt to different settings and circumstances, identifying new knowledge, skills, and perspectives needed to practice proficiently.
- ✓ Solve problems, think critically and creatively, and respond to clinical complexity.
- ✓ Make independent and shared decisions, considering costs and involving clients and their families as partners.
- ✓ Meet deadlines, demonstrating responsibility, self-esteem, self-confidence, self-management, sociability, and integrity.
- ✓ Collaborate with professionals, peers, patients, families, and other health care workers by cultivating communication, interpersonal, and group-thinking skills.
- ✓ Think holistically, looking after the entire patient, considering both disease process and the impact of the disease and associated problems on individual lifestyles.
- ✓ Promote wellness through education, health screening, reduction of risk factors, and control of symptoms and causative factors.
- ✓ Make ethical decisions based on ethical principles (see page 20).
- ✓ Teach and learn efficiently by taking advantage of individual learning style preferences.
- ✓ Assess and respond to the diverse needs and values of various cultural and ethnic groups, as well as to reach out to diverse personalities through personality sensitivity.
- ✓ Advocate for clients and families, with the ability to present a case and listen to needs of others and a commitment to promote access to health care for all people, regardless of ability to pay.
- ✓ Lead, supervise, and listen to and grasp the needs of followers.
- ✓ Manage information, and organize and maintain files using computers to assist in interpretation and processing of information.
- ✓ Use technology: select equipment and tools, maintain and troubleshoot equipment, apply technology to tasks, and evaluate the appropriateness of complex and costly equipment.
- ✓ Use resources: allocate time, money, materials, space, and human resources in the development of programs and delivery of care.
- ✓ Assess social and organizational systems; monitor and correct performance; design or improve systems.
- ✓ Determine the role of community services in health care delivery, providing support as needed.
- ✓ Provide customer service with a clear understanding of what's important to consumers.

---

*This is a compilation of skills addressed in the following publications: U.S. Department of Labor. (1992). Washington, DC: Author; *Learning a Living: A blueprint for high performance, a SCANS report for America 2000; A Vision for Nursing.* [On-line]. Available: *http://nln.org/info-vision.htm.* Accessed September 1, 2000.

New Illnesses and Treatments Emerge. As worldwide travel becomes easier, there is more international concern about the spread of diseases. For example, U.S. citizens need to be concerned about new illnesses emerging in Africa because they may be transmitted readily by travelers. Concern for prevention of new and resistant bacteria grows. Researchers study new diagnostic and treatment modalities such as the use of vaccines and genetic manipulation to prevent illness and find new cures.

Lifelong Learning Required. Speed of change requires commitment to lifelong learning and professional development. Nurses are required to be knowledge workers who are able to manage information and technology as well as make complicated clinical judgments. Independent learning, often through the use of computers and the Internet, becomes commonplace.

Health Care Driven by Consumer and Community Needs. Health care organizations aiming to succeed recognize that they must compete for their clients' dollars: services must be driven by consumer needs and customer satisfaction. Insurance companies and consumers alike want to know that they are getting the best value for their dollar.

Healthy People 2010. National health promotion and disease prevention initiatives bring together national, state, and local government agencies; nonprofit, voluntary, and professional organizations; businesses; communities; and individuals to achieve two major goals: (1) to help people of all ages increase life expectancy and improve their quality of life, and (2) to eliminate health disparities among different segments of the population. Specific focus areas and objectives are targeted (Display 1–4, next page).

DISPLAY 1–3   Promoting Consumer Satisfaction*

To promote consumer satisfaction, consider the following:

- ☐ **Symptom Severity:** Degree to which individuals subjectively experience symptom variation; that is, whether symptoms improve or worsen in frequency, duration, and intensity.
- ☐ **Level of Functioning:** Ability to perform activities of daily living (impact on physical, psychosocial, and cognitive function).
- ☐ **Therapeutic Alliance:** Degree of positive relationship between consumer and nurse.
- ☐ **Use of Services:** Quantity and appropriateness of nursing services used.
- ☐ **Client Satisfaction:** Consumer's satisfaction with various aspects and outcomes of the nurse–client experience (see Display 1–2).
- ☐ **Risk Reduction:** Type and quality of positive behaviors adopted by consumers and caregivers that reduce risk of illness, injury, and disease complication or progression.
- ☐ **Protective Factors:** Type and consistency of changes in the client's or caregiver's environment that protect the client from deteriorating health.

*Data from Mastal, 2000.

DISPLAY 1–4   *Healthy People 2010* Focus Areas*

The following 28 focus areas will be monitored through 467 objectives targeted for improvement by the year 2010. Some objectives focus on interventions designed to reduce or eliminate illness, disability, and premature death among individuals and communities; others focus on broader issues, such as improving access to quality health care, strengthening public health services, and dissemination of information.

- Access to Quality Health Services
- Arthritis, Osteoporosis, and Chronic Back Conditions
- Cancer
- Chronic Kidney Disease
- Diabetes
- Disability and Secondary Conditions
- Educational and Community-Based Programs
- Environmental Health
- Family Planning
- Food Safety
- Health Communication
- Heart Disease and Stroke
- HIV

- Immunization and Infectious Diseases
- Injury and Violence Prevention
- Maternal, Infant, and Child Health
- Medical Product Safety
- Mental Health and Mental Disorders
- Nutrition and Overweight
- Occupational Safety and Health
- Oral Health
- Physical Activity and Fitness
- Public Health Infrastructure
- Respiratory Diseases
- Sexually Transmitted Diseases
- Substance Abuse
- Tobacco Use
- Vision and Hearing

*Available: *http://web.health.gov/healthypeople/prevagenda/focus.htms*. Accessed November 1, 2000.

Evidenced-Based Care and Best Practices. Thanks to research and clinical studies, we continue to see an accumulation of evidence that can be analyzed to come to a consensus about what are the best approaches to specific conditions from outcome and cost perspectives. These best approaches often are referred to as *benchmarks* or *best practices*. Today's consumer wants to know the answer to, "What evidence can you give me that this is the best approach for me?"

Managed Care and Reimbursement Challenges. Managed care aims to reduce cost by providing services within a group of providers who network to give quality care in the most cost-effective manner. Nurses, physicians, and therapists working in a managed care environment are challenged to deliver the highest standard of care with the best value. By continuing to track patient outcomes and provide evidence for what really works in the long run, we can build cases for reimbursement for essential diagnostic and treatment modalities.

Shift to Predictive Model. Health care delivery moves from a *diagnose-and-treat* (DT) approach to patient care to one of *predict, prevent, and manage* (PPM). The DT approach implies that we wait for evidence of problems before beginning treatment, whereas PPM stresses the importance of preventing problems before they begin. In many cases, this approach is based on evidence from clinical studies that shows that certain health problems follow an orderly sequence of events. By close monitoring, early detection, and preventive treatment, we often can alter that sequence and prevent or minimize associated problems. For example, with HIV exposure, we treat patients who have had significant exposure rather than waiting to find out if there is evidence of the HIV virus in the blood. The PPM approach also stresses the importance of improving health through management of symptoms. For instance, in asthma management, we have set a national goal of getting as many asthma sufferers to be symptom-free as possible—too many have come to accept symptoms as a part of their daily lives.

Refinement of Critical Paths and Protocols. Critical paths (also known as critical pathways, clinical pathways, and CareMaps™), which are standard multidisciplinary plans used to predict and determine care for specific problems, are refined and improved (see example, page 252 in the Appendix). As we continue to track treatment and outcome data, we have more evidenced-based protocols. For example, if you have pneumonia, you'll be likely to receive a specific antibiotic proven to be effective from human and cost perspectives.

Standards and Practice Guidelines. Federal, state, local, managed care, and private organizations set standards, protocols, and guidelines that aim to reduce useless or harmful practices. For example, nursing homes are required to follow specific guidelines for monitoring, prevention, and treatment of pressure ulcers.

More Elderly and Chronically Ill. People live longer with diseases and disabilities. Nurses must focus on promoting health in spite of existing health problems; for example, how to help people with lung disease maximize exercise tolerance. They also must be equipped to deal with patients with multiple health problems; for example, a patient who has diabetes, hypertension, chronic lung disease, and arthritis.

Patients' Rights and Cultural Needs. Standards require that patients have the right to have their cultural and communication needs addressed. For example, statements of patients' rights (see page 18) must be given to clients; nurses must assess cultural influences such as beliefs, values, and spiritual orientation. Nursing and health care organizations mandate that we identify cultural needs that may affect how someone responds to a plan of care; for example, if someone who is Muslim wants his bed turned toward Mecca five times a day, this request must be respectfully accommodated (ANA, 1991; Joint Commission on Accreditation of Hospital Organizations [JCAHO], 1997).

Computers and Technology. New technology facilitates diagnosis, decision making, and research. Although these technologies create constant learning challenges for all, the ultimate improvements save time and improve care quality. More documentation is being done directly on the computer, often at patients' bedsides. Computerized records, informally called CPR (computerized patient records), CMR (computerized medical records), or OLPR (On-Line Patient Records), are common.

Informatics and Quest to Standardize and Unify Language. Informatics, the study of how to use computers to capture data better for clinical and research purposes, grows. Because having adequate computerized records is impossible without agreement

PATIENTS' RIGHTS*

Dear Consumer:

State law requires that your health care provider or facility recognize your rights while receiving health care and that you respect their right to expect certain behavior on the part of patients. You may request a copy of the full text of this law from your health care provider or facility.

YOU HAVE THE RIGHT TO:

☐ Be treated with courtesy and respect with appreciation of dignity and protection of your need for privacy.

☐ Prompt and reasonable response to questions and requests.

☐ Be informed of:
  - who is providing health care services and who is responsible for your care
  - what patient support services are available, including whether an interpreter is available if you have communication problems.
  - your diagnosis, planned course of treatment, alternatives, risks, and prognosis.
  - whether treatment is for purposes of experimental research (and to give or refuse your consent to participate in such research).

☐ Refuse treatment, except as otherwise provided by law.

☐ Have impartial access to treatment or accommodations, regardless of race, national origin, religious, physical handicap, or source of payment.

☐ Be given treatment for any emergency condition that will deteriorate from failure to receive treatment.

☐ Express any grievances about any violation of your rights as stated by state law, through the grievance procedure of your health care provider or facility and appropriate state licensing agency.

☐ File complaints against a health care professional, hospital, or ambulatory surgical center with the Agency for Health Care Administration. (Appropriate information for how to reach each state's agency must be listed here).

☐ Receive (upon request):
  - full information and necessary counseling on the availability of financial resources for your care.
  - a reasonable estimate of charges for medical care before treatment.
  - information about whether your health care provider or facility accepts the Medicare assignment rate before treatment.

☐ Be given a copy of a resonably clear and understandable, itemized bill, and upon request, to have charges explained.

AND YOU HAVE THE RESPONSIBILITY TO:

☐ Provide your health care provider, to the best of your knowledge, accurate and complete information about your complaints, past illnesses, hospitalizations, medications, and other matters relating to your health.

☐ Follow the treatment plan recommended by your provider.

☐ Report unexpected changes in your condition to the health care provider.

☐ Keep appointments. And, if you're unable to do so for any reason, notify your provider or facility.

☐ Assure that the financial obligations of your health care are fulfilled as soon as possible.

☐ Comply with health care provider and facility rules and regulations affecting patient conduct.

---

* This is an example form and summary of rights. Rights may vary from state to state. Forms may vary from facility to facility.

on use of common terms, several organizations work to standardize the terms used by health care professionals. These methods of standardizing terms also are known as nomenclatures, classifications systems, and taxonomies. For example, what some nurses may call *shortness of breath* might be called *dyspnea* by others. Efforts to link similar terms like this in computer data bases become crucial from research and clinical perspectives, especially as we work to identify nursing-sensitive outcomes (outcomes that are clearly improved by nursing care). Chapter 3 addresses classifying and standardizing terms in more depth (see pages 84–85).

New Ethical Concerns. End-of-life care and technologic advancements in the treatment of infertility, illness, and disease challenge traditional ethical and societal values regarding conception, birth, death, and dying. Society is more concerned with the ethics of palliative care (care that alleviates pain and suffering and promotes a sense of physical and spiritual well-being, but doesn't cure). Nurses often find themselves "in the trenches" with ethical dilemmas, helping patients and families make informed ethical decisions or advocating on their behalf.

Case Management. Case management—the use of collaborative approaches to ensure that the best available resources are used to reach outcomes efficiently—becomes essential to promote quality and efficiency of care. This approach is firmly grounded in prevention and early intervention and requires understanding of how complex systems operate, as well as excellent critical thinking and people skills.

Wellness Centers, Holistic and Alternative Therapies. There is a greater focus on promoting health and triggering the body's natural healing powers through holistic and alternative therapies (eg, diet, exercise, acupuncture, massage, and other ways to manage stress such as meditation and aromatherapy).

Educated Consumers. Nurses are called on to help consumers at both ends of the "knowledge spectrum," from those who are illiterate to those who travel the Internet, becoming experts on the latest information on their problems. Many consumers today are well informed and expect to participate in decisions affecting their care.

Think About It

Cutting Costs, Not Corners. *Cutting costs doesn't mean "cutting corners." Rather, it means working to get equal results within a budget. For example, you may recommend that a patient ask the pharmacist or primary care provider about taking a generic antibiotic, which needs to be taken five times a day, instead of a brand-name drug, which needs to be taken only three times a day but is significantly more expensive. Conversely, if you're not getting the results you want because of compliance problems, you might point out that it may be cheaper in the long run to change from the less-expensive generic drug that must be taken frequently to a comparable brand drug that's more expensive but convenient to take.*

Ethics: Protecting Client Rights

A key part of using the nursing process is that of recognizing your role as a client advocate and acting in a professional, ethical manner. It's your responsibility to make sure that decisions and actions performed on behalf of clients are determined ethically. Display 1–5 addresses your responsibilities related to giving care in an ethical manner according to the American Nurses Association (ANA).

As you use the nursing process, keep in mind the importance of upholding the following ethical principles:

- **Autonomy.** People have the right to make decisions based on (1) their *own* values and beliefs, (2) adequate information given free from coercion, and (3) sound reasoning that considers all the alternatives.
- **Beneficence.** Aim to do the greatest good and avoid harm.
- **Justice:** Treat people equally and fairly.
- **Fidelity:** Keep promises and don't make promises you can't keep.
- **Veracity (Truth Telling):** Be honest with patients, families, and peers.
- **Confidentiality.** Respect the privacy of information.
- **Accountability.** Be accountable for the consequences of your actions.

> N O T E : About the critical thinking exercises throughout this book—the point of the critical thinking exercises is to allow you to master content and practice critical thinking skills, not to make you do time-consuming writing exercises. You may either write your answers, explain them to someone else, verbalize them out loud to yourself, or tape record them. If you feel you don't need the practice, skip the session entirely. The answers provided in the back of the book are example responses—they aren't the only answers. They are provided to allow you to evaluate and correct your own thinking. If you doubt whether your response is acceptable, ask your instructor.

DISPLAY 1-5   Ethics: Protecting Client Rights*

As a nurse, you're responsible for:
- ✓ Following the *Code of Ethics* (ANA, 1985; see Appendix, page 249).
- ✓ Maintaining client confidentiality.
- ✓ Acting as a client advocate.
- ✓ Seeking available resources to help formulate ethical decisions.
- ✓ Delivering care in a way that is
  Nonjudgmental, nondiscriminatory, and sensitive to client diversity
  Preserves and protects client autonomy, dignity, and rights.

*From: American Nurses Association. (1991). *Standards of clinical nursing practice: Standards of professional performance*. Washington, DC: Author.

CRITICAL THINKING EXERCISE 1

Nursing Process in a Changing World

To complete this session, read pages 4–20. Example responses can be found on page 243.

1. Using terms a layperson can understand, explain:

   a. The steps of the nursing process.

   b. Five advantages of using the nursing process.

   c. How it complements what other disciplines do.

2. Give three reasons why learning to apply the nursing process is an essential requirement of nurses.

3. Explain why the accuracy of each step of the nursing process depends on the accuracy of the preceding step.

4. Imagine you work on an acute care unit. Consider Display 1–6 (Patient Satisfac-

DISPLAY 1–6   Patient Satisfaction: Top 10 Issues*

The 10 issues that most closely correlated with the likelihood that patients will recommend your hospital to others.

☐ Staff sensitivity to the inconvenience that health problems and hospitalizations cause
☐ Overall cheerfulness of the hospital
☐ Staff concern for patients' privacy
☐ Amount of attention paid to patients' special or personal needs
☐ Degree to which nurses took patients' health problems seriously
☐ Technical skill of nurses
☐ Nurses' attitudes toward patients calling them
☐ Degree to which the nurses kept patients adequately informed about tests, treatment, and equipment
☐ Friendliness of nurses
☐ Promptness in responding to the call button

*From McIntosh, T. (1997). Empathy: Why patients recommend hospitals. *Healthcare Benchmarks, 4,* 39.

tion: Top 10 Issues) on page 21 and think of three ways you could help nurses stay focused on the little things that mean a lot to patients.

Try This on Your Own

Scan the list of focus areas addressed by Healthy People 2010 *in Display 1–4 (page 16). Choose one area that you happen to encounter in your personal life (eg, you may have asthma or know someone who has it). Then go to the web site listed in the box and compare where you or your friends are in relation to the listed focus goals.*

Knowledge, Skills, and Caring: The Heart of Nursing Process

The following diagram shows that when knowledge and critical thinking (what to, why to), technical, and interpersonal skills (how to), and caring (willing to, able to) come together, the nursing process becomes a driving force for quality care.

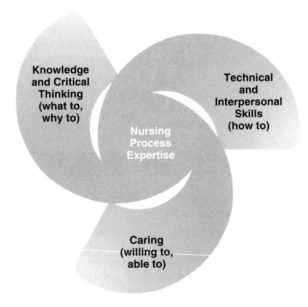

Nursing Knowledge: Broad and Varied

The knowledge base that guides nursing actions is broad and varied, including all of the following:

Health promotion

Growth and development

Mental health/psychiatry

Anatomy and physiology

Epidemiology

Nursing diagnosis/nursing process

Community and public health

Culture/ethics/law

Research/leadership

Group and organizational dynamics

Teaching/counseling

Communication/negotiation/conflict resolution

Problem solving/critical thinking

Computers/technology

Nursing care management

Disease process/treatment

Diagnostic/monitoring modalities

Pathophysiology/pharmacology

Microbiology/chemistry

Physical and social sciences

Practice wisdom (knowledge gained from experience)

Critical Thinking

Unlike the mindless thinking we do when going about our daily routine, critical thinking is careful, deliberate, outcome-focused (results-oriented) thinking. Display 1–7 defines critical thinking in nursing.

How to Become a Critical Thinker

In one way, critical thinking is like any other skill: if you practice it, it becomes more automatic. The exercises throughout this book are intended to help you develop, refine, and practice your ability to think critically in the context of nursing situations. As you complete each chapter, learning and applying the principles and rules that guide you to use the nursing process, you'll begin to develop habits that will help you be more automatic in your approaches to nursing situations. For now, take a few moments to look at Display 1–8, which lists characteristics of critical thinkers, and evaluate your current habits of thinking. Check each characteristic and ask yourself, "Is this me?" Put a mark next to the ones you want to develop or improve.

DISPLAY 1–7   What Is Critical Thinking in Nursing?*

Critical Thinking in Nursing:

- Entails purposeful, outcome-directed (results-oriented) thinking.
- Is driven by patient, family, and community needs.
- Is based on principles of nursing process and scientific method.
- Requires knowledge, skills, and experience.
- Is guided by professional standards and ethics codes.
- Requires strategies that maximize *human potential* (eg, using individual strengths) and compensate for problems created by *human nature* (eg, the powerful influence of personal perspectives, values, and beliefs).
- Is constantly re-evaluating, self-correcting, and striving to improve.

*From Alfaro-LeFevre (1999). *Critical thinking in nursing: A practical approach.* Philadelphia: W.B. Saunders.

DISPLAY 1–8   Characteristics of Critical Thinkers

Critical Thinkers Are:

- **Aware of their strengths and capabilities:** They're confident that they can reason to find answers and make good decisions.
- **Sensitive to their own limitations and predispositions:** They know their weaknesses, values, and beliefs and recognize when these may hamper their ability to assess a situation or solve a problem.
- **Open minded:** They listen to new ideas and viewpoints and consider the situation from many perspectives.
- **Humble:** They overcome their own tendency to feel that they should have all the answers.
- **Creative:** They are constantly looking for better ways to get things done. They follow recommended procedures; however, they continually examine whether these are the best way to meet goals and objectives.
- **Proactive:** They accept responsibility and accountability for their actions. They study situations, anticipate problems, and find ways to avoid them *before* they happen.
- **Flexible:** They recognize the importance of changing priorities and interventions when planned approaches don't seem to be getting results.
- **Aware that errors are stepping-stones to new ideas:** They turn mistakes into learning opportunities, reflecting on what went wrong and identifying ways to avoid the same mistake in the future.
- **Willing to persevere:** They know that sometimes there are no easy answers and that there may be time-consuming struggles to find the best answer.
- **Cognizant of the fact that we don't live in a perfect world:** They realize that sometimes the *best* answer may not be the *perfect* answer.
- **Introspective:** They evaluate and correct their own thinking.

Critical Thinkers also:

- **Maintain a questioning attitude:** They ask questions like, "What's going on here?"; "What does it mean?"; and "What else could it mean, and how else could it be interpreted?"
- **Ask for clarification when they don't understand:** For example, they say, "I'm not clear about this. Can you tell me more?" *or* ask questions like, "What do you mean by *better,* better in what way?"
- **Apply previous knowledge to new situations:** They see similarities and differences between one experience and another, between one concept and another.
- **See the situation from many perspectives:** They value all viewpoints and watch that their judgments are based on *facts,* not personal feelings, views, or self-interest.
- **Weigh risks and benefits (advantages and disadvantages) before making a decision:** They avoid risky decisions and find ways to reduce adverse reactions before putting a plan into action.
- **Seek help when needed.**
- **Put first things first:** They ask, "What's the most important thing to do here?"

(continued)

DISPLAY 1–8   Characteristics of Critical Thinkers (Continued)

Critical Thinkers Use Logic. They:

- **Test first impressions to make sure they are as they appear:** They double-check the logic of their thinking and the workability of their solutions.
- **Distinguish between fact and fallacy:** They take the time to verify important information to be sure it's true.
- **Distinguish fact from inference (what they *believe* the fact means):** For example, they recognize that because someone is sitting quietly in a corner may not mean that the individual is *withdrawn;* it means that they are sitting quietly in a corner and that it would be helpful to find out why.
- **Support views with evidence:** They wouldn't state that the person above is withdrawn without providing additional supporting evidence, such as the individual saying he wants nothing to do with anyone.
- **Determine what's relevant and what's irrelevant:** They recognize what's important for understanding a situation and what's unimportant. For example, the fact that you're a nurse or studying to be a nurse is relevant to how I should write this book; the fact that you are female or male is irrelevant.
- **Apply the concept of "cause and effect":** They look for what's causing a problem to more fully understand the problem itself. They anticipate responses to their actions before performing the action. For example, critical thinkers would attempt to find out the *cause* of pain before deciding how to *treat* it. They would determine how someone might *respond* to a medication before *administering* it.
- **Withhold judgment until all the necessary facts are in:** They realize the dangers of jumping to conclusions.

Think About It

Rethinking the Rules. *Critical thinking is contextual (it happens within a set of circumstances for a specific purpose). The ability to think critically must be mastered within each different context or situation. For example, moving from working in a hospital (where you're in charge and equipment and resources are plentiful) to working in home care (where you're a guest in someone else's home and often have to improvise) requires you to re-think the rules.*

Technical Skills

Mastering technical skills, such as giving injections, monitoring intravenous lines, and other skills involving equipment and coordination, is an important part of developing an ability to think critically in the clinical area. Once you're familiar with the principles and manual skills involved in using new equipment, it frees you to direct your brain power to think more about what you're doing with *the patient* than *the equipment*. Making time to practice using equipment and mastering nursing procedures before seeing patients clinically will greatly improve your clinical reasoning ability.

Interpersonal Skills

Developing interpersonal skills is as important as developing critical thinking skills. If you're unable to establish positive interpersonal relationships, you're unlikely to get the real facts, understand the real problems, get others to help, or be an effective team player.

Many believe that communication skills are the key to positive interpersonal relationships. However, good communication skills really are only half of what's required to build sound interpersonal relationships. Relationships are developed as much by how we *behave* as by how we communicate: actions speak louder than words. To establish positive interpersonal relationships, you must develop behaviors that send messages like, *I'm reliable . . . , I respect you . . . , You can trust me . . .* , and *I want to do a good job.*

In the next chapter, you'll practice specific communication techniques in the section on interviewing. For now, think about the messages sent by behavior. Look at Table 1–3, next page, which describes behaviors that promote or inhibit interpersonal relationships. Consider some behaviors you'd like to develop or improve.

VOICES

It Pays to be Nice. "[Our studies show that] patients who come away from a positive encounter with a nurse are more likely to follow prescribed directions, take medications, and seek follow-up care . . . [however, if] a patient encounters a health care worker who's in a negative emotional state, it becomes a springboard into other negative behaviors. Down the road, their own outcomes suffer, and they just don't fare well. . . . Try to make the work environment as fun as possible. If you see a staff member in a bad mood, jump in and try to derail it before it becomes contagious."—*Howard Weiss, PhD*

(Farella, C. [2000]. Cooling the cauldron on your unit. *Nursing Spectrum, 10* [13FL], p. 9.)

Willingness and Ability to Care

Let's look at the third component of nursing process expertise, *caring*.

Willingness to Care

Being willing to care means making the choice to do what it takes to help others. This includes choosing to

- Keep the focus on what's best for the consumer (patient, family, community).
- Respect the values and beliefs of others.
- Stay involved, even when problems become chronic or more severe.
- Maintain a healthy lifestyle so you're able to help.

In addition to these points, the ANA addresses standards of professional performance, or professional behaviors, that enhance the use of the nursing process (Display 1–9). Being willing to care involves being willing to work toward making these behaviors habits of performance. The case study on page 28 shows how applying these behaviors can make a significant difference in the quality of patient care and job satisfaction.

TABLE 1–3 Behaviors Affecting Interpersonal Relationships

Behaviors That Enhance Interpersonal Relationships	Behaviors That Inhibit Interpersonal Relationships
Conveying an attitude of openness, acceptance, and lack of prejudice.	Conveying an attitude of doubt, mistrust, or negative judgment.
Being honest.	Giving false information.
Taking initiative and responsibility; responding to others' concerns.	Conveying an "it's not my job" attitude.
Being reliable.	Not meeting commitments, only partially meeting commitments, or not being punctual.
Demonstrating humility.	Demonstrating self-importance.
Showing respect for what others are, have been, or may become.	"Talking down" or assuming familiarity.
Accepting accountability.	Making excuses or placing blame where it doesn't belong.
Being confident and prepared.	Being unsure and trying to "wing it."
Showing genuine interest.	Acting like you're only doing something because it's a job.
Conveying appreciation for others' time.	Assuming others have more time than we do.
Accepting expression of positive *and* negative feelings.	Demonstrating discomfort when negative feelings are expressed.
Taking enough time.	Rushing.
Being frank and forthright.	Sending mixed messages, saying things just because we think it's what the other person seems to want to hear, or talking behind others' backs.
Admitting when we've been wrong.	Denying or ignoring when we've made an error.
Apologizing if we've caused distress or inconvenience.	Acting like nothing happened or making excuses.
Being willing to forgive and forget.	Holding grudges.
Showing a positive attitude.	Conveying an "it'll never work" attitude.
Conveying a sense of humor.	Acting like there's no room for anything but "serious business."
Allowing others control.	Trying to control others.
Giving credit where credit is due.	Ignoring achievements or taking credit that doesn't belong to us.

DISPLAY 1-9   ANA Standards of Professional Performance*
(Professional Behavior)

Standard   I **Quality of Care:** The nurse systematically evaluates the quality and effectiveness of nursing practice.

II **Performance Appraisal:** The nurse evaluates his/her own nursing practice in relation to professional practice standards and relevant statutes and regulations.

III **Education:** The nurse acquires and maintains current knowledge in nursing practice.

IV **Collegiality:** The nurse contributes to the professional development of peers, colleagues, and others

V **Ethics:** The nurse's decisions and actions on behalf of clients are determined in an ethical manner.

VI **Collaboration:** The nurse collaborates with the client, significant others, and health care providers in providing client care.

VII **Research:** The nurse uses research findings in practice.

VIII **Resource Utilization:** The nurse considers factors related to safety, effectiveness, and cost in planning and delivering client care.

*From American Nurses Association. (1991). *Standards of clinical practice*. American Nurses Association. Washington, DC: Author.

C A S E   S T U D Y
How Using Resources, Applying Research, and Using a Collegial Approach to Collaborating Can Make a Difference in Care Quality and Job Satisfaction

Mr. Moran has chronic lung disease and has been on nasal oxygen at home for the last 6 months. He's been admitted for evaluation of possible heart problems. Bruce Franklin is Mr. Moran's nurse. Dr. Kenny is his physician. Bruce notes that Mr. Moran continues to have extreme difficulty breathing any time he moves around, even when using his oxygen. Although Dr. Kenny is aware of this, she has had some other major priorities and hasn't been able to focus on Mr. Moran's chronic breathing problems.

Bruce begins to wonder if something could be done to improve the situation. He asks Dee Baker, the respiratory clinical nurse specialist, if she would discuss Mr. Moran's care with him. They set aside time to discuss Mr. Moran's care. Dee mentions that she's read about the benefits of transtracheal oxygen delivery. She asks the librarian to do a computer search on transtracheal oxygen delivery, and two research articles are found. Dee and Bruce review the articles and learn that transtracheal oxygen delivery may be more effective than nasal cannula oxygen delivery. Bruce asks for a copy of the research articles for his files.

Bruce and the clinical specialist discuss the findings with Dr. Kenny, resulting in new orders of transtracheal oxygen delivery. Mr. Moran demonstrates a significant improvement in ability to tolerate activity. Bruce has the satisfaction of knowing that he made a difference and gained knowledge of treatment modalities. Dee has the satisfaction of knowing she's made a difference in two lives, Mr. Moran's and Bruce's. The next time she sees the librarian, she lets her know that her computer search benefited all involved. Dr. Kenny is pleased to know that she has two dependable colleagues who are independent thinkers, use resources, and are willing to work as a team to make a difference.   ■

Display 1–10 lists some behaviors you can use to show patients and families you care.

Being Able to Care

Being able to care requires understanding ourselves and understanding others.

Understanding Ourselves

Learning to understand ourselves is a lifelong pursuit. Gaining insight into ourselves involves learning about our tendencies, reactions, and habits, and these tend to change as we grow and mature. By making a commitment to learn about ourselves and recognize how our values and frame of reference might influence our thinking and ability to understand others, we can take deliberate steps to be more objective in our thinking.

Understanding Others

Understanding others takes learning how to listen empathetically, or to listen with the intent to enter into another's way of thinking and viewing the world (Covey, 1989). Some use the analogy of trying to view the world through someone else's glasses or trying to walk in another's shoes. (Both often are almost impossible!) Listening empathetically takes letting go of how we, ourselves, view the world and connecting with an-

DISPLAY 1–10   Ten Caring Behaviors

1. Inspiring someone, or instilling hope and faith (creating a vision of what is or could be).
2. Demonstrating patience, compassion, and willingness to persevere.
3. Offering companionship (eg, listening, or being with someone for no other reason than to listen or *be* with the person).
4. Helping someone stay in touch with positive aspects of his life (eg, inquiring about significant others, pets, special interests, or hobbies).
5. Demonstrating thoughtfulness (eg, calling or visiting someone for no other reason than knowing it will let the person know you're thinking of him).
6. Bending the rules when it really counts (eg, arranging for a pet to visit).
7. Doing the "little things" and the "extra things."
8. Taking the time required rather than hurrying through just to get things done.
9. Keeping someone informed.
10. Showing your human side by sharing "stories" (exchanging tales of special interests and activities).

DISPLAY 1-11   Steps for Listening Empathetically

1. Eliminate thoughts about how *you* see the other person's situation.
2. Listen carefully for *feelings* and try to identify with how the *other* person perceives his situation. Don't allow yourself to think about how you're going to respond; think only about the *content* of what you're hearing.
3. Reflect on what you've been told, then rephrase the *feelings.*
4. Seek validation that you've understood the message, content, and emotion correctly. Keep trying until you're sure you understand.
5. Detach, and come back to your own frame of reference.

other's feelings and perceptions. It takes identifying with another's struggles, frustrations, and desires. And then it takes detaching from the feelings and returning to our own frame of reference. Once we've detached, we're likely to be more objective and still be able to understand what's important to the person. We'll be more able to identify needs, prioritize problems, and find common goals. Display 1–11 provides steps for listening empathetically. The following case study demonstrates how these steps might be used in a real situation.

C A S E   S T U D Y
Example of How Listening Empathetically Promotes Understanding of the Real Issues, Fostering Caring for Human Responses

Today Pat is caring for Sharon, who's just given birth to her fifth child, a healthy baby girl. Pat never has been able to conceive, has always wanted children, and feels a little envious of Sharon's family of two boys and (now) three girls.

Pat notes that Sharon seems very quiet. Recognizing the importance of being an empathetic listener, Pat has the following conversation with Sharon.

Pat: "You've been pretty quiet since I came on."

Sharon: "I can't help it. I'm supposed to be happy, but I'm really disappointed—I was so sure I'd have a boy."

Pat (making a conscious effort to eliminate thoughts about the fact that she'd be happy with any child, and rephrasing what Sharon seems to be feeling): "You feel like you're supposed to be happy, but you really feel sort of sad?"

Sharon: "Yes."

Pat pauses to reflect on the feeling of sadness and encourage Sharon to continue.

Sharon: "I was going to name this baby after my father. He died 2 months ago."

Pat (connecting to what Sharon must be feeling): "I'm sorry. That would be a disappointment. Being able to name the baby after him would have been a lovely thing to do."

Sharon (crying): "Yes. I had it all pictured in my mind."

Pat, conveying acceptance and understanding, sits quietly, allowing Sharon to cry.

Pat (detaching and coming back to her own frame of reference): "Sharon, I think you needed to cry and you may need to cry again. But right now you've got a beautiful baby girl with the longest hair I've ever seen waiting to meet her mother. How would you feel if I brought her in to you?"

Sharon: "Yes. I really haven't seen her for more than 5 minutes (smiling). It's not her fault she's a girl. I've got to admit, I've always gotten along better with my girls than my boys." ■

CRITICAL THINKING EXERCISE II

Knowledge, Skills, and Willingness and Ability to Care

To complete this session, read pages 22–31. Unless an asterisk is placed after the number, an example response to each question can be found on page 243.

1. List five critical thinking characteristics you'd like to acquire or improve.

2. Complete the following sentence, using as many words as you choose: *If I were to tell someone how I think, I would say that I . . . .*

3. In five sentences or less, describe what critical thinking means to you.*

4. Give three examples of caring behaviors.

5. Choose three of the statements below, summarized from *Nursing's Social Policy Statement* (ANA, 1995) and explain how they relate to this chapter.*

- Health and illness are human experiences (p. 4).
- The presence of illness does not preclude health nor does optimal health preclude illness (p. 4).
- An essential feature of contemporary nursing practice is the provision of a caring relationship that facilitates healing (p. 6).
- Humans manifest an essential unity of mind, body, and spirit (p. 3).
- Human experience is contextually and culturally defined (p. 3).

Try This on Your Own

1. **Improve your interpersonal skills by learning how to get along with "difficult" people.** Check out my article, *Don't Worry! Be Happy! Harmonize Diversity Through Personality Sensitivity.* Available at: *http://nsweb.nursingspectrum. com/ce/ce236.htm.**

2. **Are you stressed out?** Managing stress is an important part of staying healthy. Take the Life Stress Test at *http://www.cliving.org/lifstrstst.htm.* Think of some things that you can do to reduce your stress level.*

3. In the case history on pages 30–31, everyone works well together and is happy with the results. However, in the real world, one or two of the people involved may come away with bruised feelings. Who might these people be? What could be done about it?

4. **Practice Empathetic Listening.** Ask someone to tell you about an upsetting experience in his childhood and listen using the steps of empathetic listening listed in Display 1–11.

Summary

The nursing process is systematic, dynamic, humanistic, and outcome-focused (results-oriented). It's required by national practice standards, provides the basis for state board exam questions, and helps you think critically in the clinical setting. Its five steps—*Assessment, Diagnosis, Planning, Implementation,* and *Evaluation*— overlap and are interrelated. The accuracy of all of the steps depends on factual, relevant, and comprehensive patient information.

Using the nursing process complements what other health care professionals do by focusing on both the medical problems and *human response* to medical problems, treatment plans, and changes in activities of daily life. The nursing process aims to promote health by maximizing independence, sense of well-being, and ability to function, regardless of the presence of illness or disability. Being competent in using the nursing process requires a broad nursing knowledge base, critical thinking, strong interpersonal and technical skills, and an ability and willingness to care.

Evaluate your knowledge of this chapter. Check to see if you can achieve the learning outcomes on page 2.
Bibliography: See pages 199–201.

2

Assessment

LEARNING OUTCOMES

After mastering the content in this chapter, you should be able to:

- Describe five phases of *Assessment.*
- Explain why having incomplete or incorrect assessment data affects the entire plan of care.
- Compare and contrast the terms *data base assessment* and *focus assessment.*
- Discuss ethical, cultural, and spiritual considerations related to performing an assessment.
- Explain how the interview and physical assessment complement and clarify each other.
- Give an example of an open-ended question, closed-ended question, leading question, and exploratory statement.
- Describe how you plan to do an interview and physical examination the next time you're in the clinical setting.
- Identify subjective and objective data in a nursing assessment.
- Differentiate between cues and inferences.
- Explain why organizing data according to more than one method (eg, both a body systems model and a nursing model) promotes critical thinking.
- Give a detailed account of how you'll do a comprehensive assessment the next time you're in the clinical setting.
- Explain how you'll decide what information to report and record the next time you're in the clinical setting.

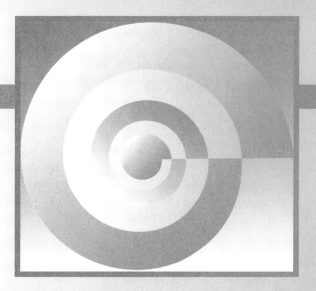

Standard I. *Assessment.* The nurse collects client health data.*

Critical Thinking Exercises

- **Critical Thinking Exercise III:** The Nursing Interview and Physical Assessment

- **Critical Thinking Exercise IV:** Subjective and Objective Data; Cues and Inferences; Validating Data

- **Critical Thinking Exercise V:** Organizing (Clustering) Data

- **Critical Thinking Exercise VI:** Recognizing Abnormal Data, Deciding What's Relevant, Applying the Principle of Cause and Effect

---

What's in this chapter?

Emphasizing the point that the entire plan of care depends on the accuracy and completeness of *Assessment,* this chapter examines how to do an assessment in a way that facilitates the next step, *Diagnosis.* It gives useful tips on interviewing and examining patients and explains the *how to's* and the *why's* of the five key activities of *Assessment* (collecting data, validating data, clustering data, identifying patterns/testing first impressions, and reporting and recording data).

---

*Excerpted from *ANA Standards of Clinical Nursing Practice* (ANA, 1998).

Assessment: The First Step to Determining Health Status

Assessment, the first step to determining health status, is when you do an interview and examination and gather information to make sure you have all the "necessary puzzle pieces" to get a clear picture of the person's health. Because the entire plan of care is based on the data collected during this phase, you need to make every effort to ensure that your information is correct, complete, and organized in a way that helps you begin to get a sense of patterns of health or illness. This chapter gives helpful strategies for interviewing and examining patients and families. It also addresses how and why you gather information to ensure you have an accurate, relevant, plan for each patient.

Here are the five key phases of assessment addressed in this chapter:

* *Collecting Data:* Gather data (information) about health status.
* *Validating (Verifying) Data:* Double-check to make sure that your data are accurate and complete.
* *Organizing Data:* Cluster the data into groups of information that help you to identify patterns of health or illness (eg, cluster data about nutrition together, the data about activity together, and so forth).
* *Identifying Patterns/Testing First Impressions:* You get a beginning idea of patterns of function and focus your assessment to gain more information to better understand the situation at hand. For example, you may start to think that someone has a pattern of poor nutrition and decide to find out what's contributing to this pattern (does the person have poor eating habits or could it be something else, like lack of available refrigeration?).
* *Reporting and Recording Data:* Report significant data (eg, a high fever) and complete the patient's record. Reporting significant data before charting ensures that other responsible members of the health care team are immediately aware of your major concerns.

Collecting Data

Collecting data is an ongoing process. It begins when you first meet the patient, and it continues until the person is discharged. Let's take a look at the resources and methods you use to gather information about someone's health.

What Resources Do You Use?

The following bullets summarize the resources to consider to ensure comprehensive assessment. However, remember that your direct examination and interview of the person requiring care are likely to provide the most significant information.

* Consumer (patient, family, community)
* Significant others

- Nursing and medical records
- Verbal and written consultations
- Diagnostic/laboratory studies

The data you collect may be classified into two categories: direct and indirect data. *Direct data* is information gained directly from the patient (eg, from your interview and examination). *Indirect data* is information gained from other sources (eg, someone's spouse, another nurse).

How Can You Ensure Comprehensive Data Collection?

Comprehensive data collection usually occurs in three phases:

1. **Before you see the person:** You find out what you can. This information may be limited (only name and age) or extensive (medical records may be available for you to read).
2. **When you see the person:** You interview the person and perform a physical examination.
3. **After you see the person:** You review the resources you've used and determine what other resources may offer additional information (eg, you may talk with a social worker or consult with a pharmacist to gain more information about a medication regimen).

Data Base (Start of Care) Versus Focus Assessment

There are two main types of assessment:

1. Data base (start of care) assessment: Comprehensive information you gather on initial contact with the person to assess *all aspects* of health status
2. Focus assessment: Data you gather to determine the status of a *specific condition* (eg, someone's bowel habits)

Data Base (Start of Care) Assessment

Most facilities have standardized their assessment tools, also called data base forms. Three major factors influence how these tools are designed and what information is required:

1. **The needs and problems commonly encountered** on the specific unit. For example, an adult assessment tool is different from an infant assessment tool (Figure 2–1, page 38) and an acute care assessment tool is different from one used in long-term care (compare Figures 2–2, page 39, and 2–3, page 43).
2. **The nursing model or theory** adopted by the facility (functional health patterns, self-care theory, human responses, and so forth).
3. **Standards of care** for assessment as defined by regulatory agencies and professional nursing associations; for example, the Joint Commission for Accreditation of Healthcare Organizations, the Community Health Accreditation Program

---

Excerpt from an Adult Assessment Tool: Health Perception-Health Maintenance

Past History

Previous illnesses/hospitalizations
History of smoking/alcohol intake?
Exercise tolerance?
Patient's statement of past health status?
Medications?

Excerpt from an Infant Assessment Tool: Health Perception-Health Maintenance

Birth History

Prenatal:	Planned pregnancy?	Emotional response?
	Weight gain?	Alcohol/Drug use?
	Complications?	
Labor:	Length?	Spontaneous delivery?
	Vaginal/Cesarean?	Anesthesia?
	Complications?	
Bonding:	Major care giver?	Other family members?

F i g u r e **2–1.** Excerpts from an adult assessment tool and an infant assessment tool showing how tools are tailor-made to meet the needs of specific populations.

(CHAP), the American Nurses Association (ANA) and other professional organizations, such as the American Association of Critical Care Nurses. Information required by insurance companies also may influence what information is required by the tool. The following is an example of how government requirements also influence data collection.

All long-term care facilities receiving Medicare and Medicaid reimbursement must[1]

• Design a comprehensive and accurate assessment system that is standardized and reproducible. These assessments are the basis for identifying problems and strengths and for developing an individualized care plan that aims to attain the highest physical, mental, and psychosocial functioning.
• Collect a minimum set of data (known as minimum data set) in a standardized way (see Figure 2–4, page 47).

Focus Assessment

You might do a focus assessment as part of a comprehensive data base assessment or by itself to monitor specific problems or aspects of care. For example, as part of a compre-

(text continued on page 48)

---

[1]Omnibus Budget Reconciliation Act of 1987.

Main Line Health
Jefferson Health System

☒ Paoli Hospital   ☐ Lankenau Hospital

☐ Bryn Mawr Hospital   ☐ Bryn Mawr Rehab

INITIAL PATIENT ASSESSMENT

Patient I.D.

(Complete shaded area if **not** admitted through Emergency Department) **OR**   ☒ See 24 Hour Flow Sheet   ☐ See CCP

Name: Rose Feterini	Date: 5-8-02	Time: 11:30	Age: 82	DOB: 5-1-20	Circle Sex: Ⓕ M

Height 5'1"   Weight 105#

Vital Signs Temp 98⁴ P 100 RR 32 BP 96/70

O2 Sat 94% O2 2 ℓ/min RA —

Patient History

Presenting Complaint/Time of Onset: Dizziness palpitations

Present History/Assessment: Felt weak for past 3 days. Passed out at beauty salon today. Paramedics called — was alert when they arrived. Monitor - rapid atrial fib - no PVC's.

Allergies: Drug/Food/Latex/Tape/Dyes

ALLERGIES	REACTION	ALLERGIES	REACTION	ALLERGIES	REACTION
☒ None Known					

ALL MEDICATIONS

☒SENT HOME ☐TO PHARMACY (include over-the-counter drugs, vitamins, and supplements currently being taken)	Dose	Route	Frequency	Last Taken	Reason for Taking/Comments
1. Multivit	ī OD	po	daily	today 10⁰	
2. Digoxin	0.25mg	po	daily	today 10A	Heart
3. ASA	ī tab	po	daily	today 10A	Heart
4. Ativan	? dose	po	prn	yesterday	anxiety
5.					
6.					
7.					
8.					
9.					

Recent Aspirin/ Ibuprofen/ Blood Thinner: Daily aspirin 500mg Procedure/Date: —

Reason for Procedure/hospitalization: ——

Advance Directives/ Organ Donation	☐ NA (Patient < 18 years old)	☐ Unable to Assess
Does the patient have an advance directive?	☒ Yes	☐ No
If "Yes" copy in chart?	☒ Yes	☐ No Follow-up action: ☐ Family to obtain copy for record ☐ Patient to formulate another advance directive (sample in "It's Up To You") ☐ Substance as stated by patient: _____ ☐ Patient declines stating substance ☐ Patient/family declines to bring, and/or complete advance directive information
If "No" does the patient wish to make an advance directive?	☐ Yes- Refer to Social Work	☐ No
Has patient completed an Organ Donor Card?	☐ Yes	☒ No

Correct ID band in place ☒ Yes

☒ Patient Handbook/Patient's Rights and Responsibilities reviewed.

☒ Patient/family oriented to room

MLH 900-177 (8/00)

F i g u r e **2–2.** Initial patient assessment.

Patient Name: _____Rose Feterini_____

HEALTH HISTORY	Check Applicable Boxes Only

NEUROLOGIC
☐CVA/TIA
☐Aphasic/Dysarthric
☐Blackouts/Fainting/Vertigo
☐Seizures
☐Migraine/Headaches
☐Numbness/Tingling
☐Confusion
☐Memory Changes
☐Swallowing/Choking
☐Head Injury
☐Other_____
☒*No identified problems*

CARDIOVASCULAR
☐Hypertension/Hypotension
☐Aneurysm
☐Myocardial Infarction
☐Heart Failure
☐Murmur
☐Chest Pain/Angina
☒Arrhythmia
☐Circulation Problem
☐Phlebitis/Clots
☐Pacemaker/Defrib.
☐Other_____
☐*No identified problems*

RESPIRATORY
☐Emphysema/Bronchitis
☒Asthma
☐Shortness of breath
☐TB
☐Pneumonia
☒Seasonal/Environmental
  Allergies
☐Snoring/Apnea
☐Breathing Devices:_____
_____
☐Other_____
☐*No identified problems*

GASTROINTESTINAL
☐Hiatal Hernia/Reflux
☐Hepatitis
☐Ulcers
☐Crohn's/Colitis
☐Gall Bladder Disease
☐Irritable Bowels
☐Diverticular Disease
☐Wt Change_____lbs. +/-
☐Recent change in bowel habits
☐Blood in stool
☐Other_____
☒*No identified problems*

Comments: _____

MUSCULOSKELETAL
☒Arthritis
☐Muscle Weakness
☐Joint Replacement _____
☐Spinal Problems
☐Other _____
☐*No identified problems*
METABOLIC
☐Diabetes Type: _____
☐Thyroid
☐Hypoglycemia
☒High cholesterol
☐Other_____
☐*No identified problems*

GENITOURINARY
☐Kidney Stones
☐Prostate Problems
☐Burning/Urgency
  Frequency
☐Blood in Urine
☐Kidney Failure
☐Dialysis
☐Breast Masses/
  Tenderness/Discharge
☐LMP _1970_____
☐Possibility of Pregnancy
☐Other_____
☒*No identified problems*

PSYCHOSOCIAL
☐Alcohol use _____
☐Drug use _____
☐Panic/Anxiety Attacks
☐Depression
☐Tobacco use _____
☐Claustrophobia
☐ADD
☐Growth and Development
  not appropiate for age
☐Other_____
☒*No identified problems*

MISCELLANEOUS
☐Vision Changes

☐Glaucoma/Cataracts
☐Blood/Bleeding Disorders
☐CA _____
☐Skin Problems
☐Hearing Deficit
☐Infectious Disease/STD
☐Head Circumference _____
  (if appropriate)
☐Immunizations up to date
☐Other_____
☒*No identified problems*

Comments: ___Family states she's very independent. Walks a mile a day.___

Assistive Devices Brought to Hospital		
☐ Orthodontic appliance	☐ Prosthesis	☐ Crutches/Walker/Cane
☐ Dentures _____	☒ Glasses/Contacts	☐ Other _____
☐ Hearing Aid	☐ Wheelchair	

Past surgical History: ___Hysterectomy 1970_____

Previous anesthesia: ☒ General   ☐ Spinal

Other: _____

Problems with Anesthesia? ___None_____

Blood Donations- This Admission   ☐ Autologous   ☐ Direct Donor   ☒ None

Needs Assessment

CURRENT PAIN		CARE OR LEARNING NEED
☒ Denies Pain		☐ Pain Management
Duration of Pain?		
_____		☐ Patient Education
What Controls the Pain:_____		
_____		*Indicate in the diagram where pain is located and label the intensity 1-10, with "1" meaning minimal pain to "10" being the worst pain.*
What is the Impact on ADL's?		
_____		
_____		

F i g u r e   **2–2.** (Continued)

COMPLETE THIS SECTION FOR INPATIENTS ONLY
UNLESS SPECIFIC ASSESSMENT IS WARRANTED

Patient Name: _Rose Feterini_

NUTRITIONAL STATUS	PROBLEM/NEED
If any of the following are present, send computer order to Nutrition Services ☐ Unintentional Weight Loss≥10 lbs in the Last 6 Months ☐ Vomiting /Diarrhea for the Last 3 Days or Longer ☐ Poor Appetite for the Last 5 Days or Longer ☐ Swallowing Difficulties resulting in inadequate intake ☐ Newly Diagnosed Pt with Diabetes Need for Education **(also notify Diabetes Educator)** ☐ Decub Ulcer Stage II or greater ☐ Dialysis ☐ New to modified Diet and Needs Education ☒ *No Identified Problems*	☐ Nutrition Referral ☐ Diabetes Educator

RESPIRATORY ASSESSMENT	PROBLEM/NEED
☐ Patient is pre-op for upper abdominal or thoracic surgery <u>and</u> has a history of Emphysema, Bronchitis, Asthma, or Pulmonary Fibrosis	☐ Respiratory Care Consult ☐ Respiratory Therapist Paged

FUNCTIONAL STATUS ASSESSMENT	Independent	Some Assist	Total Assist	PROBLEM/NEED
Feeding	X			☐ Assist with ADL's
Bathing	X			
Dressing	X			
Toileting	X			
Transfers(bed to chair, to/from toilet)	X			☐ Patient / Family Education
Walking/ Use of Wheelchair	X			

If any of the following are present, refer as follows:

OCCUPATIONAL THERAPY
☐ Condition Resulted in Impairment of One or Both Upper Extremities.
☐ Diminished Capacity for Self-Care That Could Be Resolved With Therapy Intervention.
☐ Physically Unable To Feed Self   ☐ **No Needs Identified**
PHYSICAL THERAPY
☐ Condition has Resulted in Decline in Gait, Transfer and/or Balance Skills That Could Be Resolved with Physical Therapy Services.
☐ Condition has Resulted in Decreased Strength and/or Range of Motion of Extremities.
☐ Condition has Resulted in Acute Increase in Musculoskeletal Pain. ☐**No Needs Identified**
SPEECH THERAPY
☐ Difficulty Swallowing or Signs of Aspiration While Drinking/Eating.
☐ Diagnosis of CVA, Myasthenia Gravis, Multiple Intubations, or At Risk for Silent Aspiration.
☐ Unable to Follow Simple Instructions for Daily Care and/or Unable to Communicate Wants and Needs.
☒ **No Needs Identified**

PROBLEM/NEED

☐ Physician Order Requested For:

❑ PHYSICAL THERAPY

❑ OCCUPATIONAL THERAPY

❑ SPEECH/LANGUAGE PATHOLOGY

FALL RISK ASSESSMENT*	Low Risk 0-20	Moderate Risk 25-60	High risk 65-100	*See Patient Safety: Fall Safety Program

Fall Assessment Indicators	Weight Score	Assessment Score
Admission or transfer	5	2
History of falls	20	0
Recent change in functional mobility	20	0
Alteration in elimination	20	0
Diagnosis/Medication which effects cognition/mobility/balance	10	0
Confusion/impairment of judgement/forgetful/agitated and or non-compliant	20	0
Sensory/Visual/Perceptual impairment (unrelated to above)	5	0
TOTAL SCORE	100	2

F i g u r e **2–2.** (*Continued*)

COMPLETE THIS SECTION FOR INPATIENTS ONLY
UNLESS SPECIFIC ASSESSMENT IS WARRANTED

Patient Name: _Rose Fetrini_

CULTURE/RELIGIOUS/SPIRITUAL	PROBLEM/NEED
Religious Preference: ☐None ☒Catholic ☐Protestant ☐Jewish ☐Other_____	☒ Cultural Needs _Daily prayer -_
Any special cultural or spiritual needs while in the hospital?	_Two hours_!
☐No ☐Yes Specify: _Prays 2 hrs/day - Rosary with her_	☒ Refer to Chaplain
Would like to see the hospital chaplain ☐No ☐Yes	

SOCIAL/DISCHARGE PLANNING	PROBLEM/NEED
☒Lives Alone	
☐Lives with spouse/significant other/family/caretaker	
☐Lives in nursing home/assisted living ❶	☐Assist With ADLs
☐Compromised in ADLs and /or lack of support network ❶	
☐Special discharge needs ❶_____	☐Patient Education
☐Insurance concerns ❶	
☐Received supports prior to admission: ☐unknown ☐home care ☐med equip ❶	❶ ☐ Refer to Case Manager
☐Patient plans to be discharged to: _____	
☐Discharge Transportation (Name) _____(Phone#)_____	
☐Unable to return to previous living arrangement ❷	
☐Financial concerns ❷	❷ ☐ Refer to Social Work
☐Evidence of physical/emotional abuse or neglect or domestic violence ❷	
☐Current substance abuse ❷	
☒No discharge planning needs identified	

EDUCATION NEEDS ASSESSMENT

Learning Readiness: ☒Willing to Learn   ☐Unable to Learn
Barriers to Learning: ☒No Barriers   ☐Cognitive   ☐Cultural   ☐Educational   ☐Emotional
☐Language   ☐Motivational   ☐Financial   ☐Physical   ☐Religious   ☐Refuses at this time
☐Comments/Other_____

Plans to Overcome Barriers to Education: ☐Family involvement   ☐Reinforcement   ☒Written Materials
☐Audiovisual Aids   ☐Interpreter   ☐Other_____

Specific Educational Needs: ☐Disease Process   ☐Activity Level   ☐Diet   ☐Procedures   ☐Hygiene
☒Medications (including Drug and Food Interactions)   ☐Medical Equipment/Assistive Devices
☐Skin/Ostomy (Enterostomal Therapist notified)
☐Other _____

Teaching to be directed primarily to: ☒Patient   ☐Family   ☐Other_____
Patient Folder Given?   ☒Yes   ☐No

Based on this assessment, the following clinical pathway/ standard of care has been implemented

Atrial Fibrillation - Arrythmia

Completed by RN: _R. Alfonso-La Fure_   Date: _5/8/02_ Time: _12 Noon_

Reviewed by RN: _Nancy Flynn_   Date: _5/08/02_ Time: _3 PM_

Figure 2–2. (Continued)

Community Nursing Service & Hospice

NURSING EVALUATION

CLIENT'S NAME _____

FID# _____

EXPECTED OUTCOME	RANKING KEY
1. Normal	
2. Abnormal but stable	
3. Abnormal but improved	
4. Abnormal	

FUNDING SOURCE: (CHECK ONE)
☐ MEDICARE   ☐ PRIVATE INS.
☐ MEDICAID   ☐ SELF-PAY
☐ OTHER _____
BRANCH _____

_____ Certification _____ Recertification   **PERIOD: FROM** _____ **TO** _____

Reason for referral (admission only): _____

☐ Y ☐ N   HOLD 485 for other disciplines? WHO? ☐ P.T. ☐ O.T. ☐ S.T. ☐ OTHER _____

☐ Y ☐ N   DELETE 485 information from other disciplines? WHO? ☐ P.T. ☐ O.T. ☐ S.T. ☐ OTHER _____

RN SIGNATURE _____ DATE _____ Casemanager?   ☐ YES   ☐ NO

Casemanager (if known): _____

EXPECTED OUTCOME	1	2	3	4

R   L   L   R

INTEGUMENT: ☐ History: _____
☐ Jaundice
☐ Petechiae
☐ Rashes
☐ Lesions
☐ Contusions   Why _____
☐ Wound/pressure sore
size   L _____   (see
        W _____   drawing)
        D _____
☐ Suture line _____
☐ Drainage _____
☐ Other _____
☐ No problems

INTERVENTION: ☐ No   ☐ Yes
Who _____ Why _____

EXPECTED OUTCOME	1	2	3	4

PAIN: ☐ History: _____
Location _____
Intensity (scale 1-10) _____
Quality _____
Frequency _____
Relief _____
   ☐ No problems

INTERVENTION: ☐ No   ☐ Yes
Who _____
Why _____
Methods _____

NEUROMUSCULAR: ☐ History: _____
☐ Weakness   ☐ Impaired gait/ROM
☐ Impaired balance   ☐ Seizures _____
☐ Impaired use of hands   ☐ Tremors _____
☐ Paresthesias   ☐ Paralysis _____
☐ Hernia   ☐ Developmental
☐ No problems   delay
                         ☐ Normal reflexes

INTERVENTION: ☐ No   ☐ Yes   Who _____
Why _____

EXPECTED OUTCOME	1	2	3	4

EXPECTED OUTCOME	1	2	3	4

CNS 132 (6/92)

TRANSCRIPTION COPY
TRAVELING COPY

F i g u r e **2–3.** Nursing evaluation. (Courtesy of Community Nursing Service, Salt Lake City, Utah).

CLIENT'S NAME _____

FID# _____

FUNCTIONAL LIMITATIONS:

- ☐ 1 Amputation
- ☐ 2 Bowel/Bladder
- ☐ 3 Contracture
- ☐ 4 Hearing
- ☐ 5 Paralysis
- ☐ Infant
- ☐ B Other _____

- ☐ 6 Endurance
- ☐ 7 Ambulation
- ☐ 8 Speech
- ☐ 9 Legally blind
- ☐ A Dyspnea with
  minimal exertion

ADL LIMITATIONS AND PRIOR FUNCTIONAL STATUS: _____
_____
_____
_____
_____

ACTIVITIES PERMITTED:

- ☐ 1 Bedrest complete
- ☐ 2 Bedrest BRP
- ☐ 3 Up as tolerated
- ☐ 4 Transfer bed/chair
- ☐ 5 Exercise prescribed
- ☐ 6 Partial weight bear

- ☐ 7 Independent at home
- ☐ 8 Crutches   ☐ 9 Cane
- ☐ A Wheelchair
- ☐ B Walker
- ☐ C No restrictions
- ☐ D Other _____
- ☐ Infant

MENTAL STATUS:

- ☐ 1 Oriented
- ☐ 2 Comatose
- ☐ 3 Forgetful
- ☐ 4 Depressed

- ☐ 5 Disoriented
- ☐ 6 Lethargic
- ☐ 7 Agitated
- ☐ 8 Other _____

PROGNOSIS: ☐ 1 Poor   ☐ 2 Guarded   ☐ 3 Fair   ☐ 4 Good   ☐ 5 Excellent

REHAB POTENTIAL: ☐ Full recovery/independent of CNS Care   ☐ Return to preacute level
☐ Will require ongoing CNS care   ☐ Endstage illness, support until death
Other _____

ALLERGIES: _____

SELF-CARE:	FEEDING	MEAL PREP	BATH/ PERS. CARE	DRESSING/ GROOMING	TRANS-FERS	AMBUL-LATION	TOILET-ING	HOUSE-KEEPING	LAUNDRY SHOPPING	MANG. FIN.
IND.	☐	☐	☐	☐	☐	☐	☐	☐	☐	☐
MECH. ASST.	☐	☐	☐	☐	☐	☐	☐	☐	☐	☐
MOD. ASST.	☐	☐	☐	☐	☐	☐	☐	☐	☐	☐
DEP.	☐	☐	☐	☐	☐	☐	☐	☐	☐	☐

INTERVENTION: ☐ No   ☐ Yes   Who _____   Why _____

EXPECTED OUTCOME	1	2	3	4

☐ CLIENT/S.O. IS INVOLVED IN CAREPLANNING.   Who _____

CAREGIVER CAPABILITY   ☐ Suff.   ☐ Inconsistent   ☐ Ltd.   ☐ None

CARDIOVASCULAR: _____
_____

- ☐ History _____
- ☐ Edema - Degree _____
  Where _____ When _____
- ☐ Chest Pain ___ c̄ ___ s̄ activity
  Degree _____ Frequency _____
  Duration _____ Relief _____
  Cyanosis - Where _____
- ☐ Murmurs
- ☐ Orthopnea
- ☐ Palpitations
- ☐ Bleeding Problems _____
- ☐ S/S Orthostatic Hypotension _____
- ☐ Cardiopulmonary monitor _____
- ☐ Juglar Venous Distention
- ☐ No problem

Cap. Refill _____ secs
Pedal Pulses R _____
L _____
Other _____

INTERVENTION: ☐ No   ☐ Yes   Who _____
Why _____

EXPECTED OUTCOME	1	2	3	4

RESPIRATORY: _____

- ☐ History _____
- Lung Sounds _____
- ☐ SOB   ☐ c̄   ☐ s̄ exertion
- ☐ Cough _____ Retractions
- ☐ Sputum Color _____
  Amt _____
- ☐ Smoker Amt _____ Yrs _____
- ☐ 02 _____ l/min per
- ☐ Other equipment _____
  _____
- ☐ Other _____
- ☐ No problems

INTERVENTION: ☐ No   ☐ Yes
Who _____
Why _____

EXPECTED OUTCOME	1	2	3	4

CNS132 (6/92)

TRANSCRIPTION COPY
TRAVELING COPY

F i g u r e **2–3.** (Continued)

CLIENT'S NAME _____

FID# _____

GI   GU   ENDOCRINE   3

GI
- ☐ History _____
- Last BM _____
- Bowel Habits _____
- ☐ Constipation
- ☐ Diarrhea
- ☐ Incontinence
- ☐ N/V
- ☐ Rectal bleeding
- ☐ Indigestion
- ☐ Appetite
- ☐ Hydration
- ☐ Ascites _____
- ☐ Liver involvement
- ☐ Breast feeding
- ☐ Bottle feeding
      amount _____
- ☐ Other _____
- ☐ No problems

INTERVENTION: ☐ No   ☐ Yes
Who _____
Why _____

| EXPECTED OUTCOME | 1 | 2 | 3 | 4 |

GU
- ☐ History _____
- Urinary Habits _____
- ☐ Incontinent ____ diapers ____ pads
- ☐ Indwelling Cath size ____ fr
      freq. of change _____
- ☐ Condom cath ____ Circumcision
- ☐ Frequency ____Urgency ____Hesitancy
- ☐ Nocturia ____ Dysuria
- ☐ Pyuria ____ Hematuria
- ☐ Other _____
- ☐ No problems

INTERVENTION: ☐ No   ☐ Yes
Who _____
Why _____

| EXPECTED OUTCOME | 1 | 2 | 3 | 4 |

ENDOCRINE
- ☐ History _____
- ☐ Hyperthyroid
- ☐ Hypothyroid
- ☐ Pancreas
- ☐ IDDM   ☐ NIDDM
- ☐ PBS _____
- ☐ Prostate
- ☐ Uterus
- ☐ Breast Lumps
- ☐ Discharge
- ☐ Performs SBE
- ☐ Other _____
- ☐ No problems

INTERVENTION: ☐ No ☐ Yes
Who _____
Why _____

| EXPECTED OUTCOME | 1 | 2 | 3 | 4 |

NUTRITIONAL REQUIREMENTS:
_____

EYES/EARS/NOSE/THROAT   ☐ History _____

- ☐ Vision Impairment
- ☐ Glasses   ☐ Contacts
- ☐ Can   ☐ Cannot see print
- ☐ Can   ☐ Cannot see television
- ☐ Can   ☐ Cannot see shadows
- ☐ Legally blind
- ☐ Inflammation   ☐ Discharge
- ☐ Cataracts   ☐ Glaucoma
- ☐ No problems

- ☐ Hearing impairment
- ☐ Hearing aides ☐ L   ☐ R
- ☐ Vertigo
- ☐ Tinnitus
- ☐ Other _____
- ☐ No problems

- ☐ Sinus problems
- ☐ Nosebleeds
      frequency _____
- ☐ Discharge
- ☐ Patent ☐ R   ☐ L
- ☐ Other _____
- ☐ No problem

- ☐ Hoarseness   ☐ Dysphagia   ☐ Difficulty chewing
- ☐ Mouth sores/irritation/bleeding   ☐ Dentures   ☐ upper   ☐ lower   ☐ partial _____
- Mouth breather   ☐ Poor suck response   ☐ No problem

INTERVENTION: ☐ No   ☐ Yes   Who _____   Why _____

| EXPECTED OUTCOME | 1 | 2 | 3 | 4 |

DME AND SUPPLIES: _____
_____
_____

REASON HOMEBOUND: _____
_____

MEDICAL/NON-MEDICAL REASONS CLIENT REGULARLY LEAVES HOME AND HOW OFTEN:
_____

CNS132 (6/92)

TRANSCRIPTION COPY
TRAVELING COPY

F i g u r e **2–3.** (*Continued*)

CLIENT'S NAME _____

FID# _____

4

PSYCHOSOCIAL:

CIRCLE ONE

(Y = Yes N = No)

	CLIENT		SO/WHO	
Cooperative	Y	N	Y	N
Willing/capable of learning	Y	N	Y	N
Communication impairment	Y	N	Y	N
Speech impairment	Y	N	Y	N
Impaired comprehension	Y	N	Y	N
Language barrier	Y	N	Y	N
Depressed	Y	N	Y	N
Anxiety	Y	N	Y	N
Grief	Y	N	Y	N
Combative	Y	N	Y	N
Hostile	Y	N	Y	N
Agitated	Y	N	Y	N
Confused	Y	N	Y	N
Interpersonal conflict	Y	N	Y	N
Illiterate	Y	N	Y	N

LIVING ARRANGEMENTS:

☐ A. Lives alone ☐ home ☐ apt.
☐ B. Lives with willing persons
   ☐ family ☐ friends
☐ C. Lives with unwilling persons
☐ D. Other

UNUSUAL HOME/SOCIAL ENVIRONMENT:

_____
_____
_____

CLIENT'S STATEMENT OF
EXPECTATIONS/OUTCOME OF HOME CARE:

_____
_____
_____
_____

ASSISTANCE FROM RELATIVES/FRIENDS:
(Support systems) _____
_____
_____
_____

INTERVENTION: ☐ No ☐ Yes

Who _____
Why _____

EXPECTED OUTCOME	1	2	3	4

IS CLIENT RECIEVING CARE PAID FOR BY OTHER THAN MEDICARE? ☐ YES ☐ NO Who _____

No. of people in household _____   Teach family/S.O.   ☐ YES   ☐ NO

Approx. length of care _____

ANY SUPPLEMENTARY TREATMENT PLANS FROM OTHER THAN REFERRING PHYSICIAN? ☐ YES ☐ NO

(Refer to orders)

Desires Home care ☐ Yes ☐ No

SAFETY: (✓ = Assessed += problem) CIRCLE ONE

			COMMUNITY RESOURCES
+ ✓ Home safe	+ ✓ Cluttered	+ ✓ Food adequate	☐ County mental health
+ ✓ Telephone	+ ✓ Pests	+ ✓ Heat adequate	☐ MOW
+ ✓ Running Water	+ ✓ Pets	+ ✓ Bedding adequate	☐ Transportation
+ ✓ Electricity	+ ✓ Stairs # _____	+ ✓ Lighting	☐ Alternatives
+ ✓ Refrigerator	where_____	+ ✓ Able to call for help	☐ WIC
+ ✓ Handrails	+ ✓ Elevator	+ ✓ Safe neighborhood	☐ Sr. companion
			☐ Other _____

INTERVENTION: ☐ No ☐ Yes   Who _____   Why _____

CLIENT IS SAFE AT HOME WITH SERVICES CNS CAN PROVIDE: ☐ Yes ☐ No

CNS132 (6/92)

TRANSCRIPTION COPY
TRAVELING COPY

F i g u r e **2–3.** (Continued)

MDS Form

MINIMUM DATA SET FOR NURSING HOME RESIDENT ASSESSMENT AND CARE SCREENING (MDS)
(Status in last 7 days, unless other time frame indicated)

SECTION A. IDENTIFICATION AND BACKGROUND INFORMATION

1. **ASSESSMENT DATE** — Month — Day — Year

2. **RESIDENT NAME** — (First) (Middle Initial) (Last)

3. **SOCIAL SECURITY NO.**

4. **MEDICAID NO. (if applicable)**

5. **MEDICAL RECORD NO.**

6. **REASON FOR ASSESSMENT**
   1. Initial admission assess.
   2. Hosp/Medicare reassess.
   3. Readmission assessment
   4. Annual assessment
   5. Significant change in status
   6. Other (e.g., UR)

7. **CURRENT PAYMENT SOURCE(S) FOR N.H. STAY** (Billing Office to indicate; check all that apply)
   - Medicaid — a.
   - Medicare — b.
   - CHAMPUS — c.
   - VA — d.
   - Self pay/Private insurance — e.
   - Other — f.

8. **RESPONSIBILITY/ LEGAL GUARDIAN** (Check all that apply)
   - Legal guardian — a.
   - Other legal oversight — b.
   - Durable power attrny./ health care proxy — c.
   - Family member responsible — d.
   - Resident responsible — e.
   - NONE OF ABOVE — f.

9. **ADVANCED DIRECTIVES** (For those items with supporting documentation in the medical record, check all that apply)
   - Living will — a.
   - Do not resuscitate — b.
   - Do not hospitalize — c.
   - Organ donation — d.
   - Autopsy request — e.
   - Feeding restrictions — f.
   - Medication restrictions — g.
   - Other treatment restrictions — h.
   - NONE OF ABOVE — i.

10. **DISCHARGE PLANNED WITHIN 3 MOS.** (Does not include discharge due to death)
    0. No   1. Yes   2. Unknown/uncertain

11. **PARTICIPATE IN ASSESSMENT**
    a. Resident   0. No   1. Yes
    b. Family   0. No   1. Yes   2. No family

12. **SIGNATURES** Signature of RN Assessment Coordinator

    Signatures of Others Who Completed Part of the Assessment

SECTION B. COGNITIVE PATTERNS

1. **COMATOSE** (Persistent vegetative state/no discernible consciousness)
   0. No   1. Yes (Skip to SECTION E)

2. **MEMORY** (Recall of what was learned or known)
   a. Short-term memory OK—seems/appears to recall after 5 minutes
      0. Memory OK   1. Memory problem
   b. Long-term memory OK—seems/appears to recall long past
      0. Memory OK   1. Memory problem

3. **MEMORY/ RECALL ABILITY** (Check all that resident normally able to recall during last 7 days)
   - Current season — a.
   - Location of own room — b.
   - Staff names/faces — c.
   - That he/she is in a nursing home — d.
   - NONE OF ABOVE are recalled — e.

▨ = Code the appropriate response   ☐ = Check all the responses that apply

Appendix B: Page B-2

---

4. **COGNITIVE SKILLS FOR DAILY DECISION-MAKING** (Made decisions regarding tasks of daily life)
   0. Independent—decisions consistent/reasonable
   1. Modified Independence—some difficulty in new situations only
   2. Moderately Impaired—decisions poor; cues/supervision required
   3. Severely Impaired—never/rarely made decisions

5. **INDICATORS OF DELIRIUM —PERIODIC DISORDERED THINKING/ AWARENESS** (Check if condition over last 7 days appears different from usual functioning)
   - Less alert, easily distracted — a.
   - Changing awareness of environment — b.
   - Episodes of incoherent speech — c.
   - Periods of motor restlessness or lethargy — d.
   - Cognitive ability varies over course of day — e.
   - NONE OF ABOVE — f.

6. **CHANGE IN COGNITIVE STATUS** Change in resident's cognitive status, skills, or abilities in last 90 days
   0. No change   1. Improved   2. Deterioriated

SECTION C. COMMUNICATION/HEARING PATTERNS

1. **HEARING** (With hearing appliance, if used)
   0. Hears adequately—normal talk, TV, phone
   1. Minimal difficulty when not in quiet setting
   2. Hears in special situations only—speaker has to adjust tonal quality and speak distinctly
   3. Highly impaired/absence of useful hearing

2. **COMMUNICATION DEVICES/ TECHNIQUES** (Check all that apply during last 7 days)
   - Hearing aid, present and used — a.
   - Hearing aid, present and not used — b.
   - Other receptive comm. techniques used (e.g., lip read) — c.
   - NONE OF ABOVE — d.

3. **MODES OF EXPRESSION** (Check all used by resident to make needs known)
   - Speech — a.
   - Writing messages to express or clarify needs — b.
   - Signs/gestures/sounds — c.
   - Communication board — d.
   - Other — e.
   - NONE OF ABOVE — f.

4. **MAKING SELF UNDERSTOOD** (Express information content—however able)
   0. Understood
   1. Usually Understood—difficulty finding words or finishing thoughts
   2. Sometimes Understood—ability is limited to making concrete requests
   3. Rarely/Never Understood

5. **ABILITY TO UNDERSTAND OTHERS** (Understanding verbal information content—however able)
   0. Understands
   1. Usually Understands—may miss some part/intent of message
   2. Sometimes Understands—responds adequately to simple, direct communication
   3. Rarely/Never Understands

6. **CHANGE IN COMMUNICATION/ HEARING** Resident's ability to express, understand or hear information has changed over last 90 days
   0. No change   1. Improved   2. Deterioriated

SECTION D. VISION PATTERNS

1. **VISION** (Ability to see in adequate light and with glasses if used)
   0. Adequate—sees fine detail, including regular print in newspapers/books
   1. Impaired—sees large print, but not regular print in newspapers/books
   2. Highly impaired—limited vision; not able to see newspaper headlines; appears to follow objects with eyes
   3. Severely impaired—no vision or appears to see only light, colors, or shapes

2. **VISUAL LIMITATIONS/ DIFFICULTIES**
   - Side vision problems—decreased peripheral vision (e.g., leaves food on one side of tray, difficulty traveling, bumps into people and objects, misjudges placement of chair when seating self) — a.
   - Experiences any of following: sees halos or rings around lights; sees flashes of light; sees "curtains" over eyes — b.
   - NONE OF ABOVE — c.

3. **VISUAL APPLIANCES** Glasses; contact lenses; lens implant; magnifying glass
   0. No   1. Yes

December, 1990

Figure 2–4. The first page of the Minimum Data Set (developed by HCFA).

hensive admission assessment, you may perform a focus assessment of the neurologic status of someone who has just had a head injury. Later, you may perform neurologic focus assessments every hour to monitor for changes in status.

Although there are some forms that guide focus assessments, you often do focus assessments without a guide, so you need to know what types of questions you should be asking. The following are four key questions to ask:

1. What is the *current* status of the problem (are there signs, symptoms, or risk factors for the problem)?
2. Compared with the baseline data (data gathered before treatment began), does the information indicate that the problem is better, worse, or the same?
3. What factors are contributing to the problem, and what has been done about these factors?
4. What's the *patient's perspective* on the current status of the problem and how it's being managed?

The following focus assessment shows how to apply the preceding questions to assessing for *Constipation.*

1. **What is the current pattern of bowel elimination?** (Is there evidence of signs, symptoms, or risk factors for *Constipation*?)
2. **Compared to the baseline data, does the current status indicate that the constipation (or risk for constipation) has changed?** (Are the signs, symptoms, and risk factors still present; are there new ones?).
3. **What factors are contributing to the *Constipation* (eg, poor diet, lack of fluid intake, medication side effects, immobility)?** How can we ensure enough roughage and fluid intake? Is there anything we can do about the immobility? What can we do about medication side effects? How can we be sure we stay on top of this problem?
4. What's the patient's perspective on his current status and preventing and managing *Constipation?* Is he able to relate how to do this? Is there a need for teaching?

Health Promotion: Screening for Prevention and Early Diagnosis

As we move more toward the predict, prevent, and manage model addressed in Chapter 1, expect to be involved in screening for prevention and early diagnosis of common health problems. When performing assessments, look for opportunities for health promotion. To meet the goals of *Healthy People 2010,* which aim to increase the length and quality of life, providers in all settings must identify health risk factors and record health promotion counseling during every patient encounter. Take a look at Tables 2–1 and 2–2, and Display 2–1, which show recommended health screening for the general population, examples of screening tests for high-risk groups, and the criteria for screening tests.

TABLE 2 – 1 Recommended Screening for the General Population

Birth to 10 Years

- ➤ Height and weight
- ➤ Blood pressure
- ➤ Vision (age 3–4 yr)
- ➤ Hemoglobinopathy (birth)[1]
- ➤ Phenylalanine (birth)
- ➤ T_4 and TSH (birth)

11–24 Years

- ➤ Height and weight
- ➤ Blood pressure
- ➤ Pap test[2]
- ➤ *Chlamydia*[3]
- ➤ Rubella serology or vaccination history[4]
- ➤ Assess for problem drinking

25–64 Years

- ➤ Height and weight
- ➤ Blood pressure
- ➤ Pap test[5]
- ➤ Total blood—cholesterol (men: 35–65; women 45–65)
- ➤ Fecal occult blood and sigmoidoscopy older than age 50
- ➤ Mammogram and clinical breast examination[7] (women 50–69 years)
- ➤ Assess for problem drinking
- ➤ Rubella serology or vaccination history[4]

65 Plus

- ➤ Height and weight
- ➤ Blood pressure
- ➤ Pap test[5]
- ➤ Fecal occult blood[6]
- ➤ Mammogram and clinical breast examination[7] (women 69 years and younger)
- ➤ Vision and hearing
- ➤ Assess for problem drinking

T_4, thyroxine; TSH, thyrotropin.

1. Whether screening should be universal or targeted to high-risk groups depends on the proportion of high-risk individuals in the screening area.

2. If sexually active at present or in the past, every 3 years or less; if sexual history is unreliable, begin Pap tests at 18 years,

3. If sexually active.

4. Serologic testing, documented vaccination history, and routine vaccination against rubella are equally acceptable alternatives.

5. All women who are or have been sexually active and who have a cervix, every 3 or less years.

6. Annually.

7. The American Cancer Society recommends an annual clinical examination with screening mammogram every 1 to 2 years between the ages of 40 and 50, and an annual mammogram every year after age 50.

From *Report of the U.S. Preventive Services Task Force: Guide to Clinical Preventive Services*. (1996). (2nd ed). Baltimore, MD: Williams & Wilkins.

TABLE 2 – 2 Examples of Screening Tests for High-Risk Groups

Examples of Screening Tests for High-Risk Groups

Risk Factor	Screening Test
Preterm or low birth weight	Hemoglobin/hematocrit
Tuberculosis contacts, immigrants, low income	PPD
Residents of long-term care facilities	PPD
Increased lead exposure	Blood lead level
High-risk sexual behavior	RPR/VDRL; HIV
Gonorrhea (female); chlamydia (female)	RPR/VDRL; HIV
Injection of street drugs	
Blood transfusion between 1978–1985	HIV screen
Cardiovascular disease risk factors	Cholesterol

Modified from *Report of the U.S. Preventive Services Task Force: Guide to Clinical Preventive Services.* (1996). (2nd ed.). Baltimore, MD: Williams & Wilkins.

DISPLAY 2 – 1   Criteria for Screening Tests

Appropriate screening includes considering specific risks, benefits, and costs involved, considering the following criteria.

- Disease represents a significant health problem.
- Disease is prevalent and affects quality of life and longevity.
- Disease has an asymptomatic period, allowing for early detection.
- Test detects the disease at an earlier stage than it would once symptoms are present.
- Disease has an acceptable method of treatment.
- Disease has better therapeutic results with early treatment, worse with delayed treatment.
- Test has a high degree of sensitivity, specificity, predictive value, and reliability.
- Test is safe, acceptable, affordable, and accessible.
- Resources are available for diagnosis, treatment, counseling, and follow-up.
- The cost of screening is balanced by the benefits of early detection and treatment.
- The screening test is relevant to the population to be screened.

Adapted from Fielo, S. (2000). *Screening: How to change world health.* Available: *http://nsweb. nursingspectrum.com/ce/ce211.htm.* Accessed January 9, 2000.

The Nursing Interview and Physical Assessment

Interviews and physical assessments complement and clarify one another, as you can see in the following example.

E X A M P L E

> You interview someone who tells you, "I feel like my breathing isn't quite right, but I can't explain exactly what I mean." You then listen to her lungs with a stethoscope. What you hear (whether the lung sounds are normal or abnormal) gives you additional information that complements and clarifies what you've been *told*.

Ethical, Cultural, and Spiritual Considerations

The success of your interviewing and examination techniques is influenced by your awareness of ethical, cultural, and spiritual concerns. As a nurse, you must:

1. Provide services with respect for human dignity and the uniqueness of the client, unrestricted by considerations of social or economic status, personal attributes, or the nature of health problems (ANA, 1985).
2. Safeguard the client's right to privacy by judiciously protecting information of a confidential nature (ANA, 1985).
3. Be honest. Tell the person the truth about how you'll use the data (eg, "I have to write a paper examining someone's eating patterns. Would you be willing to tell me about your eating habits?").
4. Respect individual cultural and religious beliefs and be aware of physical tendencies related to culture. This includes being aware of:
   - **Biologic variations.** For example, differences among racial and ethnic groups (eg, skin color and texture, and susceptibility to diseases like hypertension or sickle cell anemia)
   - **Comfortable communication patterns.** For example, how language and gestures are used, whether eye contact or touching is acceptable, and whether the person is threatened by being in close proximity to another
   - **Family organization and practices.** We have diverse family units and practices we must understand to gain insight into factors that influence health status.
   - **Beliefs about whether people are able to control nature and influence their ability to be healthy** (eg, whether blood transfusions are allowed, whether rituals are required)

V O I C E S

Spiritual Needs Matter.
Spirituality encompasses the whole of a person's being. Although many people do not subscribe to a recognized, organized system of beliefs—an established religion—virtually all humans are spiritual beings and uphold certain individual principles. These principles shape their view of themselves, the world, and God or a higher power.—*Susan Richardson, RN, MS, CS*

(Richardson, S. [2001]. Making a spiritual assessment. *Nursing Spectrum, 11*[2FL],12–15.)

- **The person's concept of "God" and beliefs about the relationship between spiritual beliefs and health status** (eg, "God gives you what you deserve").

The Nursing Interview

Your ability to establish rapport, ask questions, listen, and observe is the key to a positive nurse–patient relationship and essential to getting the facts. People who seek health care, whether they're well or acutely ill, are in an extremely vulnerable position; they need to know that they're in good hands and that their main concerns will be addressed. This is where you come in. Consider the following guidelines that can help you to establish trust, create a positive attitude, and reduce anxiety.

Guidelines: Promoting a Caring Interview
How to Establish Rapport

Before you go into the interview

- **Get organized:** When you know what you're going to do, you're more confident and able to focus on the person.
- **Don't rely on memory:** Have a written or printed plan to guide the questions you'll be asking. Some nurses use the nursing data base as a guide (see page 39).
- **Plan enough time:** The admission interview usually takes 30 minutes to 1 hour.
- **Ensure privacy:** Make sure you have a quiet, private setting, free from interruptions or distractions.
- **Get focused:** Take a minute to clear your mind of other concerns (other duties, worries about yourself). Say to yourself, "Getting to know this person is the most important thing I have to do right now."
- **Visualize yourself as being confident, warm, and helpful:** Seeing yourself in this light helps you to *be* confident, warm, and helpful; your genuine interest comes through.

When you begin the interview

- **Give your name and position** (if the person can read, give it in writing). This sends the message that you accept responsibility and are willing to be accountable for your actions.
- **Verify the person's name and ask what he or she would like to be called** (eg, "I have your name listed here as Michael Riley. Is that correct? What would you like us to call you?"). Verifying the name sends the message that you want to make sure things are correct. Using the preferred name helps the person to feel more relaxed and sends the message that you recognize that this person is an individual who has likes and dislikes.
- **Briefly explain your purpose** (eg, "I'm here to do the admission interview to help us plan your nursing care").

During the interview

- **Give the person your full attention:** Avoid the impulse to become engrossed in your notes or reading the assessment tool.
- **Don't hurry:** Rushing sends the message that you're not interested in what the person has to say.
- **Sit down.** This communicates that you're willing to take the time needed to collect information.

How to Listen

- **Be an empathetic listener** (see page 29).
- **Use short, supplementary phrases** that let the person know you understand and encourage the person to continue. Some examples are, "I see," "Mm-hm," "Oh, no," "And . . . ," and "Then what?" A nod of the head also lets the person know that you're listening.
- **Listen for feelings** as well as words. For example, the person who sighs, looks away, and says, "I think I'll be okay with this," might be telling you, "I doubt this is going to work."
- **Let the person know when you see body language that sends a message that conflicts with what is being said** (eg, "You say that you aren't having pain, but you look uncomfortable to me").
- **Allow the person to finish sentences.** Be calm and don't rush him.
- **Be patient if the person has a memory block.** This information may be remembered later when you ask related questions.
- **Avoid the impulse to interrupt.** If the interview is getting off track, allow the person to finish his sentence, then say, "We seem to be getting off track. Can we get back to . . . ?"
- **Allow for pauses in conversation.** Silence gives both you and the person time to gather thoughts.

How to Ask Questions

- **Ask about the person's main problem first** (eg, "What is the main reason you're here today?").
- **Focus your questions to gain specific information about signs and symptoms.** For example: Show me where the problem is. Can you describe how this feels more specifically? When did this start? When does this seem to happen? Is there anything that makes it better? What makes it worse?"
- **Don't use leading questions** that are likely to lead the person to a specific response (eg, "You don't drink alcohol, do you?" leads the person to a "no" answer).
- **Do use exploratory statements** (statements that begin with words like *tell, describe, explain,* and *elaborate*) to direct the person to tell you more about a specific condition (eg, "Tell me more about your sleeping patterns"). (Some authors call these types of statements *leading statements.* I use *exploratory statements* to avoid confusion with *leading questions,* which shouldn't be used.)

- **Use communication techniques that enhance your ability to think critically and get the facts:**
  - ○ Use phrases that help you see the other person's perspective (eg, "From your point of view, what are the biggest problems?" or "What are the problems as you see them?").
  - ○ Restate the person's own words. This clarifies meaning and encourages the person to expand on what's been said (eg, "When you say . . . , what are you saying?" or "When you say . . . , does this mean . . . ?").
  - ○ Ask open-ended questions (questions requiring more than a one-word answer, such as "How are you feeling?" rather than "Are you feeling well?").
- **Avoid closed-ended questions** (those requiring a one-word answer) unless the person is too ill to elaborate or you're trying to clarify a response by getting a yes or no answer. The following are some examples of appropriate use of closed-ended questions: Asking someone who is short of breath, "Are you having pain?" Asking, "You've told me you've had pain for 2 weeks, but not all of the time. Are you saying it comes and goes?" Asking, "Is there a history of hypertension in your family?" Table 2–3 gives more examples of open-ended and closed-ended questions. Table 2–4 summarizes the advantages and disadvantages of using each of these types of questions.

How to Observe

- **Use your senses.** Do you see, hear, or smell anything unusual?
- **Note general appearance.** Does the person appear well groomed, healthy, well nourished?
- **Observe body language.** Does the person appear comfortable? Nervous? Withdrawn? Apprehensive? What behaviors do you see?
- **Notice interaction patterns.** Be aware of the person's responses to your interviewing style (eg, sometimes cultural and personal differences create communication barriers).

How to Terminate the Interview

- **Ask the person to summarize her most important concerns,** then summarize the most important concerns as you see them. For example, say, "OK, we've talked about

TABLE 2–3 Examples of Open-Ended and Closed-Ended Questions	
Closed-Ended	Open-Ended
Are you happy about this?	How does this make you feel?
Do you get along with your husband?	How is your relationship with your husband?
Does this make you sick to your stomach?	How does this affect your stomach?

TABLE 2-4 Advantages and Disadvantages of Open-Ended and Closed-Ended Questions

Advantages	Disadvantages
Open-Ended Question	
Brings forth more information than a question that requires only a one-word response.	May allow the person to sidestep the question.
Gives people a chance to verbalize and involves them in dialogue.	Requires a more wordy response. This may be undesirable in an emergency situation or if the individual is confused, in pain, or having difficulty breathing.
Tends to bring forth a more honest reply.	
Usually less threatening and less likely to convey negative judgment.	Allows opportunity to ramble and get off the track.
Often interpreted to imply sincere interest.	
Closed-Ended Question	
Helps clarify responses to open-ended questions.	May be more threatening.
Saves time in emergency situations.	Limits the amount of information offered.
Can be helpful in focusing the interview on specific data (eg, following a checklist that asks for history of specific illnesses, such as high blood pressure, heart attacks).	Does not encourage the person to express concerns from his or her point of view.
	Does not encourage active dialogue between the nurse and the person.
May be helpful for those who are confused, in pain, or having difficulty breathing.	

a lot of things. To make sure I have it right, tell me the most important things I can help you with."

- **Ask if there are concerns that weren't discussed.** For example, "Is there anything else you want me to know about you?" or, "What do you want to tell me that we haven't already talked about?"
- **Offer yourself as a resource and answer any questions that arise.** For example. "I want to be kept informed on how you're doing. Let me know if something changes or if you have any questions."

- **Explain care routines and provide information about who is accountable for nursing care decisions.** Remember that consumers often are confused about who is responsible for what.
- **End on a positive note** and encourage the person to become an active participant. For example, "We have a good start here. I want you to be actively involved in making decisions about your care. Don't hesitate to offer suggestions or ask questions at any time."
    Display 2–2 lists common communication errors to avoid.

Think About It

Learning to Ask Relevant Questions. *Having a holistic assessment tool that's tailor-made to gain specific information in specific situations (eg, in labor and delivery) can be the key to getting relevant, complete data. Asking yourself* why *every piece of information that the tool guides you to collect is required helps you to master the critical thinking skills of* recognizing what's relevant *and* asking relevant questions.

Physical Assessment

The key to performing a physical assessment is being thorough, systematic, and skilled in technique. Physical assessment skills include the following:

- *Inspection:* Observing carefully by using your fingers, eyes, ears, and sense of smell.
- *Auscultation:* Listening with a stethoscope.
- *Palpation:* Touching and pressing to test for pain and feel inner structures, such as the liver.
- *Percussion:* Directly or indirectly tapping a body surface to determine reflexes (done with a percussion hammer) or to determine whether an area contains fluid (done by tapping fingers over surface).

DISPLAY 2–2   Common Communication Errors

- **Using first names without permission.** For some, being called by their first name by someone other than a close friend or family member is disrespectful.
- **Using endearing names.** Most people feel degraded when called "honey, deary, sweetie, pop, grandma" by anyone other than close family.
- **"Talking down."** For example, "So you've had a pain in your tummy?"
- **Using medical terminology with laypeople.** Many people don't know common medical terms such as void, vital signs, BM.
- **Using communication techniques you're comfortable with, without paying attention to the person's response.** For example, touching someone to offer support and not noticing that he withdraws, sending the message that he doesn't want to be touched.

The best way to become thorough and systematic in physical assessment is to choose a good way to organize your approach and use it consistently so it becomes automatic.

How you organize your assessment is influenced by two things:

1. **The person's condition:** If the person is ill or has a specific complaint, begin by examining the problem areas before going on to other parts of the body. For example, if there is abdominal pain, examine the abdomen first; if someone is unconscious, assess neurologic, respiratory, and cardiovascular status first.
2. **Your own preference:** For example, you may choose a head-to-toe approach, beginning by assessing the head and neck, and continuing down the body to the thorax, abdomen, legs, and feet, in that order. Or you may choose a systems approach, starting with the respiratory system (nose, mouth, throat, lungs) and continuing with cardiac, circulatory, neurologic, gastrointestinal, genitourinary, musculoskeletal, and skin status.

The following guidelines can help you to develop habits that promote a thorough and systematic physical assessment.

Guidelines: Performing a Physical Assessment

- **Promote communication between yourself and the person you're examining.** Provide for privacy, establish rapport, and use good interviewing techniques (rather than working in silence).
- **Respect privacy.** Uncover only the body parts being examined, keeping the rest of the body draped. Tell the person before touching a part of the body that she can't see. For example, "I'm going to feel this cyst on your back."
- **Don't rely on memory.** Jot down notes to be sure of accuracy.
- **Choose a method of organizing your assessment** and use it consistently. For example, use the following method, which is a modified head-to-toe approach.

> **Neurologic status:** Mental status; orientation; pupillary reaction; vision and appearance of the eyes; gag reflex; ability to hear, taste, feel, and smell; gait; coordination; presence of pain/discomfort.
>
> **Respiratory status:** Airway, breath sounds, rate and depth of breathing, cough, symmetry, presence of pain/discomfort.
>
> **Cardiac status:** Apical rate, rhythm, heart sounds, presence of pain/discomfort.
>
> **Circulatory status:** Rate, rhythm, and quality of pulses (radial, brachial, carotid, femoral, dorsalis pedis); presence of pain/discomfort.
>
> **Gastrointestinal status:** Condition of the lips, tongue, gums, teeth; presence of bowel sounds; presence of abdominal distention or tenderness; impaction; hemorrhoids.
>
> **Genitourinary status:** Color and amount of urine, presence of distended bladder, discharge (vaginal, urethral), presence of pain/discomfort; breast examination, condition of the vulva; testicular examination.
>
> **Skin status:** Color, temperature, turgor, edema, lesions, hair distribution, presence of itching/pain/discomfort.

Musculoskeletal status: Muscle tone, strength, range of motion, presence of pain/discomfort.

Think About It

> **Pain and Cough—The Fifth and Sixth Vital Signs.** *Pain is the fifth vital sign. When doing routine vital signs (temperature, pulse, respirations, and blood pressure), ask about the presence of pain or discomfort and assess closely as indicated. Cough is the sixth vital sign. Although thorough lung assessment is important, you also can learn a lot from brief encounters even if you have only a few minutes. You can say something like, "Can you cough for me so I can hear how it sounds?". The person's ability (or inability) to comply with this request gives you a lot of information; for example, whether the person has pain with coughing, whether there's congestion, or whether the person's cough effort is enough to clear the lungs. This brief encounter can flag patients who need more in-depth assessment.*

Checking Laboratory and Diagnostic Studies

Checking laboratory and diagnostic studies is essential to doing a comprehensive assessment. These studies are like a "report card" on how the body is functioning. They often provide key evidence that helps you to determine health status. For example, you may find that assessment data are perfectly normal and then note a low potassium level, which needs evaluation and treatment because it creates a risk for heart problems. Or you may have some suspicions about the presence of a health problem, such as dehydration, which may be confirmed by laboratory studies such as a high hematocrit.

CRITICAL THINKING EXERCISE III

The Nursing Interview and Physical Assessment

To complete this session, read pages 36–58. Example responses can be found on page 243.

Part One: The Interview

1. **Practice making open-ended questions.** Restate each question below so it's an open-ended question.

   a. "Are you feeling better?"

   b. "Did you like dinner?"

   c. "Are you happy here?"

   d. "Are you having pain?"

2. **Practice clarifying ideas by using reflection (restating what you hear) and making open-ended questions.** For each statement below, write a reflective statement and an open-ended question that would help you to clarify what has been said.

   a. "I've been sick off and on for a month."

   b. "Nothing ever goes right for me."

   c. "I seem to have a pain in my side that comes and goes."

   d. "I've had this funny feeling for a week."

3. **Test your knowledge of communication techniques.** Read each sentence below and identify whether it is an open-ended statement (O), a closed-ended statement (C), a leading question (L), an exploratory statement (E), or a supplementary phrase or statement intended to help the person continue (S).

   a. _____ Are you afraid of dying?

   b. _____ Tell me when this first started.

   c. _____ I see.

   d. _____ You're not still afraid to feed Hector, are you?

   e. _____ How do you think you'll be doing this at home?

   f. _____ Do you have a history of hypertension in your family?

   g. _____ And . . .?

   h. _____ You do want your family to visit, don't you?

   i. _____ How do you feel about being here?

   j. _____ You don't need more practice, do you?

   k. _____ Explain what you mean by "a long time."

4. Rephrase each leading question that you identified in number 3 to ask an open-ended question.

Part Two: Physical Assessment

1. Because physical assessment and interviewing go hand in hand, use the following situations to practice focusing your interview questions on areas of concern noted during the physical examination.

   a. You examine and find: The patient's hands and fingernails are filthy with ground-in dirt, although the rest of him is clean. You may state or ask:

   b. You examine and find: The patient has a lump on the back of his head. You may state or ask:

   c. You examine and find: The patient's respirations are 40. You may state or ask:

   d. You examine and find: The patient's right eye is red, teary, and inflamed. You may state or ask:

2. Now practice focusing your physical examination on areas of concern voiced by the patient.

   a. Patient states: "I have had a rash that comes and goes." You may reply and examine:

b. Patient states: "My stomach has been hurting me." You may reply and examine:

c. Patient states: "I find it burns when I urinate." You may reply and examine:

d. Patient states: "I feel like I'm heavier than usual, like I'm bloated with fluid." You may reply and examine:

Try This on Your Own: Practice Combining Interview and Physical Examination Techniques

Practice combining interviewing techniques with a physical examination by doing a mock interview and physical examination on a peer, friend, or family member using the assessment tool on page 39. Be sure you can explain *why* the form requires you to collect each piece of data.

Identifying Subjective and Objective Data

Separating information into subjective data (what the person *states* verbally or in writing) and objective data (what you *observe*) aids critical thinking because each complements and clarifies the other. For example, your notes might look like this:

Subjective data: States, "I feel like my heart is racing."
Objective data: Pulse 150 beats, regular, and strong.

The objective data above *support* the subjective data: what you observe confirms what the person is stating.

Sometimes, what you observe and what the person states are *different*. For example, your notes might look like this:

Subjective data: States, "I feel fine."

Objective data: Color pale, becomes easily short of breath.

What the person states above *isn't supported* by what you observe. You have to do more investigating to understand the full scope of the problems. The following can help you to remember the difference between these two types of data:

S—S: **S**ubjective data = **S**tated

O—O: **O**bjective data = **O**bserved

Remember that you should chart objective data using as specific (measurable) terms as possible. For example *a temperature of 100.6°F* is more specific and measurable than *feverish*. Chart subjective data by putting the person's own words in quotation marks.

The following shows examples of subjective and objective data:

Subjective Data	Objective Data
"I feel sick to my stomach."	Blood pressure 110/70
"I have a stabbing pain in my side."	Rash on right arm
"I wish I were home."	Walks with a limp
"I feel like nobody likes me."	Urinated 150 mL clear urine

Identifying Cues and Making Inferences

The subjective and objective data you identify act as *cues*. Cues are data that prompt you to get an initial impression about patterns of health or illness. For example, consider the following cues:

Subjective Data: "I just started taking penicillin for a tooth abscess."

Objective Data: Fine rash over trunk.

The above gives you cues that may lead you to infer (suspect) that there is an allergic reaction to penicillin. How you interpret or perceive a cue—the conclusion you draw about the cue—is called an *inference*. In the above case, you make an inference about the rash: you decide the rash may indicate a penicillin allergy.

Your ability to identify significant cues and make correct inferences is influenced by your observational skills, your nursing knowledge, and your clinical expertise. Your values and beliefs also affect how you interpret some cues, so make a conscious effort to avoid making value judgments (for example, inferring that a person who bathes only once a week needs to be taught better hygiene when this practice may be part of his culture).

To clarify your understanding of cues and inferences, study the following examples of cues and corresponding inferences.

Cues	Corresponding Inference
"I have trouble moving my bowels."	May be constipated
(With sad face) "I don't want to talk"	May be depressed
Blood pressure 60/50.	The person is in shock
"I can't stand this pain any more."	The person is experiencing unbearable pain.

Think About It

More Evidence Means Better Judgments. *Critical thinking requires making judgments based on evidence (fact) as much as possible. When making inferences, or drawing conclusions, the more cues (evidence) you have, the more likely you are to be correct. For example, if you have two cues—the patient just started penicillin and there's a fine rash over the trunk—additional cues, like finding out that the person had a rash before when taking penicillin, can help you confirm what you suspect.*

Validating (Verifying) Data

Validating, or verifying that your information is factual and complete, is an essential step in critical thinking. It helps you to avoid:

- Making assumptions
- Missing pertinent information
- Misunderstanding situations
- Jumping to conclusions or focusing in the wrong direction
- Making errors in problem identification.

For example, suppose you ask a woman whether she might be pregnant, and she responds, "No." If that's all you ask and you don't verify this by seeking more information (eg, asking *"When was your last period?"* or finding out the results of a pregnancy test), you may operate under the assumption that the woman isn't pregnant when indeed she is, which can be dangerous (eg, drugs might be ordered that harm the fetus). Consider the following guidelines.

Guidelines: Validating (Verifying) Data

- Data that can be measured accurately can be accepted as factual (eg, height, weight, laboratory study results). There's always the possibility of laboratory error or other factors that may alter the accuracy of the laboratory studies (eg, a fasting blood sugar test that is done even though the person has eaten 1 hour before). Rechecking gross abnormalities should verify whether the studies are valid.
- Data that someone *else* observes (indirect data) may or may not be true. When the information is critical, verify it by directly observing and interviewing the patient yourself.

- Validate questionable information by using the following techniques, as appropriate:
  - Double-check that your equipment is working correctly.
  - Recheck your own data (eg, take a patient's blood pressure in the opposite arm or 10 minutes later).
  - Look for factors that may alter accuracy (eg, check whether someone who has an elevated temperature and no other symptoms has just had a hot cup of tea).
  - Ask someone else, preferably an expert, to collect the same data (eg, ask a more experienced nurse to recheck a blood pressure when you're not sure).
  - Double-check information that's extremely abnormal or inconsistent with patient cues (eg, use two scales to check an infant who appears much heavier or lighter than the scale states; repeat a extremely high or low laboratory result).
  - Compare subjective and objective data to see if what the person is stating is congruent with what you observe (eg, compare actual pulse rate with perceptions of "racing heart").
  - Clarify statements and verify your inferences (eg, saying, "To me, you seem tired.").
  - Compare your impressions with those of other key members of the health care team.

CRITICAL THINKING EXERCISE IV

Subjective and Objective Data; Cues and Inferences; Validating Data

To complete this session, read pages 58–64. Example responses can be found on page 244.

Part I. Subjective and Objective Data

Case History

Mr. Michaels is 51 years old. He was admitted 2 days ago with chest pain. His physician has ordered the following studies: electrocardiogram, chest x-ray, and complete blood studies including a blood sugar. Results of these studies were just posted on the chart. When you talk with him, he states, "I feel much better today, no more pain. It is a relief to get rid of that discomfort." You think he appears a little tired or weary; he seems to be talking slowly and sighs more often than you think is normal. He denies being weary. His vital signs are as follows:

T: 98.6 P: 74 (regular) R: 22 BP: 140/90

1. List the subjective data noted in the case history above (what were you told directly by Mr. Michaels?).

2. List the objective data noted in the case history above (what information can be readily observed?).

Part II. Cues and Inferences

1. List the cues in the case history just given.

2. List the inferences that you might make about the cues that you've identified.

Part III. Validating Data

1. From the cues and inferences that you identified in Part II, indicate in three separate columns those that you feel are *certainly valid, probably valid,* and only *possibly valid.*

2. For the data listed in the *possibly valid* and *probably valid* columns, identify some methods of clarifying whether they are indeed true (eg, what other questions might you ask?).

Try This on Your Own

In a clinical conference or with another student, choose data from a real patient, identify cues, then discuss the inferences that you might make from the cues. Discuss the validity of the cues and inferences and how you might clarify or validate the information.

Organizing (Clustering) Data

Clustering related data together is a critical-thinking principle that enhances your ability to get a clear picture of health status. Just as putting puzzle pieces with similar colors together helps you to see parts of a picture puzzle, clustering health status data into related groups helps you to begin to get a picture of various aspects of health status.

If you use a well-designed assessment tool, a lot of the organizing already is complete because the tool guides you to record related cues together (eg, information about nutrition is mostly in one place, information about activity is mostly in one place, and so on). However, because assessment tools don't organize *all* the information, and because ongoing assessment often is done *without* an assessment tool, this section describes different ways to cluster data for different purposes.

Clustering Data According to a Nursing Model

When identifying nursing diagnoses, it's helpful to cluster data according to a holistic model rather than a medical model. For example, many nurses use Gordon's functional health patterns, North American Nursing Diagnosis Association's human response patterns, Maslow's theories, or a combination of these to cluster data to maintain a holistic approach. (Table 2–5 compares these methods.) These methods are helpful when identifying nursing diagnoses because they have a holistic focus and bring together related data about patterns of human responses and functioning, rather than giving only patterns of organ or system function.

Clustering Data According to Body Systems

When aiming to identify data that may indicate possible medical problems, the body systems approach (Display 2–3, on page 68) is helpful because medical problems often are caused by abnormalities in system or organ function.

The following diagram shows the relationship between clustering data and identifying health problems.

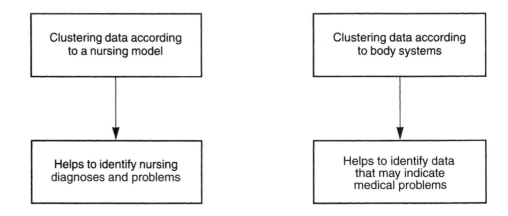

TABLE 2 – 5 Holistic Models for Clustering Data (Different methods are used by nurses according to preferences)

Human Needs (Maslow)	Functional Health Patterns (Gordon)	Human Response Patterns (Unitary Person)
Physiologic (survival) needs: Food, fluids, oxygen, elimination, warmth, physical comfort. **Safety and security needs:** Things necessary for physical safety (eg, a cane) and psychological security (eg, a child's favorite toy) **Love and belonging needs:** Family and significant others. **Self-esteem needs:** Things that make people feel good about themselves and confident in their abilities (eg, being well groomed, having accomplishments recognized). **Self-actualization needs:** Need to grow, change, and accomplish goals.	**Health perception/health management:** Perception of general health status and well-being. Adherence to preventive health practices. **Nutritional–metabolic:** Patterns of food and fluid intake, fluid and electrolyte balance, general ability to heal. **Elimination:** Patterns of excretory function (bowel, bladder, and skin), and client's perception. **Activity/Exercise:** Pattern of exercise, activity, leisure, recreation, and ADL; factors that interfere with desired or expected individual pattern. **Cognitive–perceptual:** Adequacy of sensory modes, such as vision, hearing, taste, touch, smell, pain perception, cognitive functional abilities. **Sleep/Rest:** Patterns of sleep and rest–relaxation periods during 24-hour day, as well as quality and quantity. **Self-Perception/Self-Concept:** Attitudes about self, perception of abilities, body image, identity, general sense of worth and emotional patterns. **Role/Relationship:** Perception of major roles and responsibilities in current life situation. **Sexuality/Reproductive:** Perceived satisfaction or dissatisfaction with sexuality. Reproductive stage and pattern. **Coping/Stress Tolerance:** General coping pattern, stress tolerance, support systems, and perceived ability to control and manage situations. **Value–belief:** Values, goals, or beliefs that guide choices or decisions.	**Exchanging:** Nutritional status, temperature, elimination, oxygenation, circulation, fluid balance, skin and mucous membranes, risks for injury. **Communicating:** Ability to express thoughts verbally; orientation, speech impairments, language barriers. **Relating:** Establishing bonds, social interaction, support systems, role performance (including parenting, occupation, and sexual role). **Valuing:** Religious and cultural preference and practices, relationship with deity, perception of suffering: acceptance of illness. **Choosing:** Ability to accept help and make decisions, adjustment to health status, desire for independence/dependence, denial of problem, adherence to therapies. **Moving:** Activity tolerance, ability for self-care, sleep patterns, diversional activities, disability history, safety needs, breast-feeding. **Perceiving:** Body image, self-esteem, ability to use all five senses, amount of hopefulness, perception of ability to control current situation. **Knowing:** Knowledge about current illness or therapies; previous illnesses; risk factors, expectations of therapy, cognitive abilities; readiness to learn, orientation, memory. **Feeling:** Pain; grieving; risk for violence, anxiety level, emotional integrity.

DISPLAY 2-3   Clustering Data According to Body Systems

Clustering in this way helps you identify data that should be referred to the physician.
1. Cluster together a brief client profile (vital statistics), including the following:
   Name, age, reason the individual is seeking health care, vital signs, any known medical problems or diagnoses, allergies, or problems with diet
2. Cluster together any data you suspect may be abnormal for any of the following systems:
   - ✓ Respiratory system
   - ✓ Cardiovascular system
   - ✓ Nervous system
   - ✓ Integumentary system (skin)
   - ✓ Gastrointestinal system
   - ✓ Musculoskeletal system
   - ✓ Genitourinary system

To recognize both medical and nursing problems, cluster your data both ways: use body systems *and* a nursing model. If you cluster data according to body systems *only*, you're likely to miss key information that helps you to identify nursing diagnoses. If you cluster data according to a nursing model *only*, you may group your data in such a way that medical problems may not be obvious.

Display 2–4 shows the same data clustered according to human needs, functional health patterns, and body systems. You don't have to memorize these; you'll learn them by using them later on.

Think About It

Organizing Data Promotes Critical Thinking by Helping You See Things in Different Ways. *Think about the following points:*
1. There are different ways of organizing assessment data. How you organize it influences how you see problems.
2. Organizing and reorganizing information promotes critical thinking by helping you to see different patterns; each organization reveals different aspects of the information while hiding others.
3. Nursing models help you to see nursing problems; medical models, or body systems, help you to see medical problems.

DISPLAY 2-4   Examples of the Same Patient Data Organized According to Human Needs, Functional Health Patterns, and Body Systems

Data

1. 21-year-old male
2. Married, no children*
3. Occupation: Firefighter*
4. Ht: 6'1"; Wt: 170 lb
5. T: 98; P: 60; R: 16
6. BP: 110/60
7. Unconscious from head injury
8. Spontaneous respirations
9. Lungs clear
10. History of seizures
11. Foley draining clear urine
12. Wife states he's always constipated
13. Tube feeding via nasogastric tube every 4 hours
14. Extremities rigid
15. Has reddened areas on both elbows
16. Allergic to penicillin
17. Wife states she feels as though she is falling apart*
18. Wife states that before the accident, he took pride in being physically fit*
19. Wife states that they were considering converting to Catholicism before the accident*

Data Organization by Gordon's Functional Health Patterns

✓ Health-perception–health-management pattern: 10, 18
✓ Nutritional–metabolic pattern: 4, 5, 6, 8, 9, 11, 13, 15, 16
✓ Elimination pattern: 11, 12, 13, 15
✓ Activity–exercise pattern: 5, 8, 9, 14
✓ Cognitive–perceptual pattern: 7
✓ Sleep–rest pattern: 7
✓ Self-perception–self-concept pattern: 18
✓ Role–relationship pattern: 1, 2, 3
✓ Sexuality–reproductive pattern: 2
✓ Coping–stress-tolerance pattern: 17
✓ Value–belief pattern: 19

Data Organization by Maslow's Needs

✓ Physical: 1, 4, 5, 6, 7, 8, 9, 10, 11, 12, 13, 14, 15, 16, 18
✓ Safety and security: 7, 10, 13, 17, 19
✓ Love and belonging: 2, 17, 19
✓ Self-esteem: 2, 3, 18
✓ Self-actualization: 3

Data Organization by Body Systems to Determine What Should Be Referred to the Physician

✓ Vital statistics (client profile): 1, 4, 5, 6, 7, 10, 16
✓ Respiratory system: 8, 9
✓ Cardiovascular system: 5, 6, 9
✓ Nervous system: 7, 10
✓ Musculoskeletal system: 14
✓ Gastrointestinal system: 12, 13
✓ Genitourinary system: 11
✓ Integumentary system: 15

*These data are more likely to be clustered according to a nursing model only and therefore are not assigned a category under the body systems organization.

CRITICAL THINKING EXERCISE V

Organizing (Clustering) Data

To complete this session, read pages 61–70. Example responses can be found on page 244.

1. Why is it important to organize data according to both a body systems framework *and* a nursing model? (Three sentences or less.)

2. On a separate piece of paper, cluster the following data according to body systems and according to any holistic nursing model you choose.

Case History

1. Age 36

2. Married, has three small children

3. Occupation: Landscape architect and homemaker

4. Religion: Episcopalian

5. Medical diagnosis: Pneumonia

6. T: 100; P: 100; R: 28; BP: 104/68

7. States she is concerned about how her husband is caring for the children, that it is "tough on him."

8. States she feels weak and tired all the time but can't seem to rest because she keeps coughing all the time

9. Appetite poor. Has eaten less than half of regular meals. Is forcing fluids well (1000 mL per shift)

10. Before illness, she smoked a pack of cigarettes a day but has not smoked since hospitalization.

11. States she always has been in good health and never had to be hospitalized (even gave birth at home)

12. States that all of the tests that have to be done make her nervous; she is worried about getting AIDS from needle sticks

13. Lungs have bilateral rhonchi; she coughs up thick yellow mucus

14. Chest x-ray shows improvement over the last 2 days

15. White blood cell count is elevated at 16,000

3. When you organized these data, you may have found that some categories had no data listed. If this happens to you in the clinical area, what should you do?

Identifying Patterns/Testing First Impressions

After you cluster your data into groups of related information, you begin to get some initial impressions of patterns of human functioning. But you must test these impressions and decide if the patterns really are as they appear. Testing first impressions involves deciding what's relevant, making tentative decisions about what the data may suggest, and focusing assessment to gain more information to fully understand the situations at hand. Like the puzzle analogy, you put some of the puzzle pieces together and you think you know what the picture looks like. However, often those last few key pieces can surprise you with essential details that change the whole picture.

Consider the following example in which a nurse clustered the following data together:

- 72-year-old man
- Blind
- States "I'm always bumping myself."
- States "I get around by using my cane to find my way."
- Has visible bumps and bruises over arms and on head

The information just given suggests that there is a pattern of frequent injury, perhaps because of blindness. However, there isn't enough data. You need to examine the information, decide what's relevant and irrelevant, and look for reasons why the injuries are happening. You may decide the following:

Irrelevant: man

Relevant: elderly, blind, says he's always bumping himself, uses a cane, has bumps and bruises over arms and on head

These data support the conclusion that the injuries are related to blindness. But you need to ask more questions, such as "Does he live alone, or is someone else responsible for his care? Are the injuries really caused by blindness?" Perhaps he's falling down because of weakness or dizziness. After all, if he's using the cane correctly, do you think he'd bump himself all the time? These questions that come to mind when identifying patterns guide you to collect additional information to test initial impressions and describe the problems more clearly. For example, with the man just described, you could use probing questions to clarify how and why he keeps hurting himself. You may find that he's hurting himself because he's fainting, doesn't use the cane properly, is a victim of abuse, has a low platelet count, or takes anticoagulants.

To focus your assessment on testing first impressions and gaining key pieces of information about patterns of health or illness, keep the following critical thinking principles in mind:

1. **Determine what's relevant and irrelevant:** Ask yourself what *relevant* information might be missing.
2. **Remember cause and effect:** Find out why or how the pattern came to be (ie, look for contributing factors).

Reporting and Recording

The final phase of *Assessment* is reporting and recording. Reporting abnormal data in a timely fashion expedites diagnosis and treatment of urgent problems. Recording data in a timely fashion promotes:

1. **Continuity:** No one can read your notes when they're in your pocket.
2. **Accuracy:** Your notes are more likely to be accurate and complete when your memory is fresh.
3. **Critical thinking:** Writing information down and then evaluating it to interpret what it means and what might be missing is a key strategy that can enhance your ability to think critically.

Reporting significant findings may take priority over recording comprehensive assessment data. For example, if you take someone's vital signs and find a temperature of 104° F, you report the vital signs immediately before taking the time to record the entire data base.

Whereas Chapter 5 discusses reporting and recording during *Implementation*, this section focuses on deciding what to report and record after doing an *initial* comprehensive data base assessment.

Deciding What to Report

Many beginning nurses have trouble deciding what to report. Until you gain enough experience to be confident in determining what data might be significant of an impending problem, follow this rule:

R U L E ▶ Report anything you *suspect* might be abnormal.

Think About It

Reporting Suspected Abnormalities Is Worthwhile. *Reporting anything you suspect might be abnormal to your instructor, preceptor, or supervisor accomplishes three things:*
1. It promotes early diagnosis even if you don't have the knowledge to diagnose the problem yourself.
2. It keeps others informed who are accountable for your patient's well-being.
3. It helps you to learn. Often, you receive help determining whether the information is significant.

Deciding What's Abnormal

There are many factors to consider when deciding what's abnormal (eg, age, disease process, culture, stress tolerance). If your knowledge is so limited that you're not certain what's abnormal, be sure that you work with a more experienced nurse (or instructor). To be safe, ask him or her to review your assessment data until you become more comfortable with identifying abnormalities.

Review Display 2–5, which lists key questions to ask to decide what's normal and abnormal, then consider the following two rules.

R U L E ▶

To decide if something is abnormal, compare the information with accepted standards for normalcy; if the information isn't within normal limits, consider it to be abnormal. For example, if you're caring for an adult and find a resting pulse of 110 beats per minute, you'd suspect this is abnormal because the normal limits for an adult resting pulse is 60 to 100 beats per minute.

R U L E ▶

Normal limits may vary from person to person and situation to situation. For example, a pulse of 110 beats per minute may be normal for a child or for someone who's anxious, but abnormal for a sleeping adult who usually has a resting pulse of 56 beats per minute.

DISPLAY 2–5   Questions to Ask to Determine What's Normal and What's Abnormal

Ask the Person
- Would you say this is normal or abnormal for you?
- What would you describe as normal for you?

Ask Yourself
- What's accepted as normal for someone who's this person's age? Physical stature? Culture? Developmental status?
- What's accepted as normal for someone who has:
    This disease process?
    This person's beliefs or cultural background?
    This occupation, this socioeconomic level, this lifestyle?
- If I compare the data I've collected with the data gathered on admission (baseline data) or the data gathered in the last 24 to 48 hours, are there changes that reflect increasing problems?
- Are there too many slightly abnormal factors that, when put together, signify an overall picture of abnormality?
- Is what the individual accepts as normal detrimental to his health?

Guidelines: Reporting Significant Findings

General Guidelines

- If you find yourself thinking, "I'm not sure if there's anything abnormal here I need to report," you probably don't have enough knowledge to make this decision and need to get help. Consult your instructor, a more experienced nurse, or a reliable text.

- Report abnormal findings as soon as possible. This prevents you from forgetting and may expedite problem identification.

- Before reporting, take a moment to be sure you have all the necessary information readily at hand (eg, patient's name, room number, vital signs, laboratory studies, intake and output, medication record). In emergencies, this may not be possible; instead, ask another nurse to contact the appropriate professional (nurse, physician) while you continue to gather your information.

- If you're nervous about giving the report, jot down the facts in order of importance, then read your list.

- Give precise information. State the facts rather than how you *interpret* the facts. This allows the other professionals to come to their own conclusions without being influenced by your interpretation of the facts.

E X A M P L E

> **Right:** Mrs. Ling is complaining of a right frontal headache. She received two Tylenol an hour ago, but she's still restless and says she has no relief. Her vital signs and neurologic status are stable.
> **Wrong:** Mrs. Ling isn't doing well. I think she has a migraine because she already got Tylenol and she's not any better.

- If the person you're talking to doesn't seem to understand the problem after hearing the facts, then state your interpretation of the data (eg, "I'm concerned that she has a migraine and needs something stronger than Tylenol for relief.").

- Chart the time you made the report, the name of the person you notified, and any actions taken on the data base or nurses' notes (eg, "Notified L. Ballard, RN. She assessed the patient and will notify Dr. Sophocles."). Documenting what you reported and to whom you reported lets others know (1) that you observed something that you believed was significant enough to notify someone with more knowledge and authority, and (2) who is aware of the information (and, therefore, whether anyone else needs to be notified).

Guidelines for Phone Reports

- Identify yourself by name and position. If you're a student nurse, you may not be allowed to take verbal orders (varies by state). Ask your instructor to listen on another line and tell the physician that she's listening (eg, "This is Ms. Pratt. I'm a student. My instructor, Ms. Rae, is listening on the other line.").

- State the patient's name, diagnosis, and location and then ask, "Do you know whom

I'm talking about?" This gives the person time to focus on the particular patient. It also helps you know how much background information might be needed.

- Double-check your interpretation of the conversation (eg, "So, you don't want to be notified unless the temperature is above 102°F. Is that correct?").

CRITICAL THINKING EXERCISE VI

Recognizing Abnormal Data, Deciding What's Relevant, Applying the Principle of Cause and Effect

To complete this session, read pages 71–75. Example responses can be found on page 244.

1. Practice identifying what's normal and abnormal by completing the exercise below. Study the following data. In the space to the left, put "N" next to the normal data, "A" next to the abnormal data.

   a. _____ States he usually has a bowel movement every other day.

   b. _____ Temperature of 101°F.

   c. _____ Pulse rate of 72 and regular (adult).

   d. _____ Pulse rate of 150 (adult).

   e. _____ Has hives over entire body.

   f. _____ Infant cries as mother leaves the room.

   g. _____ Patient complains of pain with urination.

   h. _____ Grandmother suddenly does not recognize favorite grandchild.

   i. _____ Grandmother says, "I can see okay as long as I wear my glasses."

   j. _____ Infant cries, pulls at ears, and cannot be consoled by his mother.

2. **Practice looking for relevant information:** Turn to the case study on page 28. Consider what questions you might ask to gain additional relevant information you'd need if you were trying to determine how Mr. Moran cares for himself at home.

3. **Practice determining contributing factors** (applying the principle of cause and effect): For the same case study, consider what questions you might ask to gain additional information to help you more fully understand factors that might be contributing to, or causing, Mr. Moran's breathing problems.

Deciding What to Record

If you think information is significant enough to report, most likely it's significant enough to record. In fact, a good rule of thumb is *record anything you report.*

How and what you chart is extremely important for the patient's sake and your own protection against malpractice suits. Remember the following rule:

R U L E ▶

> Record anything you report and always follow facility policies and procedures for charting. Policies and procedures vary from one facility to another, but follow them closely—they're designed to guide you to create a complete data base that provides legal documentation of accepted standards of care.

The following guidelines can help you form good charting habits.

Guidelines: Recording the Nursing Data Base

(Additional guidelines for charting during *Implementation* are on page 176).

* **Follow policies and procedures for charting carefully.** They are designed to meet legal and regulatory requirements.
* **When using handwritten charting systems, use ink and write or print legibly, even when pressed for time.** Your notes are useless to others if they can't be understood, and they'll be useless to you if you're asked 5 years later in a court of law to recall what happened at a given time. Sloppy or illegible notes also can work against you in court; it's easy for a jury to interpret sloppy handwriting as sloppy care.
* **Complete the data base as soon as you can.** Late charting may lead to omissions and errors that can later be interpreted as care that was substandard. If you have to leave the unit before completing the data base, make sure that the most important information (eg, vital signs, allergies, medications) is charted before you leave.
* **Chart objectively without making value judgments;** record subjective data by using direct quotes.

E X A M P L E

> **Right:** States, "I don't go to church."
> **Wrong:** Not religious.

* **Avoid terms that have a negative connotation** (eg, "drunk," "disagreeable"). In court they may convey a negative attitude on your part.
* **Keep all information confidential.** In addition to inaccurate or unrecorded information, breach of confidentiality also is a common reason for malpractice suits. If you have accessed computerized patient data, follow policies for electronic charting, including "logging off" to prevent access to sensitive, confidential information by unauthorized users.
* **Keep it short;** record the facts and be specific about the problems at hand.

E X A M P L E

> **Right:** Breath sounds diminished at left lower base. Complains of "piercing pain" with inspiration at the lower left base. Respirations 32, pulse 110, BP 130/90.
> **Wrong:** Seems to be having breathing problems. Also complains of chest pain.

• **If you make an inference, support it with evidence.**

> **Right:** Seems upset. When questioned, he states he's "fine" and that he's "not upset," but he doesn't make eye contact, uses only one-word answers, and states he doesn't "feel like talking."
> **Wrong:** Seems upset about something.

• **If you make a mistake, correct it without covering up the original words.** Instead, draw a line through the original words, write "error" and enter your initials. Never alter a chart without following this procedure; it may imply intent to cover up the facts, which is considered malpractice.

• **If the patient chooses not to answer a question, record "chooses not to answer."** If you gain information from significant others that you think you should record, list the name and relationship of the person to the patient (eg, "Wife states he's allergic to morphine.").

Think About It

What Lawyers and Regulatory Agencies Look For. *Lawyers, regulatory agencies, and insurance companies examine your charting specifically for evidence of the following: (1) skilled observation and evaluation with notification of physician if warranted, (2) risks for injury and corresponding safety precautions, (3) educational needs and teaching given, (4) discharge planning, (5) need for direct skilled nursing care, and (6) use of appropriate resources (multidisciplinary approaches).*

Summary

Assessment—the first step to determining health status—consists of five key activities: collecting data, validating data, organizing (clustering) data, identifying patterns/testing first impressions, and reporting and recording data. These activities are designed to help you be accurate, complete, and organized as you prepare for the next step, *Diagnosis.* How you organize your data influences how you see problems. To avoid missing nursing or medical problems, use *both* a body systems framework and a holistic nursing model to cluster data. Report and record abnormal data in a timely fashion. It ensures early detection of patient problems and helps you to learn (because you find out what data are abnormal enough to indicate a problem).

Evaluate your knowledge of this chapter. Check to see if you can achieve the learning outcomes on page 34.
Bibliography: See pages 199–201.

3

Diagnosis

LEARNING OUTCOMES

After mastering the content in this chapter, you should be able to:

- Give three reasons why *Diagnosis* is a pivotal point in the nursing process.
- Compare and contrast the *diagnose and treat* model with the *predict, prevent, and manage* model.
- Address the pros and cons of using critical paths and computer-assisted diagnosis.
- Discuss the legal implications of the term *diagnosis.*
- State your responsibilities in relation to nursing diagnoses, medical diagnoses, and other problems.
- Give two reasons why we need a uniform nursing language.
- Explain the possible consequences of diagnostic errors.
- Identify resources that can assist you to recognize diagnoses.
- Develop diagnostic statements for actual, risk, and possible diagnoses.
- Use diagnostic reasoning—including taking specific steps to avoid diagnostic errors—the next time you're in the clinical setting.

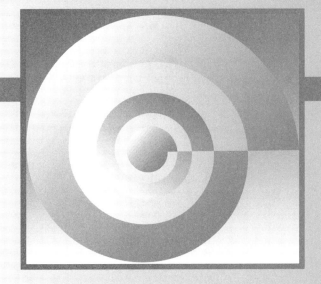

Standard II: *Diagnosis.* The nurse analyzes assessment data in determining diagnoses.*

Critical Thinking Exercises

■ **Critical Thinking Exercise VII:** Nurses' Responsibilities as Diagnosticians

■ **Critical Thinking Exercise VIII:** Recognizing Nursing Diagnoses

■ **Critical Thinking Exercise IX:** Diagnostic Statements for Nursing Diagnosis

■ **Critical Thinking Exercise X:** Predicting Potential Complications

■ **Critical Thinking Exercise XI:** Identifying Nursing Diagnoses, Potential Complications, and Strengths

What's in this chapter?

This chapter focuses on the importance of *Diagnosis,* a pivotal step in the nursing process. It addresses how nursing's diagnostic responsibilities are growing, what your responsibilities are in the face of the rapidly changing health care environment, and how to accurately diagnose and record health problems. Emphasis is given to the implications of moving from a *Diagnose and Treat* (DT) model to a more proactive *Predict, Prevent, and Manage* (PPM) model. The impact of computerized medical records and decision support is addressed together with need for a uniform nursing language (UNL).

*Excerpted from ANA Standards of Clinical Nursing Practice (ANA, 1998).

From Assessment to Diagnosis: A Pivotal Point

The following diagram shows how the activities of *Assessment* lead to what many consider to be a pivotal point in the nursing process: *Diagnosis*.

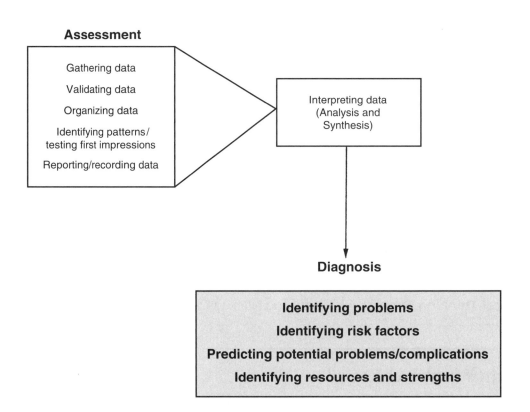

Assessment

Gathering data

Validating data

Organizing data

Identifying patterns/
testing first impressions

Reporting/recording data

Interpreting data
(Analysis and
Synthesis)

Diagnosis

Identifying problems

Identifying risk factors

Predicting potential problems/complications

Identifying resources and strengths

Diagnosis is a pivotal point for three reasons:

1. **The accuracy and relevancy of the entire plan depends on your ability to clearly and specifically identify both the problems and what's causing them.** Incorrectly diagnosing the problems or what's causing them is likely to send you and everyone else in the wrong direction, resulting in inefficient, perhaps even dangerous care. For example, imagine what could happen if you decide someone's left shoulder pain is related to his arthritis when the pain is actually related to cardiac problems.

2. **Creating a proactive plan that promotes health and prevents problems *before they begin* depends on your ability to recognize risk factors (things that we know cause problems, such as sedentary lifestyle).** Even when there are *no* problems, you must ask, "Are there risk factors that need to be addressed?" For example, you assess an overweight businessman and learn that both of his parents had hypertension.

Knowing that obesity and family history of hypertension are risk factors for hypertension, you stress the importance of preventing hypertension through exercise, weight control, and decreased salt intake.

3. **The resources and strengths you identify are the key to reducing costs and maximizing efficiency.** Be sure you identify and use one of your most valuable resources: the person requiring care and his or network of support. For example, in the case of a diabetic individual, you may have time only to do the minimally acceptable amount of teaching and follow-up. But if you take a few moments to motivate the person to get involved with the local Diabetic Association to learn more and give him the appropriate phone numbers to call, he's likely to expand and re-enforce what he learns from you.

Nurses' Growing Responsibilities as Diagnosticians

Laws and standards continue to change to reflect how nursing practice is growing. For example, nurses in the acute care setting continually gain more responsibilities for managing complex situations. As a beginning nurse, you're responsible for:

- Recognizing common health problems.
- Reporting signs and symptoms that may indicate the need for more expert diagnosis.
- Identifying those at risk and anticipating and preventing problems and complications.
- Initiating actions and referrals to ensure appropriate and timely treatment.
- Identifying factors that maximize the health of both healthy and chronically ill people (of all health care professionals, consumers and patients look the most to nurses for help with improving the quality of their lives).

Keeping this in mind, let's look at five major factors that impact on your diagnostic role today. These are summarized here and are addressed in more depth in the subsequent paragraphs.

1. The shift from *Diagnose and Treat* (DT) to *Predict, Prevent, and Manage* (PPM)
2. The development and refinement of critical pathways (also called *critical paths, clinical pathways,* or *CareMaps*™)
3. Computer-assisted diagnosis
4. More emphasis on the importance of collaborative and multidisciplinary practice
5. Greater awareness that nursing's scope of practice has a flexible boundary that responds to the changing needs of society and its expanding knowledge base (ANA, 1995)

Diagnose and Treat Versus Predict, Prevent, and Manage

As addressed briefly earlier, the DT approach implies that we wait for evidence of problems before beginning treatment. The PPM approach focuses on *early intervention* to control problems and prevent or manage their potential complications. This approach often is based on research or clinical evidence. We now know the typical course of many health problems, and we also know how to alter their course through early intervention.

Using a PPM approach requires you to do two things:

1. **In the presence of known problems,** you predict the *most likely and most danger-ous* complications and take immediate action to (a) prevent them and (b) manage them in case they can't be prevented.

E X A M P L E

> As a beginning nurse working in the emergency department, you encounter a woman with a possible heart attack. Knowing that you're inexperienced, you quickly report this problem so immediate steps can be taken to control the problem and its potential com-plications (eg, an intravenous [IV] line may be inserted, and medications may be given to improve blood flow to the heart and prevent arrhythmias).

2. **Whether problems are present or not,** you *look* for evidence of *risk factors* (things that we know may cause problems, such as risky sexual behaviors). If you identify risk factors, you aim to reduce or control them, thereby preventing the problems themselves.

E X A M P L E

> You're performing an assessment and find a teenage boy to be in excellent health. How-ever, you identify that he has risky sexual behaviors. You recognize that this puts the young man at risk for contracting HIV and other sexually transmitted diseases, and you focus on reducing his risk factors for these serious potential problems (eg, you may con-tact a peer counselor to discuss the need for safe sex).

Using the PPM model requires knowledge of disease process, treatment, and prog-nosis (prognosis is the usual course and outcome of injury or disease). Keep in mind that *predict* in PPM doesn't mean that a complication *will* happen (eg, "my patient has this problem, so we can predict that he also will have these complication." This is an as-sumption). It means you *anticipate* the possibility of certain complications and be pre-pared to detect, prevent, and manage them.

Point-of-Care Testing

Another result of moving to the PPM approach is that there is an increase in the use of point-of-care testing—diagnostic testing done by nurses on the unit—to improve effi-ciency and ensure early detection. Examples of point-of-care tests are blood glucose measurement, testing stool for blood, and urine testing. In specialty units (eg, intensive care), nurses may be accountable for more complicated point-of-care tests. Be sure you check with policies and procedures to know what tests you are responsible for doing and which ones are done by the laboratory. Be sure that you're prepared for point-of-care testing by practicing performing the tests if you're not doing them on a frequent basis.

Critical Pathways (Clinical Pathways, CareMaps™)

Through research and collaborative practice, most facilities continue to develop and re-fine critical pathways. Critical pathways are standard plans that predict the day-by-day care required to achieve outcomes for specific problems within a certain time frame. (See page 252 in the Appendix for an example critical path.)

When working in facilities that use critical paths, you're often alerted to major diagnoses and predicted care, even before meeting the patient. Knowing major diagnoses and predicted care has advantages and disadvantages. It can be helpful in that you quickly learn the usual course of treatment for common problems through repeated experience. It can be a problem in that you may be so influenced by knowing major diagnoses and predicted care in advance that you may be tempted to take shortcuts. For example, it's easy to become complacent ("I already know the problems, so I don't have to worry too much about assessment."). This type of attitude can make you miss key information that significantly changes the whole picture of patient care. When using critical pathways, keep an open mind and think independently. Always determine your patient's *specific* needs rather than assume he or she "fits" the typical critical path.

Computer-Assisted Diagnosis

Computer-assisted diagnosis also can help or hinder the diagnostic process. Computerized diagnostic programs are designed to help you identify problems. You enter data, and the computer organizes them and suggests diagnoses to consider based on the data. Computers are valuable tools that can facilitate problem identification and help you learn. But, you must use them with an active, critical mind, asking yourself questions like, "How does this compare with my patient's situation, down to the last detail?" and "What could be missing from this computer data?"

Think about the following benefits and limitations of computer-assisted diagnosis.

Benefits of Computer-Assisted Diagnosis

Computers can:

- Process large amounts of data much faster than humans.
- Perform at a consistent level (not affected by human factors like fatigue, distractions, concerns over being rushed, boredom, or complacency related to repeatedly doing the same functions).
- Store large amounts of data, keeping them all available for recall as needed.
- Prompt nurses for data entry, ensuring accuracy and completeness of documentation and diagnosis.
- Flag potential problems or mistakes, such as drug interactions or incorrect dosages.
- Facilitate diagnostic reasoning by suggesting possible diagnoses, depending on matching assessment data.

Limitations of Computer-Assisted Diagnosis

Computers:

- Assume that entered data are true, simply shuffling the information around.
- May not be up to date with minute-to-minute changes in patient status.

- Don't replace humans (computers have no common sense); they require humans to analyze and interpret the information they generate in context of current situations.
- Don't relieve you of the responsibility of learning principles and rules of diagnostic reasoning. Knowing this helps you to recognize when computers make mistakes.

Think About It

Computers Can't Think for You. *Computer and digital information is only as useful as your ability to interpret and analyze it in the context of real situations. For example, a few years ago, a jet filled with Christmas travelers crashed into a mountain in South America. The computer told the pilots they were flying at a safe altitude, well above the ground. What the computer didn't know was that the pilot made a left turn, pointing straight toward mountains. The pilots relied on the computer's information, neglecting to consider the change in the plane's direction, causing a disaster. As a nurse, you're like the pilot of an airplane, responsible for navigating your patients through the health care maze. Be careful not to rely too much on computer-generated or digital data. Use your own brains and knowledge, especially in critical situations. For example, if a digital blood pressure reading states that your patient's blood pressure is 70/40, double-check the information by taking the blood pressure manually.*

Multidisciplinary Practice

Increased awareness of the importance of multidisciplinary approaches also impacts on your role as a diagnostician. As a nurse, you must be keenly aware that you don't work in isolation. Many problems require more than nursing resources to be resolved in a timely manner. As you'll see later in this chapter, you must know when "you're out of your league," so to speak. You have to be able to recognize not only nursing problems but also problems that require management by a physician, an advanced practice nurse (APN), or another member of the health care team.

Capturing, Organizing, and Using Nursing's Expanding Knowledge Base

Nurses continue to study nursing roles and expand nursing's knowledge through research and publication of best practices (proven ways to effectively treat a condition based on outcome and clinical studies; visit the Best Practice Network site at: *http://www.best4health.org/startbp.cfm*). Specialty organizations such as the American Association of Critical Care Nurses and the American Association of Operating Room Nurses continue important work to address the various roles in specialty practices.

Acknowledging that working to develop a Unified Nursing Language (UNL) is crucial to using computerized records and facilitating research, the American Nurses Association (ANA) recognizes several nursing vocabularies (Table 3–1). As nursing organizations work to develop a UNL, another group is developing a reference terminology that incorporates terms from various disciplines (eg, medicine, nursing, occupational therapy) and links them in ways that enable computers to better connect data from different practice areas and countries (Box 3–1).

TABLE 3–1 Examples of Groups Developing Standard Nursing Language*

Group Name	Focus	Purpose
North American Nursing Diagnosis Association (NANDA)	Diagnoses	Identify, label, validate, and classify health problems that nurses diagnose and treat (for listing, see Nursing Diagnosis Quick Reference Section). (NANDA, 20001). **Web site:** *http://www.nanda.org/html/about.html*
Nursing Interventions Classification (NIC)	Interventions	Identify, label, validate, and classify actions nurses perform, including interventions directly with patients (eg, teaching) and those done indirectly (eg, obtaining laboratory studies) (see page 000). (McCloskey & Bulechek, 2000). **Web site:** *http://coninfo.nursing.uiowa.edu/nic/overview.htm*
Nursing-Sensitive Outcomes Classification (NOC)	Outcomes	Identify, label, validate, and classify nursing-sensitive patient outcomes and indicators to evaluate the validity and usefulness of the classification, and define and test measurement procedures for the outcomes and indicators (see pages 000–000). (Johnson, Maas, & Moorhead, 2000). **Web site:** *http://coninfo.nursing.uiowa.edu/noc/index.htm*
Omaha Nursing Classification System for Community Health	Diagnoses, Interventions, Outcomes	Facilitate practice, documentation, and information management in home care and community health nursing by describing and measuring health-related problems, interventions, and outcomes of care. (Martin & Scheet, 1992). **Web site:** *http://con.ufl.edu/omaha/omahas.htm*
Perioperative Nursing Data Set (PNDS)	Diagnoses, Interventions, Outcomes	Develop, refine, and validate a structured nursing vocabulary that reflects nursing responsibilities and patient outcomes related to perioperative patients' experience from preadmission until discharge. (Beyea, 2000). **Web site:** *http://www.aorn.org/research/pnds.htm*
Home Health Care Classification (HHCC)	Diagnoses, Interventions, & Outcomes	Provide a structure for documenting and classifying home health and ambulatory care. **Web site:** *http://www.sabacare.com*
International Classification for Nursing Practice (ICNP®)	Diagnoses, Interventions, & Outcomes	Capture nursing's contributions to health and provide a framework into which existing vocabularies and classifications can be cross-mapped, enabling comparison of nursing data from various countries throughout the world. **Web site:** *http://www.icn.ch/icnp.htm*

*The terms *uniform nursing language, standard nursing language,* and *structured nursing vocabularies* often are used interchangeably.

> Box 3–1 SNOMED® RT (Systematized Nomenclature of Medicine—
> Reference Terminology)
> **Purpose.** To provide a computer readable terminology that integrates, links, and
> maps health care terms used by various health care providers. The aim is to en-
> able patients, researchers, and health care professionals of all disciplines to share
> a common understanding of health care concepts across sites of care and com-
> puter systems (most comprehensive system available; first nomenclature recog-
> nized by ANA; working to integrate, link, and map concepts from NANDA, NIC,
> NOC, PNDS, ICNP, Omaha, as well as other standardized languages). The next
> generation of this program will be SNOMED® CT, a global terminology, merging
> US concepts with those from the National Health Service in the United Kingdom.[1]
> **Web site:** *www.snomed.org.*
>
> ───────────
> ([1]E-mail communication with Debra Konicek, RN, BSN, SNOMED® Research Analyst, No-
> vember 14, 2000).

The diagram below shows the importance of continuing to expand, organize, and capture nursing's knowledge base.

Study of nursing roles related to
diagnoses, interventions, and outcomes

⬇

Clearer identification of the body of
nursing knowledge

⬇

More professional autonomy

⬇

Improved patient outcomes

Think About It

Job Satisfaction Related to Autonomy. *Notice that the end results of the preceding diagram are* more professional autonomy *and* improved patient outcomes. *Studies show that having professional autonomy and being able to make an impact on patient outcomes are key factors that improve job satisfaction. Working to expand nursing knowledge base will not only help your patients, it will improve job satisfaction.*

Thinking Critically About Using Standard Languages in Practice

Developing standard nursing languages and naming and classifying the diagnoses, interventions, and outcomes used by nursing (see Table 3–1) is a challenging process. We have an excellent beginning—a big step toward being able to have a common language that facilitates computerized records and research—but there still is work to do. Leaders from various nursing specialties continue to work to answer questions like, "What are the best terms to use to facilitate practice?" and "How do we agree on how we should link terms such as NANDA (North American Nursing Diagnosis Association), NIC (Nursing Interventions Classification), and NOC (Nursing-Sensitive Outcomes Classification) together?"

To help you make decisions about how to use standard languages (ie, NANDA, NIC, NOC) in practice, remember the following points.

- Recognize that the work of researching and standardizing nursing language is important, both because of the need to facilitate use of computers and because of the need to capture and name nursing's contribution to health care.
- Not all terms are *clinically* useful (some are too broad, others work best for research purposes), and most of them are in various stages of development. An example of a term that may be problematic from a clinical perspective is the NOC term *immune hypersensitivity control:* some clinicians would rather use a more familiar, specific term such as allergy management.
- Look to expert clinicians and clinical specialty references for the most up-to-date clinical application. These resources can help you decide what is or isn't applicable to each particular practice setting. For example, Displays 3–1 and 3–2 list diagnoses commonly encountered in Rehabilitation and Perioperative Nursing.
- Terminology and use of nursing diagnoses vary from one facility to another. Use the terms recommended by your instructors or the facility where you work.

DISPLAY 3–1   Diagnoses Commonly Used in Rehabilitation Nursing

Risk for Injury	Impaired Physical Mobility
Impaired Swallowing	Activity Intolerance
Pressure Ulcer	Knowledge Deficit
Reflex Incontinence	Pain
Urinary Retention	Impaired Thought Processes
Colonic Constipation	Body Image Disturbance
Feeding Self-Care Deficit	Impaired Verbal Communication
Bathing or Hygiene Self-Care Deficit	Caregiver Role Strain
Dressing and Grooming Self-Care Deficit	Ineffective Individual Coping
Toileting Self-Care Deficit	Ineffective Family Coping
	Risk for Disuse Syndrome

Source: American Association of Rehabilitation Nurses.

DISPLAY 3–2	Diagnoses Commonly Used by Perioperative Nurses

Type of Diagnosis	Diagnostic Label	
Critical nursing diagnoses[1]	Risk for perioperative positioning injury	
	Risk for infection	
Primary nursing diagnoses[2]	Impaired protection	Risk for fluid volume deficit
	Pain	Knowledge deficit
	Risk for peripheral neuro-vascular dysfunction	Ineffective airway clearance
	Risk for aspiration	Impaired skin integrity
	Risk for impaired skin integrity	Impaired gas exchange
		Impaired tissue perfusion
	Risk for imbalanced body temperature	Decreased cardiac output
		Ineffective breathing pattern
	Risk for injury	Fluid volume deficit
	Anxiety	Fluid volume excess
	Fear	Impaired urinary elimination
	Hypothermia	Impaired physical mobility
	Impaired tissue integrity	
	Inability to sustain spontaneous respirations	
Secondary nursing diagnoses[3]	Impaired verbal communication	Urinary retention
	Sensory perceptual alterations	Social isolation
	Ineffective individual coping	Activity intolerance
	Acute confusion	Sexual dysfunction
	Powerlessness	Risk for caregiver role strain
	Impaired thought process	Hopelessness
	Hyperthermia	Ineffective thermal regulation
	Post-trauma response	Imbalanced nutrition; less than
	Risk for impaired parent/child attachment	Imbalanced nutrition; more than
	Spiritual distress	Caregiver role strain
	Body image disturbance	Ineffective therapeutic regimen
	Impaired role performance	
	Decisional conflict	Self-esteem disturbance
	Anticipatory grieving	Impaired growth and development
	Noncompliance	
	Ineffective family coping	Impaired sexuality patterns
	Impaired home maintenance management	Sleep pattern disturbance
		Ineffective denial
		Impaired family processes

[1]Occurring in more than half the patients on a daily basis with a high priority for immediate nursing attention.
[2]Occurring in less than half the patients with a moderate to high priority for nursing attention.
[3]Occurring in less than half the patients with a low to moderate priority for nursing attention.
Source: Reprinted with permission from AORN *Perioperative Nursing Data Set*, p. 9. Copyright © AORN, Inc., 2170 South Parker Road, Suite 300, Denver, CO 80231.

• Remember the importance of *individualizing care* by making sure your plans are tailored to meet your patients' particular situations. Each patient is a person, not a group of linked diagnoses, interventions, and outcomes chosen from a book or computer.

To individualize nursing care, remember the following key concepts.

Mastering Diagnoses, Interventions, and Outcomes in Practice: Key Concepts

1. **Diagnosis.** Because accurate and specific assessment and diagnosis encompasses about 50% to 60% of the task of problem solving, master the principles and rules of diagnosis (pages 100–106). Become competent in identifying common health problems and risk factors encountered in the practice areas where you work (see Displays 3–2, Diagnoses Commonly Used in Rehabilitation Nursing, and 3–3, Diagnoses Commonly Used by Perioperative Nurses). Also, become competent at detecting signs and symptoms that may indicate problems that must be referred in each particular practice setting (examples of common potential complications are listed in Display 3–3).

2. **Interventions:** Become familiar with the common interventions that are used to treat *specific* health problems in your particular practice setting. As discussed in the next chapter in depth, be as specific as possible when describing the interventions required for the real patient problems you face. For example, if you have a patient with *Impaired Communication,* look up that diagnosis in a reference, discriminating between interventions that are applicable to your patient's particular situation. Keep in mind that many of the NIC terms are broad terms that work well for research purposes (see list of NIC terms, pages 255–259 in the Appendix). In practice, you must identify specific, individualized interventions, as we'll discuss in the next chapter, *Planning.*

3. **Outcomes:** Learn the principles and rules of identifying specific, individualized patient outcomes (addressed in the next chapter). Remember that many of the NOC terms also are broad terms that work well for research but may be too broad for practice (see list of NOC terms, pages 259–261 in the Appendix).

Think About It

Using Standard Languages—Practice versus Research. *Many nurses have difficulty understanding the value of developing structured nursing vocabularies: standard languages that are organized in specific ways (see Table 3–1). Remember that this ongoing work is essential to facilitating the use of computers in patient care. In the clinical setting, avoid becoming overwhelmed by trying to learn long lists of diagnoses, interventions, or outcomes. Rather, use clinical references and experts to help you narrow the information down and learn the terms you must know in specific clinical situations. Use research courses to study and analyze how structured vocabularies are evolving and what needs to happen next to move this important work forward.*

DISPLAY 3-3   Common Potential Complications (More detailed list on inside front cover)

Problem	Potential Complications
Intravenous therapy	Phlebitis Extravasation Fluid overload
Nasogastric suction	Nasogastric tube malfunction Vomiting/aspiration Electrolyte imbalance
Skeletal traction and casts	Poor bone alignment Bleeding Embolus Neurovascular compromise
Medications	Side effects Adverse reaction/allergy Overdosage/toxicity
Foley catheter	Catheter malfunction Infection/bleeding
Chest tubes	Chest tube malfunction Hemo/pneumothorax Bleeding/infection Atelectasis
Surgery or trauma	Atelectasis Bleeding, shock/hypovolemia Electrolyte imbalance Paralytic ileus Oliguria/anuria Fluid overload/congestive heart failure
Head trauma	Bleeding/shock Brain swelling Increased intracranial pressure Coma/respiratory depression

Definitions and Discussion of Key Terms Related to Diagnosis

Having an understanding of key terms related to diagnosis is essential to becoming a competent diagnostician, to acting in your patients' best interest, and to protecting your-self from legal problems. Study the following terms, which are listed in the order in which you need to learn them (you need to know the first term to understand the second, and so on). Then test your knowledge by completing the critical thinking exercise on page 97.

Competency. Having the knowledge and skills to perform actions safely and efficiently in various situations (also used to refer to the ability to clearly identify problems and their cause; for example, "She is a competent diagnostician.").

E X A M P L E

After the first semester of nursing, the student had demonstrated competency in giving medications. **Discussion:** You're considered competent to perform an action or diagnose health problems once you've completed appropriate courses and passed tests (clinical and theoretical), demonstrating competency.

Qualified. Being competent and having the authority to perform an action or make a diagnosis.

E X A M P L E

Although you know you're competent to give IV medications in one hospital, when you go to another hospital, you check policies to determine whether you still have the authority to do so before you can consider yourself qualified to give IV medications. Based on experience, you may be able to diagnose a urinary tract infection, but unless you've been given the authority to do so, you must refer the problem. **Discussion:** Authority to perform assessments and make diagnoses is derived from the following: laws, licensure, and certification; national, state, and community standards; institutional standards, policies, procedures, and protocols; and other health care professionals (eg, instructors, supervisors, APNs, physicians).

Nursing Domain. Actions a nurse is legally qualified to perform. May also refer to diagnoses a nurse is qualified to make.

E X A M P L E

Inserting a nasogastric tube prescribed by a physician is in the nursing domain as long as the nurse is qualified to do so. **Discussion:** The nursing domain includes actions that nurses perform independently (eg, monitoring function of a nasogastric tube) and activities that nurses perform when delegated by a physician or APN (eg, inserting a nasogastric tube). As you progress with your education and clinical experience, your nursing domain will include a wider range of activities. You're responsible for maintaining competency within your practice domain.

Medical Domain. Activities and actions a medical doctor is legally qualified to perform.

E X A M P L E

Performing surgery is in the medical domain as long as it's allowed by law and the physician is qualified to do so. **Discussion:** Some expert nurses now perform some actions (eg, pelvic examinations, removing invasive lines) that used to belong exclusively to the medical domain. When nurses take on responsibility for actions that used to belong only to the medical domain, the actions must be approved by their state board of nursing. Boards of nursing usually issue position statements that describe what nurses can or can't do related to a specific problem or procedure.

Accountable. Being responsible and answerable for something.

E X A M P L E

> If you perform an assessment and you miss problems, you're *accountable* for what happens (eg, if you miss an area of skin redness and the area becomes ulcerated because of lack of treatment, you're accountable).

Definitive Interventions. The most specific treatment required to prevent, resolve, or manage a health problem.

E X A M P L E

> If a patient has *bacterial pneumonia,* you might encourage fluids, assist with coughing, and administer oxygen. However, if you don't have the definitive intervention of giving an antibiotic that's effective against that specific bacteria, you're highly unlikely to get a cure.

Outcome. The result of prescribed interventions or plan of care. Usually refers to the desired result of interventions (ie, that the problem is prevented, resolved, or managed); includes a specific time frame for when the outcome is expected to be achieved.

E X A M P L E

> "By three days after surgery, the person who has had a total knee replacement will have stable vital signs, no signs of infection, an ability to ambulate with a walker, and will be ready to be discharged to a rehabilitation facility."

Diagnose. To make a judgment and name actual and potential health problems or risk factors based on evidence from an assessment.

E X A M P L E

> After performing an assessment, the nurse diagnosed *Risk for Aspiration related to decreased level of consciousness and poor cough reflex.*

Diagnosis. In addition to referring to the second step of the nursing process, *diagnosis* can mean two things: (1) the *process* of analyzing data and putting related cues together to make judgments about health status (eg, the skill of diagnosis is learned through education, practice, experience, and application of critical thinking principles); or (2) the *result* of the diagnostic process.

E X A M P L E

> After careful analysis of all the data, the diagnosis of *Ineffective Breathing Pattern related to pain from the right chest incision* was made. **Discussion:** It's important to remember the legal implications of the word *diagnosis:* it implies that there's a situation or problem requiring appropriate, qualified treatment. This means if you identify a problem, you must consider whether you're *qualified* to treat it and willing to *accept responsibility* for treating it. If you're not, you're responsible for acquiring qualified help.

Definitive Diagnosis. The most specific, most correct diagnosis.

E X A M P L E

> If you identify signs and symptoms you suspect indicate a myocardial infarction, you begin giving oxygen, take vital signs, and immediately call the physician so a *definitive diagnosis* can be made. **Discussion:** Being very specific about the diagnosis enables you to plan very specific treatment. Would you be satisfied with a diagnosis of "lung disease," or would you want a more definitive diagnosis that clearly identifies both the problem and its cause?

Life Processes. Events or changes that occur during one's lifetime (eg, growing up, aging, maturing, becoming a parent, moving, separations, losses).

Nursing Diagnosis. A clinical judgment about an individual, family, or community response to actual or potential health problems and life processes. Nursing diagnoses provide the basis for selection of nursing interventions to achieve outcomes for which the nurse is accountable (NANDA, 1994). Nursing diagnoses often are called *human responses* because we, as nurses, focus on how people *are responding* to changes in health or life circumstances; for example, how they're responding to illness or to becoming a parent. Some specialty practice organizations use a different definition to reflect specific practice roles. For example, the American Association of Perioperative Nurses uses the following definition: *A nursing diagnosis is a concise clinical judgment label of a perioperative patient problem formulated for the purpose of directing nursing actions intended to achieve the expected outcomes* (Beyea, 2000).

E X A M P L E

> *Risk for Injury related to poor balance.* **Discussion:** The quick-reference section beginning on page 000 provides information on many of the nursing diagnoses accepted for clinical testing. However, you don't have to know all the diagnoses. Some diagnoses are in the early stages of development; some you'll never use, depending on where you work and what terminology is recommended. When first learning about nursing diagnoses, focus on the ones most commonly used in the particular setting in which you work. For examples, see Displays 3–1 and 3–2.

Medical Diagnosis. A health problem that requires definitive diagnosis by a qualified primary care provider (physician, APN, or physician's assistant). Medical diagnoses usually refer to problems with organs or systems (diseases, trauma) and don't always require nursing care (eg, hypertension in an otherwise healthy person often is managed by the patient and primary provider without nursing care).

E X A M P L E

> Acute myocardial infarction (MI). **Discussion:** As stated earlier, some nurses in advanced practice now are qualified to diagnose and treat some medical diagnoses.

Potential Complications: Organ or system problems that may arise because of the presence of certain diagnoses or treatment modalities. Carpenito (2000) uses the term *collaborative problem* to address potential physiologic complications.

> See Display 3–3 and inside front cover. **Discussion.** You're responsible for knowing how to monitor for signs and symptoms of potential complications and for being prepared to manage them (addressed in the next chapter). Table 3–2 compares the terms nursing diagnoses and medical diagnosis.

Multidisciplinary Problem. A problem requiring treatment by more than one discipline, for example, nursing, medicine, physical therapy, and occupational therapy.

> Care management of someone with a fractured hip. **Discussion.** All disciplines are accountable for independent and physician prescribed actions within their domain of practice. Increasingly in acute care and rehabilitation, problems are treated by multidisciplinary approaches. Figure 3–1 shows key questions to ask to determine whether you've identified a nursing diagnosis or medical or multidisciplinary problem.

T A B L E 3 – 2 Comparison of Nursing Diagnoses and Medical Diagnoses

Nursing Diagnoses	Medical Diagnoses
Main Focus	*Main Focus*
1. Human responses to disease, trauma, or life changes 2. Problems with functioning independently	Diseases, trauma, problems with organ or system function
Primary Manager of Problem	*Primary Manager of Problem*
Nurse (may use other resources such as physical therapy or physician expertise, but the nurse accepts primary responsibility for monitoring status and allocating resources)	Physician or advanced practice nurse (APN)
Definitive Diagnosis	*Definitive Diagnosis*
Authority to diagnose is within the nursing domain.	Nurse is required to seek physician or APN diagnosis.
Nursing Responsibilities	*Nursing Responsibilities*
1. Identification of signs, symptoms, and risk factors 2. Early detection of actual and potential problems 3. Initiation of a comprehensive plan to prevent, correct, or control the problems (nurse is the primary manager of the problems)	1. Identification of risk factors, anticipating potential complications 2. Monitoring to detect and report early signs or symptoms of potential complications or change in status 3. Initiating actions within the nursing domain to prevent or minimize the problems and their potential complications 4. Implementing medical orders (physician or APN is primary manager of the problems)

Related Factor. Something known to be *associated with* a specific health problem (eg, *history of frequent falls* is a related factor for *Risk for Injury*).

Risk Factor. Something known to cause, or *contribute to,* a specific problem (eg, *decreased vision* is a related factor for *Risk for Injury*). **Discussion:** The terms *related factor* and *risk factor* often are used interchangeably.

Etiology. Something known to cause a disease or problem. The terms *risk factor* and *etiology* sometimes are used interchangeably. **Discussion.** To completely understand a problem, you need to determine its cause or related factors.

Risk (Potential) Diagnosis. A health problem that may develop if preventive actions aren't taken.

E X A M P L E

> *Risk for Injury related to poor balance and history of frequent falls.* **Discussion:** Risk (potential) diagnoses are made when you identify risk factors for a specific problem but have *no* actual evidence of the problem.

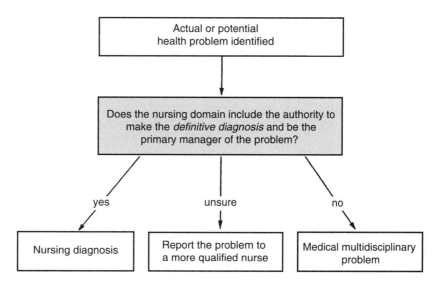

F i g u r e **3–1.** Key question to determine whether you've identified a nursing diagnosis or multidisciplinary problem.

Wellness Diagnosis. A clinical judgment about an individual, family, or community in transition from a specific level of wellness to a higher level of wellness (NANDA, 2001).

E X A M P L E

> *Readiness for Enhanced Parenting.* **Discussion:** The NANDA taxonomy (2001), uses *"readiness for enhanced"* as a prefix for wellness diagnoses. In most acute care settings, for efficiency's sake, the plan of care addresses only actual and risk (potential) diagnoses, which are considered the most important immediate concerns. In the community and home care, more opportunities are present to focus on wellness diagnoses.

Recognizing Risk Factors: The Key to Proactive Approaches

As we shift to the more proactive PPM model, the importance of recognizing and managing risk factors becomes clear. In many cases, there are no actual problems, but there *are* risk factors that indicate a need for close monitoring. For example, suppose you're caring for a pregnant woman who is healthy but smokes. Knowing that smoking contributes to low birth weight in infants and also puts the mother at risk for other problems such as clot formation, hypertension, and lung disease, you know to monitor this woman more closely and to continue to work with the woman to stop smoking (at least during the pregnancy).

Make the shift from having only a problem-solving mentality to a proactive, preventive way of thinking. Move from asking only "Have I missed any problems?" to also asking, "Have I missed any risk factors that need attention?"

VOICES

Predicting, Preventing, and Managing Violence. The most significant factor that will help to predict, prevent, and manage violence is asking about history of previous violent episodes. With angry or high-risk patients, ask questions like, "Have you ever felt out of control or been violent in the past?". . ."What do you do when you feel like you're getting out of control?". . ."What can we do when you're feeling like this?"—*Nico Oud, RN, MNSc, Dipl.N.Adm*

(E-mail communication, February 12, 2001.)

CRITICAL THINKING EXERCISE VII

Nurses'
Responsibilities as
Diagnosticians;
Key Terms
Related to
Diagnosis;
Differentiating
Between Nursing
Diagnoses and
Other Problems

To complete this session, read pages 80–96. Example responses can be found on page 244.

1. Short answer:

   a. How do you know if an action is within your domain of practice?

   b. List two key nursing responsibilities related to nursing diagnoses and two related to medical diagnoses.

2. Check your knowledge of key terms. For each definition (numbers 1–17), place the letter of the word that best matches the definition. Use each letter only once.

   a. diagnose
   b. diagnosis
   c. medical domain
   d. wellness diagnosis
   e. definitive diagnosis
   f. risk diagnosis
   g. accountable
   h. competency
   i. being qualified

   j. life process
   k. nursing domain
   l. outcome
   m. legal implications of *diagnosis*
   n. medical diagnosis
   o. nursing diagnoses
   p. definitive interventions
   q. risk (related) factor

   1. _____ Something known to contribute to (or be associated with) a specific problem.
   2. _____ A health problem for which someone is at risk.
   3. _____ The judgment that's made after drawing conclusions about assessment data. Also may refer to the skill of analyzing data to make a judgment.
   4. _____ To make a judgment and identity and name risk factors, problems, or strengths based on evidence from an assessment.
   5. _____ Being responsible and answerable for something.
   6. _____ Range of activities and actions that a physician is legally qualified to initiate or prescribe.
   7. _____ Range of activities and actions that a nurse is legally qualified to initiate or prescribe.
   8. _____ Implies that there's a situation or problem that requires appropriate qualified treatment.
   9. _____ Usually refers to the desired or expected result of interventions (ie, the problem is prevented, resolved, or minimized).

10. _____ Usually referred to as *human responses*. These provide the basis for selection of nursing interventions to achieve outcomes for which the nurse is accountable.

11. _____ A clinical judgment about an individual, family, or community in transition from a specific level of wellness to a higher level of wellness.

12. _____ Events or changes that occur during one's lifetime (eg, becoming a parent, aging, separations, losses).

13. _____ The most *specific* diagnosis.

14. _____ The most specific actions required to prevent, resolve, or control a problem.

15. _____ A problem requiring definitive diagnosis and treatment by a qualified physician. APNs also may treat some of these problems.

16. _____ Having the knowledge and skill to perform an activity or give opinions.

17. _____ Having the competency *and authority* to perform an activity.

3. Differentiating between nursing diagnoses and medical diagnoses.

   a. Place "N" in front of the phrases that describe characteristics of nursing diagnoses. Leave the ones that do not blank.

      1. _____ Deals mostly with problems with structure or function of organs or systems.

      2. _____ Includes health problems as identified from patients' perspectives.

      3. _____ Definitive diagnosis is validated by medical diagnostic studies.

      4. _____ Deals mostly with actual or potential problems with human responses to disease or life changes.

      5. _____ Related signs and symptoms don't respond to nurse-prescribed interventions.

      6. _____ Related signs and symptoms respond to nurse-prescribed interventions.

   b. For each of the following problems, write "N" in front of those that are nursing diagnoses.

      1. _____ Potential complication: hemorrhage related to clotting problems

      2. _____ Ineffective Airway Clearance related to copious secretions

      3. _____ Risk for Injury related to generalized weakness

      4. _____ Intravenous therapy

      5. _____ Fluid Volume Deficit related to insufficient fluid intake due to sore throat

      6. _____ Impaired Skin Integrity (right heel) related to unrelieved pressure point

7. _____ Potential complication: cardiac arrhythmias related to low potassium level

8. _____ Diabetes

9. _____ Diversional Activity Deficit related to prescribed bed rest

10. _____ Potential complication: malnutrition related to prescribed NPO (nothing by mouth)

11. _____ Imbalanced Nutrition: Less than Body Requirements related to poor appetite

12. _____ Impaired Physical Mobility related to prescribed bed rest

13. _____ Pneumothorax (collapsed lung)

14. _____ Potential complication: thrombus formation related to venous shunt placement

4. Compare and Contrast: List one way the *DT* and the *PPM* models are the same and one way that they're different.

Try This On Your Own

Together with at least one other classmate, discuss the implications the statement below has for using critical paths.

Think About It

No Patient is a Critical Path. *Critical paths are developed for specific problems, not specific people.*

Diagnostic Reasoning: Applying Critical Thinking

Diagnostic reasoning, or applying critical thinking to identifying actual and potential health problems, requires knowledge, skills, and experience. At the big picture level, diagnostic reasoning involves the steps listed in the following box (Box 3–2).

Once you have repeated experiences in various clinical situations, diagnostic reasoning becomes almost automatic. However, until then, it's important to be clearly aware of basic principles and rules of diagnostic reasoning. The following principles, rules, and steps are based on sound critical thinking skills like *recognizing assumptions, being systematic and complete,* and *making judgments based on evidence.* They're designed to help you form habits that help you avoid common pitfalls and increase your ability to make accurate diagnoses.

> **Box 3–2 Diagnostic Reasoning (Big Picture Level)**
> - Analyzing cue clusters
> - Creating a list of suspected problems
> - Ruling out similar diagnoses
> - Choosing the most specific diagnostic labels
> - Stating the problems and their cause
> - Identifying strengths, resources, and areas for improvement

Fundamental Principles and Rules of Diagnostic Reasoning

- **Recognizing diagnoses requires you to be familiar with the diagnoses themselves.** For example, how can you decide whether your patient has *Ineffective Airway Clearance* or pneumonia if you don't know the associated signs and symptoms. Until you've had repeated experiences with a variety of different health problems, keep references handy. **Rationale:** By keeping references handy, you begin to recognize problems by comparing your patient's data with the signs, symptoms, and risk factors of the problems listed in the references.

- **Keep an open mind.** Avoid tendencies to be overly influenced by past experiences or by information you gain from patient charts or others (eg, you may assess someone whose chart reports a history of chronic back pain related to arthritis and fail to consider that an increase in back pain could signify something else like a kidney problem). **Rationale:** Keeping an open mind prevents you from seeing the problems from a narrow perspective, a common critical thinking error.

- **When you make a diagnosis, back it up with evidence.** Provide the cues (signs, symptoms, risk factors) that led you to make the diagnosis. **Rationale:** Others need to know your evidence so they can evaluate the accuracy of your diagnosis. Cues (signs, symptoms, risk factors) are like "key puzzle pieces"; if you don't have them, you can't complete the puzzle and label the problem. Display 3–4 clarifies the definitions of sign, symptom, defining characteristics, and cues.

- **Although intuition is a valuable tool for problem identification, never make diagnoses on intuition alone: look for evidence to verify your intuition.** Display 3–5 describes how to use intuition safely. **Rationale:** You may intuitively know the diagnosis. However, because diagnosis is based on evidence, you need to validate your intuition.

DISPLAY 3 – 4   Definitions of Diagnostic Terms

✓ **Sign:** *Objective data* that have been known to signify a health problem (eg, fever is a sign).
✓ **Symptom:** *Subjective data* that have been known to signify a health problem (eg, pain is a symptom).
✓ **Defining Characteristics:** A cluster of signs, symptoms, and risk factors usually present in patients with a specific nursing diagnosis.
✓ **Cues:** Signs, symptoms, and defining characteristics noted in a patient.

DISPLAY 3-5   How to Use Intuition Safely

1. Recognize that although you have no evidence that a problem exists, your intuition is sending up a red flag that says, "There is a problem here; watch this patient closely," or "This patient needs help." Assess closely for existing signs and symptoms that validate the presence of the problem that you suspect. (You should say to the patient, physician, or another nurse, "My intuition tells me that . . . " or "I have the feeling that. . . .")
2. If you know that something is wrong but can't put your finger on any specific problem, increase the frequency and intensity of nursing assessment to monitor closely for early detection of signs and symptoms.
3. Before you act on intuition alone, weigh the risks of the possibility of your actions causing harm (either aggravating the situation or creating new problems) against the risk of not acting at all (other than to actively monitor more closely).

- **If you miss a problem, mislabel a problem, or identify a problem that isn't there, you've made a diagnostic error,** which may result in inappropriate, perhaps dangerous treatment. **Rationale:** An error in diagnosis is likely to cause an error in treatment. Display 3–6 lists common causes and possible consequences of diagnostic errors.

- **Just because other nurses have more experience, it doesn't mean they're always right.** When making important decisions, be an independent thinker, ask for rationale, and double-check with reliable resources (references, other qualified professionals). **Rationale:** No one is immune to error; the more experienced nurse may misinterpret your question or be preoccupied with other duties.

- **Know your qualifications and limitations. Rationale:** People have the right to be assessed by a qualified health care professional. Although you may feel that you have the knowledge to perform an assessment and diagnose the problems, you must determine (for your patient's health and your own legal protection) whether you have the authority to do so.

Ten Steps for Diagnosing Health Problems

1. Start by asking the person (and significant others) to identify their three biggest problems or concerns. **Rationale:** Often, the person requiring care and significant others are the ones best able to identify problems. Asking them to choose three problems helps them and you to prioritize.
2. Be sure you've completed the five phases of assessment, using both a nursing model and body systems model to cluster your data. **Rationale:** Systematic, comprehensive assessment is essential to diagnosis.
3. Determine normal, impaired, at risk, or possible impaired functioning (Display 3–7) and create a list of suspected, actual, and potential problems. **Rationale:** This helps reduce the amount of information you're dealing with and helps you begin to focus on problem areas.

DISPLAY 3–6   Diagnostic Errors

Causes of Diagnostic Errors

- Overvaluing the probability of one explanation or failing to consider all of the data because of a *narrow* focus.
  Example: Deciding that anxiety is related to psychological stress rather than considering whether there might be some physical problem, such as poor oxygenation, causing the anxiety.
- Continuing to *analyze* when you should be *acting* to get help.
  Example: Continuing to see if repositioning and emotional support help a breathing problem, even though they make no difference.
- Failing to recognize personal biases or assumptions.
  Example: Assuming that someone who doesn't bathe daily has a poor self-image.
- Making a diagnosis that's too general (not being specific enough in choosing a diagnostic label to name the problem).
  Example: Using *Impaired Urinary Elimination* instead of *Stress Incontinence related to weakness of bladder sphincter muscles.*
- Failing to include the correct diagnosis in the initial list of possible problems.
  Example: Listing the problems of *Noncompliance* but not including the possible problems of *Ineffective Coping* or *Ineffective Management of Therapeutic Regimen.*
- Rushing to get done, either when collecting or analyzing data.
  Example: Rushing through assessment or choosing any diagnosis that's close so you get to report on time, rather than communicating the problem with time to your supervising nurse or the oncoming nurse.

Risks of Diagnostic Errors

When you miss a problem, mislabel a problem, or fail to fully understand a problem, you run the risk of any of the following:

- Initiating interventions that actually aggravate the problems.
- Omitting interventions that are essential to solving the problems.
- Allowing problems to exist or progress without even detecting they are there.
- Initiating interventions that are harmless but wasteful of everyone's time and energy.
- Influencing others that problems exist as described incorrectly.
- Placing yourself in danger of legal liability.

4. Consider each suspected problem and look for other signs and symptoms associated with the problem. For example, if you suspect infection because of localized pain and swelling, look for other signs of infection (fever, redness, heat, drainage). **Rationale:** Diagnosis is based on evidence; the more evidence (cues) you have, the more likely you are to be correct.

5. Rule in and rule out problems (when you *rule in* a problem, it means you decide that the problem is present; when you *rule out* a problem, it means you decide it's *not* present), looking for flaws in your thinking:

DISPLAY 3–7   Checklist for Identifying Problems

List any history of allergies, disease, surgery, or trauma.

List current medications (include over-the-counter and herbal drugs) and past intolerance to medications.

	(Circle those that apply)			
Is there a problem with breathing or circulation?	Yes	No	AR*	Pos†
Is there a problem with nutrition or elimination?	Yes	No	AR	Pos
Is there a problem with fluid balance?	Yes	No	AR	Pos
Is there a problem with safety (risk for injury)?	Yes	No	AR	Pos
Is there a problem with rest or exercise?	Yes	No	AR	Pos
Is there a problem with ability to think or perceive environment?	Yes	No	AR	Pos
Is there a problem with communication?	Yes	No	AR	Pos
Is there high risk for infection transmission?	Yes	No	AR	Pos
Is there high risk for impairment of skin integrity?	Yes	No	AR	Pos
Is this admission going to cause difficulties at home?	Yes	No	AR	Pos
Is there a problem with coping or stress?	Yes	No	AR	Pos
Is there a psychological, developmental, or sociocultural problem?	Yes	No	AR	Pos
Is there a problem with personal or religious beliefs?	Yes	No	AR	Pos
Is there a problem with health maintenance at home?	Yes	No	AR	Pos
Is there a problem with role, relationships, or sexuality?	Yes	No	AR	Pos
Does the person have a problem with taking medications?	Yes	No	AR	Pos
Does the patient require teaching?	Yes	No	AR	Pos

*AR, At risk for problem (no signs and symptoms present, but risk factors are evident).
†Pos, Possible problem (insufficient data, but examiner suspects a problem).

- **What other problems could the cues represent?** For example, if someone tells you he's been having increasing episodes of left shoulder pain from an old injury, consider the possibility that this pain also could represent a cardiac problem.
- **What other data could be influencing the status of your suspected problems?** For example, you may have *ruled out* the possibility of infection because there is no fever, but when you check all the data, you realize that acetaminophen has been taken, reducing body temperature.

Rationale: Looking for flaws in thinking is a critical thinking principle that helps reduce diagnostic errors.

6. Name the problems by using the labels that most closely match assessment cues. For example, if you suspect *Anxiety* or *Fear,* compare the cues with the defining characteristics of *Anxiety* and *Fear*. If the cues are most similar to *Anxiety,* name the problem *Anxiety*. If the cues are most similar to the defining characteristics of *Fear,* label the problem *Fear*. **Rationale:** Diagnosis is based on recognizing when cues are consistent with the signs and symptoms (defining characteristics) of a specific diagnosis.

7. Determine the causes of the problem. **Rationale:** Knowing what's causing the problems helps you to determine *specific* interventions. For example, note how "*a*" below can help you to determine interventions, whereas "*b*" tells you very little.

    a. *Fear related to previous bad experience with general anesthesia*

    b. *Fear*

8. If you identify *risk factors* for a problem but have *no evidence* (no signs and symptoms) of the problem, list it as a Risk (potential) problem (eg, *Risk for Impaired Skin Integrity related to obesity and confinement to bed*). **Rationale:** Identifying potential problems is the key to the *PPM* model.

9. Share your diagnoses with the person requiring care and ask him whether the diagnoses seem appropriate. **Rationale:** The person has the right to be informed of diagnoses and must be a key player in developing the plan of care.

10. Ask the person if there's anything else that should be listed as a problem. Add these problems to the list. **Rationale:** Whatever the person perceives as a problem *is* a problem.

Three Steps for Diagnosing Strengths

1. Ask the person (and significant others) two questions:

    "Can you tell me some things about yourself that you view as strengths, as healthy aspects?"

    "Can you think of any things that aren't really problems but you'd like to manage better?"

    Rationale: Answers to these questions help everyone to recognize assets and areas that could be improved.

2. Cluster together data that indicate normal or positive functioning. Label these areas as strengths and share them with the person and significant others. For example, you might say, "You've made the decision to seek help, which is a healthy thing to do." **Rationale:** This helps both you and the person requiring care to focus on strengths as well as problems.

3. List the strengths that will assist you in preventing, resolving, or controlling the identified problems. **Rationale:** These are the strengths that you use to develop an efficient care plan.

EXAMPLE

> **Physical Strengths:** In good health; exercises daily and has excellent cardiac and respiratory reserve; eats a balanced diet; demonstrates physical adaptation; upper torso and arms are powerful (compensating for paraplegia). **Psychological and Personal Strengths:** Demonstrates effective coping; copes with chronic pain by using guided imagery and judicious use of pain medications; motivated; wants to be independent and healthy; knowledgeable; relates understanding of health care management and available resources; demonstrates good problem-solving skills; able to adjust daughter's therapy schedule for optimum results and convenience; has strong support systems.

Avoiding Diagnostic Errors

No one is immune to error, but each of us can work to develop habits that help us to avoid mistakes. Display 3–8 lists questions to ask to evaluate whether you're developing habits that reduce the likelihood of making diagnostic errors.

Considering Lifestyles and Coping Patterns

Because nursing is concerned with medical problems *and* how the problems affect someone's daily life, it's important to consider usual lifestyles and coping patterns. When you're attempting to determine how someone is responding to a change in health status or lifestyle, ask the following questions:

- How does this problem change your life?
- How do you feel you're coping with these changes?
- Tell me how you usually adapt to change.
- Can you think of anything you can do to better adapt?
- What resources (personal, community) might be able to help you cope better?

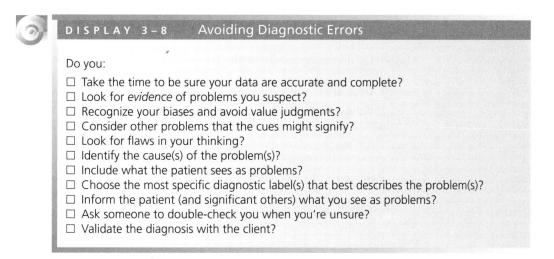

DISPLAY 3–8   Avoiding Diagnostic Errors

Do you:
- ☐ Take the time to be sure your data are accurate and complete?
- ☐ Look for *evidence* of problems you suspect?
- ☐ Recognize your biases and avoid value judgments?
- ☐ Consider other problems that the cues might signify?
- ☐ Look for flaws in your thinking?
- ☐ Identify the cause(s) of the problem(s)?
- ☐ Include what the patient sees as problems?
- ☐ Choose the most specific diagnostic label(s) that best describes the problem(s)?
- ☐ Inform the patient (and significant others) what you see as problems?
- ☐ Ask someone to double-check you when you're unsure?
- ☐ Validate the diagnosis with the client?

Determining Causative and Risk (Related) Factors

Ability to identify causative and risk (related) factors depends on your knowledge, experience, and analytical skills. However, there are some questions you can ask to help you identify these factors:

- What factors does the person (or significant others) identify as causing or contributing to the problem?
- Are there factors related to developmental age, disease, or changes in lifestyle that may be contributing to the problem?
- Are there cultural, socioeconomic, ethnic, or religious factors that may be contributing to the problem?
- Do your other resources for data collection (eg, medical records, other health care professionals, literature review) identify factors that might be causing or contributing to the problem?

Having discussed the importance of considering usual lifestyles, coping patterns, and causes of problems, let's look at how to recognize nursing diagnoses and determine potential complications.

NANDA's List of Diagnoses Accepted for Clinical Testing

NANDA is the main organization for developing and refining nursing diagnosis terms (see the *Quick-Reference to Nursing Diagnoses* section). NANDA officially updates its list every 2 years. As stated earlier, remember that some of the diagnoses on the list have been used and studied only minimally (eg, *Personal Identity Disturbance*), whereas others have had extensive use and study (eg, *Risk for Injury*).

Diagnostic Label Components

Most of the diagnostic labels on NANDA's list have three components:

Title (Label) and Definition: A concise description of the problem.
Defining Characteristics: The cluster of signs and symptoms often associated with the diagnosis. (Risk diagnoses don't list defining characteristics because risk diagnoses are those someone is *at risk for developing*. There are no signs and symptoms evident.)
Related (Risk) Factors: Factors that can cause or contribute to the problem.

To clarify the above, turn to the quick reference section beginning on page 203, which lists all the diagnoses, their defining characteristics, and related factors. Note that if there are no defining characteristics listed, it's because the diagnosis is a *risk* diagnosis.

Actual, Risk, and Possible Nursing Diagnoses

Recognizing actual, risk, and possible nursing diagnoses requires you to compare the person's assessment data with the definition, defining characteristics, and related (risk) factors of the diagnoses that you suspect. Use the following rules to help you to identify actual, risk, and possible diagnosis on NANDA's list.

R U L E ▶ | Actual Diagnoses: The person's data base contains evidence of signs and symptoms or defining characteristics of the diagnosis.

R U L E ▶ | Risk Diagnosis: The person's data base contains evidence of the related (risk) factors of the diagnosis but no evidence of the defining characteristics. (If there were evidence of defining characteristics, it would be an *actual,* rather than *risk* diagnosis.)

R U L E ▶ | Possible Diagnosis: The person's data base doesn't demonstrate the defining characteristics *or* related factors of the diagnosis, but your intuition tells you that the diagnosis may be present (eg, *Possible Ineffective Individual Coping*).

Table 3–3 compares the nursing responsibilities for actual, risk, and possible diagnoses.

Wellness Diagnoses

Being able to diagnose wellness diagnoses is based on recognizing when healthy clients indicate a desire to achieve a higher level of functioning in a specific area (eg, "I wish I were a better parent" may lead you diagnose *Readiness for Enhanced Parenting*).

Syndrome Diagnoses

There are only two syndrome diagnoses currently on the NANDA list (*Disuse Syndrome* and *Rape Trauma Syndrome*). You use a syndrome diagnosis when the diagnosis is associated with a cluster of other diagnoses. For example, Display 3–9 shows the cluster of diagnoses seen with *Disuse Syndrome,* often seen in bedridden nursing home residents.

TABLE 3 – 3 Comparison of Actual, Risk, and Possible Nursing Diagnoses

Diagnosis Type	Signs and Symptoms Present?	Etiologic or Contributing Factors Present?	Nursing Responsibilities
Actual Diagnosis **Example:** *Constipation* R/T poor roughage and fluid intake as evidenced by hard, dry stool.	Yes	Yes	Monitor signs and symptoms to determine improvement or deterioration in condition. Identify interventions to reduce or eliminate the cause of the problem.
Risk Diagnosis **Example:** *Risk for Constipation* R/T poor roughage and fluid intake	No	Yes	Perform daily focus assessments to determine if signs and symptoms have appeared to change status from risk to actual. Identify interventions to prevent, reduce, or remove risk factors.
Possible Diagnosis **Example:** *Possible Constipation*	Unsure	Unsure	Gather more data to clarify vague cues and determine if the signs and symptoms or risk factors actually are present.

R/T, related to.
Adapted with permission from Carpenito, L. (1985). Unpublished workshop notes.

DISPLAY 3 – 9   Nursing Diagnoses Associated With Disuse Syndrome

- Impaired Physical Mobility
- Risk for Constipation
- Risk for Impaired Respiratory Function
- Risk for Infection
- Risk for Activity Intolerance
- Risk for Injury
- Risk for Impaired Thought Processes
- Risk for Body Image Disturbance
- Risk for Powerlessness
- Risk for Impaired Tissue Integrity

Nursing Diagnoses Not on NANDA's List

If you identify a problem you think is a nursing diagnosis, but you aren't able to find a label on the list that describes it appropriately, check to make sure you're not making any of the errors listed on page 113 (Guidelines: Avoiding Errors When Developing

Diagnostic Statements). If you haven't made any of these errors, describe the problem, its cause, and the evidence that leads you to believe the problem exists. For example, for a child, you might identify *Bowel Movement Holding related to fear as evidenced by child's statements that she's holding stool because she's afraid it will hurt, refusal to try to have a bowel movement, and only bowel movement coming at night when the child is asleep.*

CRITICAL THINKING EXERCISE VIII

Recognizing Nursing Diagnoses

To complete this session, read pages 99–109. Example responses can be found on page 245.

This session is designed for you to practice recognizing nursing diagnoses by comparing data with the defining characteristics and related factors of specific diagnoses. Listed below are eight common nursing diagnoses (letters *a* to *h*). After the diagnoses are eight different people who have been admitted to the hospital (numbers 1–8). For each number, place the letter of the diagnosis that best matches the available patient data. To make the diagnosis: (1) study the data; (2) choose a possible nursing diagnosis from the available choices; (3) look up the diagnosis in the section on quick-reference to nursing diagnosis starting on page 203 and compare the data with the defining characteristics and related factors for the chosen diagnosis. Each letter should be used only once. To get you started, I have given you the first answer.

a. *Risk for Aspiration*
b. *Activity Intolerance*
c. *Anxiety*
d. *Risk for Impaired Skin Integrity*

e. *Fear*
f. *Ineffective Breathing Pattern*
g. *Ineffective Airway Clearance*
h. *Impaired Skin Integrity*

1. _____b_____ Assessment data for Mrs. Ballard.
   Subjective data (SD): Says she feels tired all the time.
   Objective data (OD): Lungs clear; becomes short of breath after walking 5 yards; heart rate increases to 130 beats per minute after walking 5 yards; anemic (hemoglobin 7 g/dL).

2. _____ Assessment data for Jim Riley.
   SD: States his jaws were wired closed yesterday; complains of nausea.
   OD: Jaws wired shut.

3. _____ Assessment data for Charles Lindsay.
   SD: States he feels "sort of nervous" but can't pinpoint why.
   OD: Restless, glances about, doesn't make good eye contact.

4. _____ Assessment data for Daryl Laird.

SD: States he's very afraid of having to learn to give himself an injection; states he lives alone and is worried that something might go wrong when he's alone giving himself an injection.

OD: Doesn't maintain good eye contact; restless.

5. _____ Assessment data for Tim Dydo.

SD: States he's had a cold for 2 weeks and now has pain in lower right rib cage; states he feels like he needs to cough but finds it too painful.

OD: Respiration 34 per minute; pulse 128 beats per minute; able to cough if rib cage is splinted by me; coughs up thick white mucus.

6. _____ Assessment data for Beth Hendrix.

SD: States she has problems with urinary incontinence.

OD: Wears perineal pad; perineal area red and excoriated.

7. _____ Assessment data for Mary Kay Eipert.

SD: States she's had mild emphysema for 5 years, but now it seems to be getting worse; states she gets out of breath when going up one flight of stairs; says she never learned adaptive breathing techniques.

OD: Expiratory wheezes heard in both lungs; unable to demonstrate pursed-lipped breathing; respiratory rate up to 48 per minute after going up one flight of stairs.

8. _____ Assessment data for Maggie Wolartowski.

SD: Says she's afraid of moving because of pain in her hip.

OD: 92 years old; very thin; had a hip pinning yesterday; skin very dry, no obvious breakdown at present.

Think About It

Why Students Have to Write Long Care Plans. *In the clinical setting, you may see diagnostic statements listed in only abbreviated forms. However, it's important to know the rules that guide the way diagnostic statements should formally be written. Paying attention to rules for writing diagnostic statements as described in the following section will help you think your way through the diagnostic process and ensure that you are developing good habits of diagnostic reasoning. Keep in mind that students often are required to follow these rules and write long care plans rather than the abbreviated ones seen in the clinical setting so that faculty can assess their students' knowledge of nursing theories and principles of nursing process.*

Diagnostic Statements for Nursing Diagnoses

Because it's important to be clear and specific, there are accepted ways to formally write diagnostic statements.

Rules for Making Diagnostic Statements

1. Actual Diagnoses (three-part statement).

   Use PES (Problem, Etiology, Signs and Symptoms) or PRS (Problem, Related [Risk] Factors, Signs and Symptoms) format.

   Use "*related to*" to link the problem and the etiology or related factors. Add "*as evidenced by*" to state the evidence that supports that diagnosis is present.

   E X A M P L E

   Impaired Communication related to language barrier as evidenced by inability to speak or understand English and by use of Spanish.

2. Risk Nursing Diagnoses (two-part statement).

   Use PE (Problem, Etiology) or PR (Problem, Related [Risk] Factors) format.

   Use "*related to*" to link the potential problem with the related (risk) factors present.

   E X A M P L E

   Risk for Impaired Skin Integrity related to obesity, excessive diaphoresis, and confinement to bed.

3. Possible Diagnoses (one-part statement). Simply name the possible problem.

   E X A M P L E

   Possible Impaired Sexuality Patterns.

4. For Wellness Diagnoses (one-part statement). Use *Readiness for Enhanced* (changed from *Potential for Enhanced* [NANDA, 2001]) before the words that describe the area that is to be improved.

   E X A M P L E

   Readiness for Enhanced Parenting.

5. Syndrome Diagnoses (one-part statement). Simply name the syndrome.

   E X A M P L E

   Rape Trauma Syndrome.

Making Sure Diagnostic Statements Direct Interventions

When possible, write nursing diagnoses in such a way that they direct nursing interventions. When someone studies your diagnostic statement, it should answer the question, *"What can nurses do about this problem?"* For example, consider the boldface portions of each of the following statements and note how the first statement directs independent interventions whereas the second one does not (what can a nurse do about pneumonia?).

> Right: Risk for Ineffective Airway Clearance related to **copious thick secretions and difficulty positioning for coughing.**
> Wrong: Risk for Ineffective Airway Clearance related to **pneumonia.**

Remember the following rule:

RULE ▶

> When writing statements for nursing diagnoses, express them in such a way that the *second part* of the statement (*risk factors*) directs nursing interventions. If this isn't possible, then be sure the *problem* directs nursing interventions. (See the following examples.)

EXAMPLE

> **Right:** *Imbalanced Nutrition: Less Than Body Requirements related to throat discomfort.* Here the related factor (throat discomfort) and the problem (*Imbalanced Nutrition*) can be treated by nurse-prescribed interventions such as providing cool, high-calorie liquids and staying with the person to offer coaching and ensure that the liquids are taken.
> **Right:** *Risk for Aspiration related to wired jaws.* Here, the problem (aspiration) can be prevented by nurse-prescribed interventions even though the related factor (wired jaws) requires physician-prescribed interventions. Nurse-prescribed interventions include assisting with clearing of oral secretions, keeping the head of the bed up, teaching how to avoid aspiration, and keeping wire cutters at the bedside.
> **Wrong:** *Imbalanced Nutrition: Less Than Body Requirements related to NPO (nothing by mouth) status.* Here both the problem and the related factor require physician-prescribed interventions (in the form of IV fluids or gastric tube feedings).

VOICES

All Problems Aren't Created Equal—Determine the Cause. To understand and treat health problems, you must identify the underlying causes. For example, surgical wounds
continued

Guidelines: Using NANDA Terminology Correctly

For consistency and clarity, NANDA recommends using the following specific terminology with certain diagnoses:

* If NANDA lists the word *"specify"* in parentheses, it means you should be specific and add the necessary descriptive words to be sure the diagnosis is clear.

E X A M P L E

NANDA lists *Impaired Skin Integrity (specify)*. If the skin problem is in the rectal area, write *"rectal"* where NANDA has written *"specify."* Your diagnosis should look like this: *Impaired Skin Integrity (rectal)*.

- If you use *Deficient Knowledge* (changed from Knowledge Deficit according to NANDA, 2001) as a diagnosis, don't use "related to." Instead, put a colon after Deficient Knowledge and specify the knowledge that needs to be gained (eg, *Deficient Knowledge: insulin injection technique*).

The following guidelines are presented to help you avoid common errors in making diagnostic statements.

Guidelines: Avoiding Errors When Making Diagnostic Statements

- Don't write the diagnostic statement in such a way that it may be legally incriminating.

E X A M P L E

Incorrect: *Risk for Injury related to lack of side rails on bed.*
Correct: *Risk for Injury related to disorientation.*

- Don't "rename" a medical problem to make it sound like a nursing diagnosis.

E X A M P L E

Incorrect: *Imbalanced Hemodynamics related to hypovolemia.*
Correct: *Hypovolemia.* (This is a medical problem rather than a nursing diagnosis. Use the correct medical terminology.)

- Don't write a nursing diagnosis based on value judgments.

V O I C E S *continued*

(called primary intention wounds) are caused by surgeons and usually are closed with sutures or staples. These types of wounds usually follow the body's "healing cascade" in a predictable and orderly way. However, think about the difference between surgical wounds and chronic wounds like pressure ulcers. Unlike surgical wounds that often heal nicely on their own, ulcers are usually "stalled" in the healing process, requiring an intensive treatment plan.

Understanding the cause (etiology) of chronic wounds is essential to appropriate monitoring and treatment. For example, consider the difference between a pressure ulcer (caused by pressure) and a venous stasis ulcer (caused by inadequate venous return due to peripheral vascular disease [PVD]). For a pressure ulcer, *relief of pressure* is an essential part of wound care. For a venous stasis ulcer, an essential part of wound care is treating the *underlying venous disease* by elevating the affected limb and *applying compression,* something you would NOT do for a pressure ulcer.

Remember that all wounds aren't created equal. Local wound care without the correct supportive care, based on etiology or cause, won't work!—*Elizabeth A. Ayello, PhD, RN, CS, CWOCN*

(E-mail communication, April 2001.)

Incorrect: *Spiritual Distress related to atheism as evidenced by statements that she has never believed in God.*
Correct: There may be no diagnosis in this situation. The person may be at peace with her beliefs (not with yours).

- Don't state the nursing diagnosis using medical terminology. Focus on the person's *response* to the medical problems.

E X A M P L E

Incorrect: *Mastectomy related to cancer.*
Correct: *Risk for Self-Concept Disturbance related to effects of mastectomy.*

- Don't state two problems at the same time.

E X A M P L E

Incorrect: *Pain and Fear related to diagnostic procedures.*
Correct: *Fear related to unfamiliarity with diagnostic procedures. Pain related to diagnostic procedures.*

Display 3–10 gives a checklist to make sure you've followed the rules for making diagnostic statements.

DISPLAY 3-10   Checklist for Writing Diagnostic Statements

Is the statement

- ☐ Based on evidence from the nursing assessment?
- ☐ Descriptive of both the problem and its cause? Is the problem written before "related to" and the cause written after? For actual diagnoses, have you added "as evidenced by . . ."?
- ☐ Specific and clear?
- ☐ Reflective of a problem that nursing has been authorized to manage?
- ☐ Written with accepted terminology, using NANDA terms for nursing diagnoses unless there's no label on the list to describe the problem?
- ☐ Free of legally inadvisable and judgmental language?
- ☐ Written in such a way that there's a high probability that others with the same knowledge and experience agree with the diagnosis?

CRITICAL THINKING EXERCISE IX

Diagnostic Statements for Nursing Diagnoses | *To complete this session, read pages 109–115. Example responses can be found on page 245.*

Part I.

1. Practice identifying problems, related factors, and signs and symptoms (PRS): Study the nursing diagnoses below. Circle the problem, underline the cause (etiology, or related factors), and let the signs and symptoms stand as is.

    a. *Urge Incontinence* related to inability to hold large amounts of urine as evidenced by voiding immediately upon realization of need to void.

    b. *Anticipatory Grieving* related to impending death of mother as evidenced by statements of extreme sadness over impending death.

2. Why don't risk diagnoses have signs and symptoms? (One sentence.)

Part II.

The data presented in each clinical situation below matches one of the following diagnoses: *Powerlessness; Imbalanced Nutrition; Less than Body Requirement; Ineffective Airway Clearance*. Study each case, choose the matching diagnosis, and write a three-part diagnostic statement using the PRS (or PES) format.

1. Mr. Stuart demonstrated the following cues (signs and symptoms):

    Subjective (SD): Asks for help clearing secretions; states he can clear airway with help from suction.

    Objective (OD): Copious secretions from tracheostomy tube.

    Nursing Diagnosis:

2. Bob demonstrates the following cues (signs and symptoms):

    SD: Reports that he's had no appetite for 2 weeks because of depression.

    OD: Ten-pound weight loss since last visit; 15 lb under recommended weight.

    Nursing Diagnosis:

3. Lilly Johns demonstrates the following cues (signs and symptoms):

    SD: Reports she's depressed and has no control over daily activities.

    OD: She is quadriplegic and has a rigorous schedule of daily physical therapy.

Nursing Diagnosis:

Part III.

The data presented in each clinical situation below match one of the following diagnoses: *Risk for Ineffective Airway Clearance; Possible Ineffective Individual Coping; Risk for Fluid Volume Deficit; Possible Sexual Dysfunction.* Study each situation, choose the matching diagnosis, and write a two-part statement, stating the problem and its cause.

1. Mr. Reardon has been confined to bed with casts on both his legs. He seems angry and has stated that he does not want to talk to anyone. You're aware that he's had a fight with his girlfriend.
   Nursing Diagnosis:

2. Mrs. Cappelli has a temperature of 101°F. She sleeps a lot and has a poor appetite. She drinks about 2000 mL a day if you offer frequent fluids and encourage her to drink.
   Nursing Diagnosis:

3. Mr. Rogers has just had his gallbladder removed today under general anesthesia. His nursing assessment form shows that he has smoked a pack of cigarettes a day for the last 20 years. He has a productive cough.
   Nursing Diagnosis:

4. You see Mrs. Jackson in clinic 3 months after a hysterectomy. She states that she feels well physically but that emotionally she just doesn't feel like herself yet. She states that she gets angry easily, cries a lot, and that she's concerned the hysterectomy is affecting her emotionally and physically.
   Nursing Diagnosis:

Part IV.

Identifying correctly stated nursing diagnoses.

A. Put a "C" in front of each nursing diagnosis that is stated correctly.

1. _____ *Risk for Constipation related to confinement to bed.*
2. _____ *Risk for Injury related to lack of side rails on bed.*
3. _____ *Pain and Anxiety related to surgery.*
4. _____ *Hopelessness related to progressive disease process.*
5. _____ *Spiritual Distress related to atheism.*
6. _____ *Mastectomy related to cancer.*
7. _____ *Impaired Skin Integrity (1" blister on heel) related to heel pressure and rubbing on sheets.*
8. _____ *Imbalanced Hemodynamics related to hemorrhage.*
9. _____ *Impaired Physical Mobility related to joint pain as evidenced by reports of pain limiting movement of joints.*
10. _____ *Imbalanced Nutrition: Less than Body Requirements related to being NPO as evidenced by inability to take food by mouth.*

B. For each diagnosis you identified as being incorrect, explain the reason it's incorrect.

Predicting and Detecting Potential Complications

Being able to predict and detect potential complications (PC) is one of the keys to the proactive PPM model. Early intervention requires early recognition of signs and symptoms that may indicate the onset of potential complications. For example, if you're caring for someone with fractured ribs, you need to look up the common related complications; that is, pneumothorax and hemothorax. Knowing this will help you focus assessments to identify early signs and symptoms of pneumothorax and hemothorax, potential complications that can lead to death if not treated.

If you're a novice, you may find it difficult to predict and detect PCs. For example, you may examine someone who has chronic respiratory problems and has wheezing, coughing, and shortness of breath even when he's well. It may be difficult for you to know whether these abnormal findings are part of the person's usual pattern of chronic illness or whether the data indicate early signs and symptoms of potential complications.

Your ability to predict and detect PCs will grow as your nursing knowledge expands and you have repeated experiences assessing people with different types of problems. Some knowledge can be gained only by clinical experience. For example, you have to listen to many lungs to clearly know what abnormal breath sounds sound like. Until you acquire this experience, the following rules and guidelines can help you act in your patients' best interest, making sure that PCs are prevented, detected, and managed in a timely way.

R U L E ▶

> Until you feel confident identifying potential complications, report all abnormal data. What may seem like an isolated cue to you may prompt a more experienced person (or someone who knows the person better) to be concerned.

R U L E ▶

> **Use critical thinking:** Onset of complications often is subtle. Signs and symptoms gradually worsen over a period of time, making changes less obvious. Always compare abnormal data with data charted over the last 24 to 48 hours (sometimes longer). If you see increasingly abnormal signs and symptoms, you may be looking at early signs and symptoms of potential complications. **Example:** You get a temperature reading of 99.6°F. You compare the reading with temperatures over the last 24 to 48 hours. If it's a new elevation, you may be detecting early complications and know you have to monitor the person more closely.

Guidelines: Identifying Potential Complications

- Look up all medications taken. Consider the likelihood of the patient experiencing side effects, toxic effects, adverse reactions, or effects of drug interactions.
- Always consider the likelihood of allergic response (to new medications, dyes, or other environmental factors).
- Read patient records (medical history and physical report, nursing history and physical report, progress reports, consultations, diagnostic studies). Often, medical diagnoses and associated complications are addressed in these records.
- Look up the most common complications associated with the person's medical problems before you begin nursing care (for examples of common potential complications, see inside cover).
- Review critical paths, policies, procedures, protocols, and standards that address your patient's situations (eg, management of chest tubes). These often guide you to assess for specific signs and symptoms you must report to monitor for potential complications.
- Be aware of recent diagnostic or treatment modalities and determine whether there are commonly associated potential complications (eg, thrombi, emboli, and bleeding are potential complications of cardiac catheterization).
- Be sure you determine not only the potential complications, but also the signs and symptoms that indicate onset of the complications. For example, if you suspect pulmonary emboli, determine what signs and symptoms may indicate pulmonary emboli (pain, shortness of breath, anxiety).
- In complex situations, check with a more qualified professional. For example, you might say to an attending physician or a clinical nurse specialist, "There's a lot going on with this patient. Are there any specific signs and symptoms we should be concerned about?"
- If you want to write a diagnostic statement for potential complications, use "PC" (potential complication), followed by a colon, then name the potential complication (Carpenito, 2000). For example, write *PC: pneumothorax*.

Identifying Problems Requiring Multidisciplinary Approaches

The key question to ask when identifying a need for a multidisciplinary approach is:

Looking at the big picture of this person's situation, is it likely that he/she will be able to reach the desired outcomes in the expected time frame using only nursing expertise for management of care?

If the answer is "no," initiate appropriate referrals. For example, if the outcome for a healthy woman having a hysterectomy is *"will ambulate the first day after surgery,"* you could expect to achieve this outcome using nursing resources alone. However, if the woman has other coexisting problems, for example, difficulty walking due to neuromuscular problems, you might want to consider requesting a physical therapist's involvement with planning and managing ambulation.

CRITICAL THINKING EXERCISE X

Predicting Potential Complications/ Identifying Problems Requiring a Multidisciplinary Approach

To complete this session, read pages 117–119. Example responses can be found on page 245.

Practice identifying potential complications. Imagine you're looking after someone with each of the problems below. After the letters **PC** (potential complications), predict the potential complications that you'll need to consider. You may use inside cover as a guide.

Part I.

1. Intravenous Therapy

PC:

2. Concussion

PC:

3. Myocardial Infarction

PC:

4. Nasogastric Suction

PC:

Part II.

How would you decide if your patient's problems are such that they may require a multidisciplinary approach (one to three sentences)?

CRITICAL THINKING EXERCISE XI

Identifying Nursing Diagnoses, Potential Complications, and Strengths

To complete this critical thinking exercise, read pages 117–119. Example responses can be found on page 245.

Study the data given for the following case history. On a separate piece of paper, list the strengths, nursing diagnoses, and potential complications that you can identify.

Case History A (Mrs. Goode, 31 years old)

Medical Diagnosis: *cerebral concussion*

Subjective Data

States she has a headache and feels dizzy when she lifts her head off the pillow.

Expresses concern about having her husband look after her two children because "he is not good with them."

States she is afraid of hospitals and needles.

States she has never worked outside the home because her children need her.

States, "I can't stay in bed and use the bedpan as the doctor said."

Objective Data

Age: 31; Ht: 5′ 8″; Wt: 160 lb

Temperature: 98.4°F

Pulse: 78 and regular

Respirations: 24 and nonlabored

Blood Pressure: 128/72

Moves all extremities with equal strength

Pupils are equally reactive to light

Large bruise over right forehead

Abdomen soft, nontender, obese

Peripheral pulses strong

IV in right arm running at 30 mL/h

Summary

Page 80 gives a visual summary of the diagnostic process, based on the PPM model. Nurses' diagnostic responsibilities continue to change and are affected by use of critical pathways, computer-assisted diagnosis, multidisciplinary practice, society's changing needs, and nursing's expanding knowledge base.

Diagnostic reasoning, or applying critical thinking to identifying problems and strengths, requires knowledge, skills, and experience. As your knowledge and clinical expertise grow, your accountability for diagnosis and treatment will also grow. To determine your diagnostic responsibilities, you need a clear understanding of all the terms listed in the critical thinking exercise on pages 97. At the big-picture level, diagnostic reasoning involves analyzing cue clusters, creating a list of suspected problems, ruling out similar diagnoses, choosing the most specific diagnostic labels, stating the diagnoses and their causes, and identifying strengths, resources, and areas for improvement.

To guide you through the diagnostic process, there are specific rules for formally writing diagnostic statements (see pages 111–115). In the clinical setting, diagnostic statements often are written in abbreviated forms. Students, however, usually are required to follow the formal rules to demonstrate their thinking to their instructors.

A key question to ask when identifying a need for a multidisciplinary approach is: *Looking at the big picture of this person's situation, is it likely that he/she will be able to reach the desired outcomes in the expected time frame using only nursing expertise for management of care?* If the answer is "no," then initiate appropriate referrals.

Evaluate your knowledge of this chapter. Check to see if you can achieve the learning outcomes on page 78.
Bibliography: See pages 199–201.

4

Planning

LEARNING OUTCOMES

After mastering the content in this chapter, you should be able to:

- Explain why every plan of care requires four components (problem list, expected outcomes, interventions, progress notes).
- Decide how you'll set priorities the next time you're in the clinical setting.
- Name five things that influence priority ratings.
- Give four reasons why specific, measurable outcomes are the key to efficient planning.
- Address the relationship of outcomes to accountability.
- Explain the importance of considering clinical, functional, and quality of life outcomes.
- Discuss how to use standards plans (eg, critical paths, guidelines, computerized plans).
- Explain the role of case management in planning efficient care.
- Discuss how to weigh risks and benefits when determining nursing interventions.
- Develop a comprehensive plan of care.
- Explain how to decide if the plan of care is adequately documented.

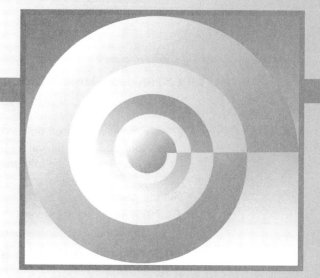

Standard III: *Outcome Identification.* The nurse identifies outcomes individualized to the client.*

Standard IV: *Planning.* The nurse develops a plan of care that prescribes interventions to attain expected outcomes.*

Critical Thinking Exercises

■ **Critical Thinking Exercise XII:** Setting Priorities and Applying Standards

■ **Critical Thinking Exercise XIII:** Planning Outcome-Focused Care

■ **Critical Thinking Exercise XIV:** Determining Interventions and Recording Nursing Orders

What's in this chapter?

Emphasizing the importance of outcome-focused care and partnering with patients to plan care, this chapter provides the how to's of establishing an initial plan of care. It guides you through the process of setting priorities and identifying realistic outcomes and interventions. It also addresses your responsibilities related to making sure the plan is adequately recorded, even when using standard plans such as critical pathways and computerized care plans.

*Excerpted from ANA Standards of Clinical Nursing Practice (ANA, 1998).

Planning: Setting Priorities, Determining Outcomes, Recording the Plan

This chapter focuses on how to develop an *initial* comprehensive plan of care. The next one addresses the daily planning required as you give nursing care.

Planning involves the following:

- Setting priorities
- Establishing expected outcomes
- Determining nursing interventions
- Ensuring the plan is adequately recorded

Let's first take a look at why care planning rules are so specific and then address how to make sure your patients' plans are specific, individualized, and able to meet today's practice standards.

Why Are Rules for Recording the Plan So Specific?

The plan of care serves four main purposes—to:

1. Promote communication between caregivers.
2. Direct care and documentation.
3. Create a record that can later be used for evaluation, research, and legal reasons.
4. Provide documentation of health care needs for insurance reimbursement purposes.

To ensure that *all key players* (eg, primary care providers, nurses, insurance providers, researchers) in health care delivery have easy access to key information they need, laws and standards mandate that patients' plans be specific, clear, and consistent.

Major Components of the Plan of Care

There are four major components to the plan of care:

1. **Expected (desired) outcomes:** What results do you expect, and by when do you expect you see these results?
2. **Actual and potential problems:** What are the actual and potential diagnoses and problems that *must* be addressed to ensure safe and efficient care?
3. **Specific interventions:** What's going to be done to prevent or manage the major problems and achieve the expected outcomes?
4. **Evaluation/progress notes:** Where can you find out how the person is responding to the plan of care?

The word **EASE** can help you remember the four main components:

E = Expected outcomes
A = Actual and potential problems
S = Specific interventions
E = Evaluation/progress notes

The following sections will help you ensure that all four components are clearly addressed on the plan of care. Let's begin by examining how to set priorities and decide which problems must be addressed in the plan of care.

Setting Priorities

Some nurses will tell you setting priorities begins with deciding what problems to deal with first. Others will tell you it begins with identifying outcomes. In a way, they're both right: First, determine urgent problems (eg, those requiring immediate medical attention). Next, determine discharge outcomes so you know what must be done first in the big picture of the whole plan.

For example, compare the two following discharge outcomes.

• Three days after surgery, will be discharged home, able to demonstrate wound care.
• Three days after surgery, will be discharged to a skilled nursing facility for wound care and medical management.

If you didn't know that the first person just listed will go home and the second will go to a skilled nursing facility, how will you know whether teaching about wound care is a high priority?

Critical Thinking and Setting Priorities

Setting priorities is an essential critical thinking skill that requires you to be able to decide:

1. Which problems need immediate attention and which ones can wait.
2. Which problems are your responsibility and which do you need to refer to someone else.*
3. Which problems will be dealt with by using standard plans (eg, critical paths, standards of care).
4. Which problems *aren't* covered by protocols or standard plans but must be addressed to ensure a safe hospital stay and timely discharge.

---

*(Deciding what to delegate to others is addressed in the next chapter, where we discuss planning on a daily basis.)

To be able to set priorities, you need to be very familiar with the following fundamental principles of setting priorities.

Setting Priorities: Basic Principles

- Choose a method of assigning priorities and use it consistently. For example, use:

    Maslow's Hierarchy of Needs:

    Priority 1. Physiologic Needs—life-threatening problems (or risk factors) posing a threat to physiologic needs (eg, problems with breathing, circulation, nutrition, hydration, elimination, temperature regulation, physical comfort).

    Priority 2. Safety and Security—problems (or risk factors) posing a threat to safety and security (eg, environmental hazards, fear).

    Priority 3. Love and Belonging—problems (or risk factors) posing a threat to feeling loved and a part of something (eg, isolation or loss of a loved one).

    Priority 4. Self-esteem—problems (or risk factors) posing a threat to self-esteem (eg, inability to perform normal activities).

    Priority 5: Personal Goals—problems (or risk factors) posing a threat to the ability to achieve personal goals.

- Assign a high priority to problems that contribute to other problems. For example, if someone has joint pain and isn't moving well, give pain management a high priority because it's likely to contribute to problems with moving.
- Your ability to successfully set priorities is influenced by your understanding of:
    - The patient's perception of priorities. If the patient doesn't agree with your priorities, it's unlikely the plan will succeed.
    - The *whole picture* of problems at hand. For example, if you have someone who is having trouble breathing, normally you correct this problem first. If, however, you look at the *whole picture* and note that the person is having trouble breathing because of an anxiety attack, you might decide that resolving the anxiety is the most important problem *right now*.
    - The person's overall health status and expected discharge outcomes. As stated earlier, teaching may have a high priority for someone who's expected to be discharged home, but it may take a lower priority for someone who's expected to be discharged to an extended-care facility (eg, a nursing home).
    - The expected length of stay. Focus on what *must* be done before what's *nice* to do, especially in short stays.
    - Whether there are standard plans that apply. For example, are there critical pathways, guidelines, protocols, procedures, or standard plans that address daily priorities for this particular patient's situation? For definitions of these terms, see Display 4–1.

Suggested Steps for Setting Priorities

Step 1. Ask, "What problems need immediate attention and what could happen if I wait until later to attend to them?" Take immediate appropriate action to initiate treatment as indicated (eg, notify the charge nurse and initiate actions to re-

DISPLAY 4-1   Definitions of Terms Related to Standards

Critical Pathways or CareMaps™: Standard plans developed to help set daily care priorities, promote timely achievement of outcomes, and reduce length of hospital stays (eg, see page 000).

Guidelines, Protocols, Policies, and Procedures: Documents that delineate how care is to be provided in specific situations.

Standards: Authoritative statements by which the nursing profession describes the responsibilities for which its practitioners are accountable (ANA, 1991). See also guidelines given earlier.

Standard of Care: A document outlining the minimal level of routine care provided for all patients in certain situations (focuses on what will be observed *in the patient* to let you know the care has been given).

Standard Care Plan: A preformulated plan that can be used as a guide to expedite development and documentation of a plan of care.

Standard of Practice: A document outlining what the *nurse will do* in giving care in specific situations. See also guidelines given earlier.

Standard of Professional Performance: Authoritative statements that describe a competent level of behavior in the professional role (see page 000).

duce the problem). **Rationale:** Identifying what could happen if you wait until later to resolve a problem helps determine what must be done now. If the patient needs expert help, notifying the appropriate people immediately as you continue to act independently ensures competent care.

Step 2. Identify problems with simple solutions and initiate actions to solve them (eg, correcting someone's position to repositioning to improve breathing). **Rationale:** Sometimes, simple things have a big impact on the person's physiologic or psychological status.

Step 3. Develop an initial problem list, identifying actual and potential problems, and their causes, if known. **Rationale:** Problem lists can show you (and everyone else) the big picture of problems, helping you decide whether something is being missed or whether one problem might be contributing to another.

RULE ▶
To communicate all major problems to the entire health care team, make sure that an up-to-date problem list with a summary of major past and current problems is in a prominent place on the patient record. See Figure 4–1 for an example.

Step 4. Study your problem list and decide what problems will be primarily managed by nursing, what problems are addressed by standard plans, and what problems require multidisciplinary planning. Check whether you have medical orders or facility guidelines to manage medical problems; notify the physician

PROBLEMS

Problem	Status	Comments
Arthritis	Since 1995	Current Meds – see list
Asthma	Since 1985	See current inhalers
Back Pain / Laminectomy	1994 –1996	Resolved ~~lamine~~ 1996
Diabetes	New 4/8/02	See diabetic teaching
Hypertension	Since 1992	Current Meds – see list
Impaired Coping R/T	current since May	Counseling ē APN current

F i g u r e **4–1.** Example ongoing multidisciplinary problem list.

or APN if you don't. **Rationale:** It's your responsibility to refer problems outside your expertise in a timely manner.

Step 5. Decide which problems *must* be addressed by the plan of care; that is, those unique patient *problems that must be controlled or resolved in order to progress to achieving the major outcomes of care*). **Rationale:** Patient records must communicate nurses' awareness of, and responsiveness to, all care priorities. Some problems may not need to be recorded on the care plan because they're addressed in other parts of the record (eg, Foley catheter care usually is addressed in policy and procedure manuals).

Step 6. Determine how each problem will be managed (eg, Medical orders? Following protocols? Nurse-developed individualized plan?). **Rationale:** Policies vary from one facility to another; you must identify where to record a problem and how to manage it according to each particular facility's policies. Figure 4–2 presents a worksheet for a problem list showing how a nurse has decided to address care management. Keep in mind that deciding what tasks will be delegated to whom is addressed in the next chapter in pages 167–168.

Think About It

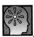

Asking Negative Questions Helps Set Priorities. *When making decisions about setting priorities, ask yourself negative questions. Negative questions begin with,* "What could happen if I **don't** . . . " *For example,* "What could happen to this person if I **don't** address this problem on the plan of care?" *or* "What could happen if I **don't** report this problem?" *Asking yourself these types of questions helps you focus on what's most important. If the answer is* "not much can happen," *you know the problem has a low priority. If the answer causes you concern, then you know the problem has a high priority.*

Applying Nursing Standards

There are guidelines and standards that you must apply when developing plans. These standards are determined by:

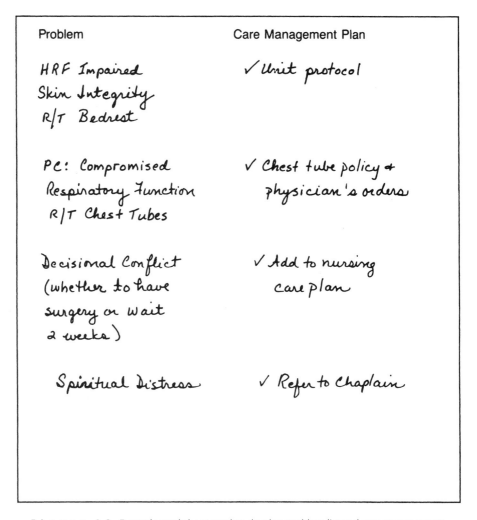

Problem	Care Management Plan
HRF Impaired Skin Integrity R/T Bedrest	✓ Unit protocol
PC: Compromised Respiratory Function R/T Chest Tubes	✓ Chest tube policy + physician's orders
Decisional Conflict (whether to have surgery or wait 2 weeks)	✓ Add to nursing care plan
Spiritual Distress	✓ Refer to chaplain

F i g u r e **4–2.** Example worksheet used to develop problem list and care management.

- **The law:** Your state's nurse practice act outlines the scope of nursing practice.
- **The American Nurses Association (ANA) and Canadian Nurses Association.**
- **Specialty Professional Organizations,** such as the Emergency Nurses Association and the Critical Care Nurses Association, develop standards for specialty practice.
- **The Joint Commission of Accreditation of Healthcare Organizations:** This powerful accrediting body has developed detailed standards that must be followed to keep accreditation.
- **The Agency for Healthcare Research and Quality:** This organization develops, reviews, and updates clinical guidelines to aid health care providers prevent, diagnose, and manage certain common clinical conditions (Display 4–2).
- **Your employer:** Each organization usually develops its own unique set of standards (standards of care, guidelines, policies, procedures, critical pathways, standard

DISPLAY 4-2   Partial List of Practice Guidelines Available From the Agency for Healthcare Research and Quality*

- ✓ Acute and chronic incontinence
- ✓ Acute low back problems
- ✓ Acute pain
- ✓ Benign prostatic hypertrophy
- ✓ Cancer screening
- ✓ Cardiac rehabilitation
- ✓ Cataracts in adults
- ✓ Colorectal cancer
- ✓ Heart failure
- ✓ Managing cancer pain

- ✓ Depression in primary care
- ✓ Otitis media with effusion
- ✓ Post-stroke rehabilitation
- ✓ Pressure ulcer treatment
- ✓ Quality determinants of mammography
- ✓ Unstable angina
- ✓ Screening for Alzheimer's disease
- ✓ Sickle cell disease
- ✓ Smoking cessation

* For comprehensive list, visit *http://www.ahcpr.gov*.

care plans, and so forth) that reflect how nursing care should be delivered in a specific situation.

Remember the following rule.

R U L E ▶ Standard plans are guides that generally, but not completely, apply to individual patient situations. You're responsible for discriminating about what does and doesn't apply and individualizing patient care accordingly.

C R I T I C A L   T H I N K I N G   E X E R C I S E   X I I

Setting Priorities and Applying Standards

To complete this session, read pages 123–130. Example responses can be found on page 246.

1. What are the four main purposes of the plan of care?

2. Name the four components of a plan of care and give an example of each.

3. List five factors that may influence how you set priorities.

4. If you had someone with the following problems, which problem would you need to treat immediately and why?

   a. Diarrhea

   b. Severe dyspnea

   c. Risk for Fluid Volume Deficit

5. Give at least three types of standards that apply to your nursing practice.

6. What is the relationship between setting priorities and identifying expected outcomes for discharge?

Planning Outcome-Focused Care

Effective health care delivery requires us to focus on client *results*, which are stated as *client-centered outcomes:* What exactly do we expect to observe *in the client* to demonstrate the expected benefits of nursing care—and by when do we expect to see these results?

    Outcomes serve three main purposes:

1. They're the measuring sticks of the plan of care. You measure the success of the plan by determining whether the expected outcomes were met.

2. They direct interventions. You need to know *what* you're trying to accomplish before you can decide *how* to accomplish it.

VOICES

Partner With Your Patients to Achieve Outcomes. Although the Nursing-Sensitive Outcomes Classification (NOC) outcomes listed on pages 259–261 provide nursing terms that help us study the impact of nursing care, remember the importance of using simple terms and partnering with patients to set outcomes and priorities. For example, if a patient expresses a desire to be more comfortable, explain that you recommend achieving better pain control by having him report when his pain level is 3 on a scale of 0-10, rather than waiting until it reaches a level of 8. Then plan the day's events with him to make that happen. If a patient expresses that he wants to be able to eat solid foods, focus on how and when it's expected that he'll to be able to eat solid foods, and what he can have in the interim.—*Ruth Hansten, RN, MBA, PhD(c)*

(E-mail communication, February 5, 2001.)

3. **They're motivating factors.** Having a specific time frame for getting things done gets everyone in motion.

Principles of Patient-Centered (Client-Centered) Outcomes

Rather than focusing on what we nurses aim to do, patient-centered (client-centered) outcomes focus on the desired *results* of treatment—that the client benefits from nursing care. Remember the following rule.

R U L E ▶

> **Outcomes and Indicators:** *Outcomes* describe what you expect to observe *in the patient or client* that will demonstrate that the patient has benefited from nursing care. Although the terms *outcomes* and *indicators* sometimes are used interchangeably, *indicators* usually are specific, measurable data that will indicate that an outcome has been achieved (see examples at the bottom of this page).

Because knowing how to develop outcomes and describe corresponding indicators is a key skill required to work in today's outcome-driven health care setting, be sure you understand the following additional principles and rules.

1. Outcomes state the benefits you expect to see *in the client* after nursing care has been given. The term *client* usually refers to the patient. In some cases, for example, with a child or elderly person, *client* may refer to a parent or caregiver.
   * Short-term outcomes describe early expected benefits of nursing interventions (eg, will be able to walk to the bathroom unassisted by tomorrow).
   * Long-term outcomes describe the benefits expected to be seen at a certain point in time after the plan has been implemented (will be able to walk independently to the end of the hall three times a day within 10 days after surgery).

Example Outcomes and Corresponding Indicators

Example Outcomes	Corresponding Indicators
Will demonstrate knowledge of medication regimen by discharge.	• Lists drug names, actions, doses, administration route, and side effects. • Explains when drugs are to be taken, including whether to take them on an empty or full stomach, and what to do if dose is missed. • Demonstrates special administration techniques (eg, injection, if applicable). • Lists reportable signs and symptoms.
Will maintain intact skin.	• Skin shows no signs of discoloration or irritation. • Risk factors managed (patient has adequate nutrition and hydration, repositioned hourly, skin care performed as specified by protocol).

2. The subject of outcome statements should be the client or a part of the client (the term *client* often is understood; eg, "demonstrates knowledge of sterile technique by 12/5). **Rationale:** You look for results *in the client*.

3. Outcomes usually are developed for *problems*. Although you usually don't develop outcomes for *interventions*, you should be able to state the benefit you expect to see in the patient after an intervention is performed. For example, if you suction someone's tracheostomy, you would expect that the lungs would be clearer after suctioning. **Rationale:** If you can't clearly identify the benefits you expect to see in the patient after nursing care, then you shouldn't be intervening.

4. At a simple level, determining outcomes requires you to simply reverse the problem. For instance, if the person has such and such a problem, your desired outcome is that the person will *not* have that problem (or at least it will be minimized; see following examples). **Rationale:** Outcomes describe what "it looks like" when the problems are corrected or controlled.

E X A M P L E

Problem or Intervention	Corresponding Expected Outcome (Expected Result)
Problem: *Impaired Skin Integrity*	Skin intact, free from signs of irritation; risk factors managed
Intervention: Irrigate N/G tube	N/G tube remains patent.

5. To develop a very specific outcome, state the broad outcome, then add the data (indicators) that will demonstrate that the outcome is achieved (see earlier). **Rationale:** Making outcomes and indicators clear helps everyone to monitor patient progress.

6. Sometimes indicators already will be developed for your patient's problems in standard plans. Carefully critique whether the indicators are appropriate to your patient's particular situation. **Rationale:** Standard plans are guides that generally, but not completely, apply to individual patient situations. Display 4–3 provides ANA standards related to identifying outcomes.

DISPLAY 4–3   Standards for Outcomes (ANA, 1998)

Outcomes are:

- Derived from the diagnoses
- Documented using measurable terms
- Mutually formulated with the client and health care providers, when possible
- Realistic in relation to client's present and potential capabilities
- Attainable in relation to resources available to the client
- Written in such a way that they include a time estimate for attainment and provide direction for continuity of care.

Think About It

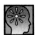

Shifting From Goals and Objectives (Intent) to Outcomes and Indicators (Results).
The terms goals *and* objectives *and* outcomes *and* indicators *often are used inter-changeably. However, goals and objectives often refer to* intent *(eg, "our goal is to teach this person about diabetes"), whereas outcomes and indicators refer to* results *(eg, "How will we know if this person actually learned what he needs to know?"). Make the shift to client-centered outcomes (results) and corresponding indicators to be sure you stay focused on the impact of care on the patient.*

7. **Make sure outcomes and indicators are measurable.** Consider the following five components to create very specific outcomes that can be used to identify interventions and monitor progress.

   Subject: Who is the person expected to achieve the outcome (eg, patient or parent)?
   Verb: What actions must the person take to achieve the outcome?
   Condition: Under what circumstances is the person to perform the actions?
   Performance Criteria: How well is the person to perform the actions?
   Target Time: By when is the person expected to be able to perform the actions?

E X A M P L E

Parents will bathe newborn in room independently by 5/8.

8. **Use measurable verbs** (verbs that describe exactly what you expect to see or hear when the outcome has been achieved). For instance, suppose you want someone to understand how to use sterile technique and you write an outcome that says, "Understands how to use sterile technique." Experts would tell you that "understand" is vague and not measurable. Ask yourself, "How can we really know if she understands?" The only way you can really know how well she understands is if she actually verbalizes or demonstrates sterile technique. Below are some examples of measurable verbs.

   Measurable Verbs (Use these to be specific)

identify	hold	exercise
describe	demonstrate	communicate
perform	share	cough
relate	express	walk
state	will lose	stand
list	will gain	sit
verbalize	has an absence of	discuss

Nonmeasurable Verbs (Do not use)

know	think
understand	accept
appreciate	feel

9. Consider affective, cognitive, and psychomotor outcomes, as described in the following bulleted list (examples are given in Table 4–1):
   * **Affective Domain:** Outcomes associated with changes in attitudes, feelings, or values (eg, deciding old eating habits need to be changed).
   * **Cognitive Domain:** Outcomes dealing with acquired knowledge or intellectual skills (eg, learning the signs and symptoms of diabetic shock).
   * **Psychomotor Domain:** Outcomes dealing with developing motor skills (eg, mastering how to walk with crutches).

10. Remember the following guidelines.

Guidelines: Determining Patient-Centered (Client-Centered) Outcomes

* Be realistic and consider:
  ○ Physical health state, overall prognosis
  ○ Expected length of stay
  ○ Growth and development
  ○ Available human and material resources
  ○ Other planned therapies for the client
* Partner with the patient, determining outcomes together with her and others involved in her health care (eg, significant others, other caregivers). If the outcomes are predetermined by standard plans, inform those involved what the outcomes are and seek agreement that the outcomes are attainable.
* In complex cases, develop both short- and long-term outcomes. Use short-term outcomes as stepping-stones to the long-term outcomes.
* Be sure the outcomes and indicators are measurable, that they describe something you can hear, see, or feel *in the person* that will demonstrate that the outcomes are achieved. Use measurable, observable verbs (see page 134).

TABLE 4 – 1 Examples of Verbs Representing the Three Domains

Cognitive	Affective	Psychomotor
Teach	Express	Demonstrate
Discuss	Share	Practice
Identify	Listen	Perform
Describe	Communicate	Walk
List	Relate	Administer
Explore		Give

- Consider the five components listed on page 134 when developing outcomes.
- Identify only one behavior per indicator. If you need to write two behaviors, write two indicators.

EXAMPLE

> **Wrong:** By 12/15, explains the role of insulin in carbohydrate metabolism and gives himself insulin.
> **Right:** By 12/15, explains the role of insulin in carbohydrate metabolism.
> By 12/15, administers own insulin.

Relationship of Outcomes to Accountability

Identifying outcomes helps you determine accountability. Look at the outcome and ask, "Who's accountable for developing a comprehensive plan to achieve this outcome?" If nursing is accountable for being the primary manager of the problem, then you're accountable for *initiating the plan*. If not, then you're accountable for *getting appropriate help*. The following diagram summarizes the decision-making process after you identify expected outcomes.

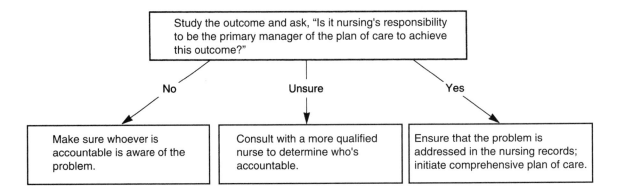

Clinical, Functional, and Quality of Life Outcomes

To ensure that we plan and evaluate care holistically, outcomes may focus on clinical, functional, or quality of life status, as explained here:

Clinical outcomes describe the expected status of medical, nursing, or multidisciplinary problems at certain points in time, after treatment has be given. They address whether the problems are resolved or to what degree they are improved. The following show some examples of clinical outcomes:

- Chest tube out third postoperative day
- Lungs clear, absence of signs of infection 2 days after admission
- Able to demonstrate wound care 3 days after surgery

Functional outcomes describe the person's ability to function in relation to desired usual activities. The following are two functional outcomes at different points in time for someone who has had a total knee replacement.

- Four days after total knee replacement, Mr. Palmer will be discharged to a rehabilitation facility able to perform straight leg raises and range-of-motion exercises twice daily.
- Six months after total knee replacement, Mr. Palmer will return to his job as a police officer, able to perform usual job description (able to walk two to three flights of stairs, participate in a chase on foot, and so forth).

Quality of life outcomes focus on key factors that affect someone's ability to be physically and spiritually comfortable. Some examples are:

- Relates successful pain management
- Absence of depression
- Usual sleep patterns
- Able to perform work and leisure activities

Discharge Outcomes and Discharge Planning

Identifying discharge outcomes and starting discharge planning early are the hallmarks of efficiency. With today's decreased length of hospital stays, you must be thinking about what will be needed when the person goes home as part of the *initial assessment*. Too often, getting equipment and services needed for care on discharge takes just as long as it takes the client to heal. Display 4–4 shows an example discharge planning questionnaire that can help you to identify discharge planning early. Discharge outcomes often are written in broad terms, describing the level of assistance the person is likely to need on discharge (eg, "will be discharged home with care managed by wife and biweekly visits by home care nurse"). These statements maybe followed with the indicators that demonstrate the expected status of various patient problems upon discharge (eg, *abdominal drains out, demonstrates wound care,* and so forth).

The following summarizes how to develop specific outcomes.

State the problem ➡ *Reverse (or control) the problem* ➡ List the indicators that will tell you the outcome is achieved

Case Management

Aiming to reduce length of—and incidence of—hospital stays through early outcome identification and optimum use of resources, case management is an essential piece of *Planning*. Today, nurses in both hospitals and communities are expected to recognize early when clients demonstrate problems that might require additional resources to achieve outcomes in a timely way. For example, suppose you assess someone who is to

DISPLAY 4-4   Discharge Planning Questionnaire

1. Is there a problem at home with any of the following?

☐ Heat	Yes	No	Possibly
☐ Hot/cold water	Yes	No	Possibly
☐ Electricity	Yes	No	Possibly
☐ Refrigeration	Yes	No	Possibly
☐ Cooking	Yes	No	Possibly
☐ Bathroom facilities	Yes	No	Possibly
☐ Stairs	Yes	No	Possibly
☐ Wheelchair accessibility	Yes	No	Possibly

2. Is necessary transportation available?   Yes   No   Possibly

3. How can the patient be reached by phone?

4. Will the person require:

☐ Assistance with activities of daily living	Yes	No	Possibly
☐ Assistance with medications	Yes	No	Possibly
☐ Assistance with treatments	Yes	No	Possibly
☐ Additional teaching	Yes	No	Possibly
☐ Ongoing nursing assessment	Yes	No	Possibly
☐ Community resources or referrals	Yes	No	Possibly

5. List available support systems (eg, family, neighbors willing to help).

have a routine cholecystectomy but also is paraplegic. This person is likely to have additional needs that an able-bodied person would not have. Consider whether you need to notify a case manager *early* to ensure comprehensive planning. Remember the following rule:

R U L E ▶ Early in the planning phase, ask yourself, "Does this person have unusual health problems or disabilities that require close monitoring by a case manager?"

  Think About It

Preadmission Discharge Planning: Good Idea. *Discharge planning is best when it begins before admission and is kept simple. For example, going over a pathway for home care (Fig. 4–3) can teach people what to expect when they leave the hospital before they're in the midst of a stressful recovery.*

'AT HOME' PATH TO RECOVERY FROM CARDIAC SURGERY: THINGS TO DO EACH DAY

Activity	*Health*	*Medications*	*Self-Care*	*Reasons to Call for More Information*
❑ Walk four times/day	Do each of the following items around the same time each day: ❑ Check your incisions ❑ Take your temperature by mouth (call if over 100°F)	❑ Take your medications as prescribed	❑ Keep your feet up while at rest ❑ Shower/bathe as instructed	The nursing station phone number is (910) 716-6658. *Call your doctor if:* ❑ your heart rate (pulse) is less than 60 beats/minute or greater than 120 at rest, or
❑ Do exercises as prescribed ❑ Rest ❑ Limit visitors the first week or so (three to four people for 30 minutes/day) ❑ Resume sexual activities when ready ❑ After two weeks, help with light housework	❑ Check your pulse for one minute (normal: 60 to 120 beats/minute) ❑ Weigh yourself (call if you gain over 2 lb. in one day)	❑ Drink several glasses of water each day	❑ Practice reading food labels for fat intake, cholesterol, and sodium levels ❑ Eat healthy! Try new recipes ❑ Wear stockings if ordered	❑ you have severe chills, or ❑ unusual shortness of breath, or ❑ fever greater than 100°F (by mouth), or ❑ weight gain over 2 lb. in one day or 5 lb. in one week, or ❑ red or draining incisions, or ❑ chest pain, or ❑ if you have *any* questions or concerns

Source: Adapted from path developed by The North Carolina Baptist Hospitals, Winston–Salem, NC.

F i g u r e **4–3.** Keeping pathways simple prevents people from being overwhelmed and promotes compliance (Wells, 1996).

C R I T I C A L   T H I N K I N G   E X E R C I S E   X I I I

Planning Outcome-Focused Care | *To complete this session, read pages 131–139. Example responses can be found on page 246.*

Part I.

1. What are the three main purposes of outcomes?

2. What four words are sometimes used interchangeably and usually mean the *desired result* of interventions?

3. Of the four terms you just listed, which two usually are considered to be *most specific?*

4. a. If you identify an outcome and decide it's not within nursing's responsibility to manage the problems to achieve the outcomes, what must you do?

   b. What must you do if it *is* within nursing's responsibility?

5. What are your responsibilities during planning in relation to case management? (Three sentences or less.)

Part II.

1. Why is it important to use measurable verbs when identifying outcomes? Give three examples of measurable verbs.

2. What are the five components of outcome statements?

3. Choose which of the following outcomes are written correctly. Identify what's wrong with the statements that are written incorrectly.
   a. Knows the four basic food groups by 1/4.

   b. Demonstrates how to use the walker unassisted by Saturday.

   c. Improves appetite by 11/5.

d. Lists the equipment needed to change sterile dressings by 9/5.

e. Walks independently in the hall the day after surgery.

f. Understands the importance of maintaining a salt-free diet.

g. Ambulates to the bathroom using her cane by 3/4.

h. Loses 5 lb by 1/9.

i. Feels less pain by Thursday.

4. For each of the following diagnosis or problem, write an appropriate outcome.
   a. *Impaired Oral Mucous Membrane related to poor oral hygiene.*

   b. *Risk for Impaired Skin Integrity related to constant diarrhea.*

   c. *Impaired Verbal Communication related to inability to speak English.*

Part III.

Identify whether each of the following outcomes is affective, cognitive, or psychomotor domain. Use "a" for affective, "c" for cognitive, and "p" for psychomotor. (Remember, there may be more than one domain for each outcome.)
   a. Demonstrates how to sterilize her baby's formula.
   b. Relates feelings concerning going home.

    c. Discusses the relationship between blood sugar levels and eating.

    d. Administers own insulin according to the results of morning blood sugar readings.

Part IV.

Once you've identified the domains of the outcomes in the examples just given, write one or two activities that would help the client to achieve the outcome. (Note the following example.)

E X A M P L E

> **Outcome:** Able to dress herself without assistance by 7/4.
> **Domain:** Psychomotor
> **Activities:** Practice buttoning buttons and tying shoes on 7/1 and 7/2.
>   Practice putting on blouse, skirt, shoes, and socks on 7/3.
>   Demonstrate dressing herself on 7/4.

Nursing Interventions

Nursing interventions are actions performed by the nurse to:

1. Monitor health status
2. Reduce risks
3. Resolve, prevent, or manage a problem.
4. Facilitate independence or assist with activities of daily living (bathing and so forth).
5. Promote optimum sense of physical, psychological, and spiritual well-being.

    Nursing interventions can be classified into two categories (McCloskey & Bulechek, 2000; ANA, 1995):

- **Direct Care Interventions:** Actions performed through direct interaction with clients. Examples include helping someone out of bed and teaching someone about diabetes.
- **Indirect Care Interventions:** Actions performed away from the client but on behalf of a client or group of clients. These actions are aimed at managing the health care environment and promoting interdisciplinary collaboration. Some examples include monitoring results of laboratory studies, transferring a client from one room to another, and contacting a social worker.

    Considering both direct and indirect interventions helps account for nurses' time. If you focus only on what the nurse does directly with the client, you miss a lot of nursing time that's spent on other crucial nursing activities.

Assessment—Monitoring Health Status

Assessment may be planned specifically to detect or evaluate certain problems or to monitor responses to interventions. In fact, *Assessment* is a part of every intervention. Your plan should reflect awareness of the need to assess *before acting* to be sure the action is safe and appropriate, to assess *while acting* to monitor for adverse reactions, and to assess *after acting* to monitor the response. For example, if you get a man out of bed, you assess him before he gets out to be sure that he's still well enough to complete the activity, you monitor him for adverse reactions (eg, dizziness) as he's getting out of bed and is out of bed, and then you determine his *response* after he gets back into bed.

Think About It

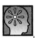

Recipe for Disaster: Skipping Assessments and Poor Planning. *Many nurses will tell you that they spend more time assessing people, simply confirming that no problems exist, than they do actually treating problems. This is as it should be. When you carefully monitor health status, you can detect risks and early signs and symptoms of potential problems. You can intervene before the problem is out of control. Monitoring health status is time-consuming, but it takes only one disaster caused by that one time someone rushed through, or skipped, an assessment to make you realize it's worth every minute. For example, in one case, a 4-year-old child recovering from hip surgery had to have additional emergency surgery to relieve compartment syndrome (pressure on blood vessels, nerves, and muscles caused by severe swelling). The nurses and hospital were found negligent because evidence presented at the trial showed that the nurses hadn't monitored the child's condition appropriately. The fact that the nurses hadn't identified their own learning needs contributed to their negligence. They were held accountable for not knowing the equipment required to test for compartment syndrome and for not knowing where the equipment was located* (Pirkov-Middaugh v. Gillette Children's Hospital *[1991]*).

Teaching—The Key to Empowerment

Teaching patients about their health and treatment plan, and motivating them to become involved in managing their care, is the key to empowering them to become their own best advocate and caregiver. Teaching may be planned specifically to enhance someone's knowledge about a specific problem (eg, teaching about diabetes) or as part of an intervention to explain why it's being done (eg, reinforcing the rationale for coughing and deep breathing as you're assisting the person to cough and breathe deeply). At every patient encounter, seize teaching opportunities. In complex situations, carefully plan what you're going to teach, and how you're going to teach it. Because teaching is a complex skill that includes paying attention to many different factors, the following guidelines are suggested to help you plan teaching.

Guidelines: Planning Teaching

• Assess readiness to learn and previous knowledge before developing a teaching plan.

VOICES

Screening and Teaching Essential to Promoting Health.
". . . Screening is a preventive strategy that can detect the likelihood of disease in its earliest stage and increase the chance of successful treatment . . . Provide consumers with clear and thorough information. Use visual materials. Encourage attendance at community-based screening activities. Be aware of screening activities scheduled in the community and workplace. . . . Refer patients for diagnostic and treatment follow-up. . . ."
—*Sandra B. Fielo, RNC, EdD, Community Health Nursing Educator*

(Fielo, S. [2000]. *Screening: How to change world health.* [On-line.] Available: *http://nsweb.nursingspectrum. com/ce/ce211.htm.* Accessed January 9, 2000.)

- Ask about preferred learning styles (for example, a person who is a "reader" might want to read a pamphlet first, whereas someone who is a "doer" might want to handle equipment first). Adapt to the patient's preferred style rather than your own.
- Plan for an environment that's conducive to learning, without interventions.
- Identify active learning experiences. Use examples, simulations, games, and audiovisuals.
- Use simple terms; it's easy to overwhelm the average person.
- Determine learning outcomes mutually with the client so that you both know what must be learned and mastered (eg, "How would you feel about learning how to give an injection by Thursday?").
- Encourage asking questions and verbalizing understanding of what is being taught (eg, "I want you to feel free to ask questions no matter how insignificant you think they are. It's not easy learning something new. It is very important that you understand this.").
- Plan to pace learning. Don't give too much information at one time; progress at the person's learning pace.
- Allow time to discuss progress (eg, to ask the person how he feels he's progressing) and to summarize what has been taught.
- Find ways to include significant others in the teaching session.

Counseling—Helping People Make Choices

Counseling people to help them make necessary changes in their lives or to help them make choices about their health care (or care of a loved one) is another important nursing intervention. Counseling includes using teaching techniques to help people acquire the knowledge to make decisions about their health care. It also includes exploring motivations and offering support during periods of adjustment to new circumstances. By using teaching and therapeutic communication techniques, you can offer valuable psychological and intellectual support, thereby reducing the stress associated with making choices about health care management. As you counsel people, apply principles of ethics (see page 20) and promote autonomy. Stress the importance of becoming informed so that they can make the best decisions based on their own values and beliefs.

Consulting and Referring—The Cornerstone of Multidisciplinary Approaches

Making appropriate consultations and referrals is the cornerstone of multidisciplinary approaches. Even when there is no need for formal consultations or referrals, with today's complex situations, you're quite likely to find yourself consulting with other experts on a fairly regular basis. For example, suppose you have someone who has trouble swallowing pills. You should be thinking, "I wonder if the pharmacist might know a better way to give medications (eg, a liquid form)." If someone isn't eating because she dislikes hospital food, think about referring this problem to the dietitian so different meals can be served. Be sure that you recognize when your patient's care would benefit by your consulting with a nurse having different or better expertise or another health care professional altogether.

Determining Specific Interventions

Determining specific interventions requires you to answer four key questions.

1. What can be done to prevent or minimize the risks or *causes* of this problem?
2. What can be done to minimize the *problem*?
3. How can I tailor interventions to meet this specific person's expected *outcomes*?
4. How likely are we to get desired versus adverse responses to the interventions, and what can we do to reduce the risks and increase the likelihood of beneficial responses? (See Fig. 4–4.)

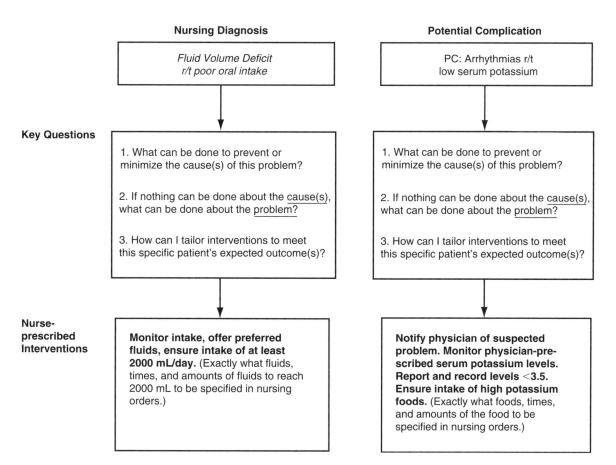

F i g u r e **4–4.** Example of how to determine nursing interventions.

Safe Practice: Weigh Risks and Benefits, Be Proactive

Safe practice requires you to weigh risks and benefits of nursing interventions and to be proactive, thinking about how to minimize risks and improve results before prescribing interventions. Weigh the risks of *causing harm* against the probability of *correcting or controlling the problem.* Ask the following questions:

1. If I prescribe this intervention, how likely are we to see the desired response?
2. What is the worst thing that can happen if this intervention is performed, and how likely is it to happen?
3. What measures can be taken to minimize the chances of causing harm?
4. What could happen to this problem if *no* interventions were prescribed?

   By answering these questions and considering the possible responses, you can *weigh the risks* (of prescribing the interventions and having an adverse reaction, or allowing the problem to go untreated) *against the benefits* (the likelihood of achieving the desired response) if the intervention is performed. Answering these four questions helps you to choose the safest interventions and be prepared for adverse reaction.

Guidelines: Determining Nursing Orders

- Determine a baseline of current signs, symptoms, and risk factors of the problem.
- Check for medical orders for nursing interventions related to the problem (eg, medications, diet, activity, diagnostic studies, and so forth).
- If you're using standard plans (eg, critical path, preprinted plan, protocol):
  ○ Use them with a critical mind. Compare the person's specific situation with the standard plan. Decide what applies, what doesn't, and what's missing.
  ○ Modify (add, delete, change) interventions as indicated, depending on your current assessment findings and what's likely to work for this specific person.
- Identify monitoring regimens for potential complications: What will you monitor? How often will you monitor it? How often will you record assessment data?
- Identify interventions that prevent or minimize the underlying causes or risk factors of the problem and help achieve the expected outcome. For example, if you have *Risk for Injury related to chronic muscle weakness* with an outcome of *demonstrates safe ambulation with the use of a walker,* tailor interventions to reflect that the person will be using a walker (eg, have the person practice using the walker for ambulation in various circumstance, like going up and down stairs and going to the bathroom).
- If you can't do anything about the *cause or risk factors,* decide if there's anything that can be done about the *problem.* For example, if someone is terminally ill and has *Death Anxiety,* you can't do anything about the fact that the person is going to die, but you can do something about the anxiety through counseling and therapeutic communication.
- Be sure the interventions are congruent with other therapies (eg, allow for rest after physical therapy).
- Consider the person's preferences; individualize as much as possible.
- Determine the scientific rationale for planned actions.

- Create opportunities for teaching (eg, explain rationale for all actions).
- Consult with other professionals when indicated (physician, APN, physical therapist).
- Before prescribing any actions:
  - Weigh the risks and benefits of performing the actions.
  - Decide whether you're willing to be accountable for the responses to the interventions you prescribe.
- Make your orders specific: Keep in mind "see, do, teach, record" (ie, what to assess [see], what to do, what to teach, and what to record). For example, suppose you're caring for someone who's had abdominal surgery and you identify *Risk for Ineffective Airway Clearance related to chronic smoking and incision pain.* Your orders might look like this:
  1. Auscultate lungs every 4 hours.
  2. Help the person to perform coughing and breathing exercises with pillow and hand over incision every 4 hours.
  3. Reinforce the importance of coughing and deep breathing.
  4. Record lung sounds and sputum production once a shift and as needed.
  5. Encourage the person to use current illness as a way to begin quitting smoking.

What to Include in Your Nursing Orders
Date: The date you write the order.
Verb: Action to be performed.
Subject: Who is to do it.
Descriptive Phrase: How, when, where, how often, how long, or how much?
Signature: Be consistent in how you sign.

Example: (Today's date) Assist patient to stand by the side of the bed for 10 minutes twice a day wearing her back brace. R. Alfaro-LeFevre, RN

Making Sure the Plan Is Adequately Recorded

Forms for, and methods of, recording the plan of care should be tailor-made to meet the needs of the nurses and clients in each unique setting. As you go from working in one place to another, become thoroughly familiar with each place's particular standards and policies for recording a plan of care: you're accountable for making sure the plan meets each faculty's specific standards. Make sure that somewhere on the patient record, people can find evidence of the four required components of the plan of care (diagnoses or problems, expected outcomes of care, prescribed interventions, and evaluation or progress notes addressing responses to interventions).

Responsibilities for Computerized and Standard Plans

Computerized and standard plans give abbreviated information, assuming that you have the knowledge to "fill in the blanks" and apply the information to each particular patient situation. For example, a critical path may state "out of bed twice a day." If your patient requires a walker to accomplish this and this is unique to your patient's situation, you're responsible for making sure it's noted in the appropriate place on the record. Policies may vary about how this is recorded, but the important thing is that it's recorded in a place where nurses are likely to check for how the patient ambulates.

Remember that standard plans aren't intended to *think* for you. They're intended to be used *as guides* to care. As the nurse, you're responsible for:

- Detecting changes in client status that may contraindicate following the plan.
- Using good judgment about which parts of the plans apply and which do not.
- Recognizing when problems aren't covered by the plan and finding other ways to address them (for example, some facilities have addendums that can be placed on the record).
- Adding unique patient requirements (eg, walker) in appropriate places.

Computerized and standard plans may be based on medical diagnoses or nursing diagnoses. If the person has more than one major problem, you may need to use more than one applicable plan, or choose the most relevant plan and modify it. The important thing to remember is that these types of plans are developed for specific *problems*, not people, and you *must* be sure you carefully adapt any standard plan to the person's *specific situation*. If you're not sure where certain unique patient needs should be recorded, check with a more qualified nurse.

Remember the following rule:

RULE ▶ It's your responsibility to make sure that any problems, diagnoses, or risk factors that are likely to impede progress toward outcome achievement are addressed somewhere on the patient record. This may require adapting a standard plan, adding a standard plan to the chart, or developing an individualized plan of your own.

Multidisciplinary Plans

Multidisciplinary plans, in which all disciplines (medicine, dietary, and so forth) work from the same plan, often are the norm today. Multidisciplinary approaches bring "the best of all worlds" together. However, keep in mind that, as the nurse, you're the one with the patient 8 hours a day. You're in the best position to be realistic about how the plan will come together *as a whole,* on a day-by-day, hour-by-hour basis. It's your job to stay focused on *human responses*, how the person is likely to *respond as a whole* to the plan of care, and to act as a client advocate.

Pages 149 through 156 at the end of this chapter show some examples of various plans of care (see Display 4–5 and Figs. 4–5 to 4–7). Remember that student plans sometimes are more theoretical and comprehensive because they're used to assess the student's knowledge of nursing theory and all aspects of nursing process.

DISPLAY 4 – 5   Multidisciplinary Record and SOAP Charting

Description: Example of a multidisciplinary record, with all disciplines charting on the same record, creating an interdisciplinary problem list (see I below) and sample of SOAP charting (see II below).

I. Sample problem list

Date of Diagnosis	Problem	Date Resolved
1/5	1. *Cerebrovascular accident* (identified by physician)	
	2. *Risk for Impaired Skin Integrity related to immobility* (identified by nursing)	
	3. Unsteady gait (identified by physical therapist)	
1/7	4. *Body Image Disturbance* (identified by nursing)	
1/8	5. *Urinary tract infection* (identified by physician)	1/13

II. Sample SOAP charting*

S: Subjective Data	"I can't feel anything on the right side."
O: Objective Data	Absent reflexes on the right side. Slouched in bed, leaning toward right. Has reddened area about 5 cm on the right hip
A. Analysis	*Risk for Impaired Skin Integrity related to right-side loss of sensation and immobility*
P: Plan	Prevent skin breakdown. Monitor back and hips for signs of decreased circulation from pressure point every 2 hours. Reposition side, back, side every 2 hours. Place air mattress and sheepskin on bed.

*After initial planning, some facilities add I (implementation) and E (evaluation), making the acronym SOAPIE.

Critical Thinking: Evaluating the Plan

Once you've completed recording the plan of care, take some time to evaluate what you've produced. Comprehensive care planning is a complicated process. Early evaluation of what you've produced promotes critical thinking by helping you detect oversights and errors early. For example, use checklist in Display 4–6 (page 157) to decide how your plan "measures up." Box 4–1 (page 157) shows 10 key questions to consider when determining if your patient's plan has been documented adequately.

Community Nursing Service & Hospice

CLIENT'S NAME PLACE LABEL HERE
FID #

INTERDISCIPLINARY CARE PLAN
(Page 1 of 4)

Physician _____   Address _____
_____

1. Diagnosis(es): Principal	2. Mental Status (check one)
	☐ Alert ☐ Lethargic ☐ Other
Secondary	☐ Semicomatose ☐ Comatose

3. Prognosis and Rehabilitation Potential	4. Diet	8. Medications
		Name Dosage Frequency
5. Homebound Status/Functional Limitations		
6. Safety Precautions		
7. Supplies/Equipment		

9. Frequency of Visits/Duration of Service
 a. Skilled Nursing _____   e. Volunteer _____
 b. Home Health Aide _____   f. Clergy _____
 c. MD _____   g. Other _____
 d. Social Service _____

	Date Recorded	Date Resolved	Person(s) Responsible
PROBLEM: Incomplete adjustment by client/S.O.(s) to effects of the terminal illness on the family unit.			

GOAL: Enhance quality of life for client/S.O.(s) during the dying process.
PLAN:
☐ 1. Present Hospice philosophy and services.
☐ 2. Assess client/S.O.(s) wishes and expectations regarding care.
☐ 3. Assess client, significant other, or caregiver resources available for care and encourage or supplement their use.
☐ 4. Assess psychosocial reaction of client/S.O.(s) to client's prognosis.
☐ 5. Encourage client/S.O.(s) to get legal and personal affairs in order.
☐ 6. Discuss and support intervention for alleviating fears, stress, etc., and encourage verbalization of feelings as family and/or client expresses the need.
☐ 7. Discuss signs and symptoms of impending death and what to do to promote comfort in dying.
☐ 8. _____
_____
_____

Cert Period from _____ to _____

12. Review Frequency:	13. Dates Plan Reviewed
	1) _____ 2) _____ 3) _____ 4) _____ 5) _____
	6) _____ 7) _____ 8) _____ 9) _____ 10) _____

Case Manager's Signature	Hospice Medical Director's Signature	Attending Physician's Signature
Date Signed:	Date Signed:	Date Signed:

CNS377 2/93

F i g u r e **4–5.** Care Plan. (Courtesy of Community Nursing Service, Salt Lake City, Utah.)

Community Nursing Service & Hospice

CLIENT'S NAME
FID #

PLACE LABEL HERE

INTERDISCIPLINARY CARE PLAN
(Page 2 of 4)

PROBLEM: Alteration in comfort. ☐ Skin ☐ HEENT ☐ Cardiopulmonary ☐ GI ☐ GU ☐ MS ☐ CNS	Date Recorded	Date Resolved	Person(s) Responsible

GOALS:
1. Client/S.O. expresses verbally or nonverbally increased level of comfort.
2. Client/S.O. will be able to apply measures to control symptom(s) effectively and safely.

PLAN:
☐ 1. Assess pain and other symptoms, including site, duration, characteristics and relief measures.
☐ 2. Teach caregiver symptom control and relief measures.
☐ 3. Teach new pain and symptom control medication regimen and effects of medications.
☐ 4. Diet counseling for patients with anorexia.
☐ 5. Assess bowel regimen and implement as needed.
☐ 6. Check for and remove impaction as needed.
☐ 7. Fleets or tap water enema as needed.
☐ 8. Rectal tube for increased flatulence.
☐ 9. Assess mental status and sleep disturbance changes.
☐ 10. Oxygen on at _____ liters per _____. Teach safety.
☐ 11. _____

PROBLEM: Self-care deficit.	Date Recorded	Date Resolved	Person(s) Responsible

GOALS:
1. Caregiver able to care for client at home.
2. ADLs and personal hygiene met through agency staff assistance.

PLAN:
☐ 1. Teach client/S.O. safety measures.
☐ 2. Teach S.O. care of weak, terminally ill client.
☐ 3. Teach care of the bedridden client.
☐ 4. Teach client/S.O. regarding techniques for energy conservation.
☐ 5. Teach catheter care.
☐ 6. HHA to assist with ADLs and personal hygiene. See care plan.
☐ 7. Teach feeding tube care to S.O.
☐ 8. Teach S.O.: ☐ p.o. ☐ s.l. ☐ topical ☐ rectal ☐ s.q. ☐ i.m. ☐ i.v. technique for medication administration.
☐ 9. _____

CNS377 2/93

F i g u r e **4–5.** *(Continued)*

Community Nursing Service & Hospice

INTERDISCIPLINARY CARE PLAN
(Page 3 of 4)

PROBLEM: Technical Deficit	Date Recorded	Date Resolved	Person(s) Responsible

GOALS: Professional disease management in the home.
PLAN:
☐ 1. Assess disease process progression and address with all involved members of the Interdisciplinary Team.
☐ 2. Assess for electrolyte imbalance.
☐ 3. Assess amount and frequency of urinary output.
☐ 4. Assess skin integrity.
☐ 5. Assess weight.
☐ 6. Assess for edema.
☐ 7. Measure abdominal girth.
☐ 8. Assess cardiovascular, pulmonary and respiratory status.
☐ 9. Assess nutrition and hydration status.
☐ 10. Measure vital signs.
☐ 11. Assess S.O.(s) knowledge and skill regarding technical procedures and care giving.
☐ 12. Administer: ☐ p.o. ☐ s.l. ☐ topical ☐ rectal ☐ s.q. ☐ i.m. ☐ i.v. ☐ injection ☐ infusion for symptom control.
☐ 13. ☐ Condom or ☐ indwelling catheter, size _____ , insertion and maintenance. Change every _____ or when leaking or plugged.
☐ 14. Decubitus care (describe): _____
_____
☐ 15. Dressing change (describe): _____
_____
☐ 16. Obtain venipuncture for _____
☐ 17. Record and report significantly abnormal findings to physician.
☐ 18. Do not attempt resuscitation.
☐ 19._____
_____
_____
_____

BEREAVEMENT

PROBLEM: Potential/actual failure of survivors to complete bereavement process.	Date Recorded	Date Resolved	Person(s) Responsible

GOALS: To provide appropriate intervention for surviving family members, S.O. and IDT members to facilitate progression of the bereavement process within one year of the client's death.
PLAN:
☐ 1. Present hospice bereavement philosophy and services to S.O.
☐ 2. Assess S.O.'s response and reactions, coping strategies, support systems available, risk of pathological grief reactions, and desire of survivors for bereavement follow-up within the first week of service.
☐ 3. Invite S.O. to bereavement support group within first month following the client's death.
☐ 4. Contact S.O. at 3, 6, 9, and 12 months following the client's death.
☐ 5. Refer S.O. demonstrating pathological grief reactions to appropriate community resources.
☐ 6. Reassess S.O.'s adjustment at 12 months following the client's death and discharge from Hospice program if appropriate.

CNS377 2/93

F i g u r e **4–5.** *(Continued)*

Community Nursing Service & Hospice

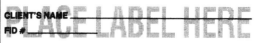

CLIENT'S NAME
FID #

INTERDISCIPLINARY CARE PLAN
(Page 4 of 4)

IN-PATIENT PAIN AND SYMPTOM MANAGEMENT AND RESPITE

PROBLEM:	Date Recorded	Date Resolved	Person(s) Responsible
☐ A. Symptoms. Specify: _____, _____, _____. ☐ B. Client care in home.			

GOALS:
1. To institute program for _____, _____,
_____, management to be continued at home.
2. To allow caregiver respite time to enhance coping ability.
3. To assure continuity of care.

PLAN:
☐ 1. Assess need through interdisciplinary team discussion.
☐ 2. Contact and coordinate care with contracted in-patient facility to assure continuity of care.
☐ 3. Establish plan of care with in-patient staff for in-patient stay.
☐ 4. Contact in-patient staff and client/S.O. regarding progression towards care plan goals daily. Visit at least every other day.
* ☐ 5. Facilitate safe return to the home setting.

*Transportation is the family's responsibility.

Case Manager's Signature	Hospice Medical Director's Signature	Attending Physician's Signature
Date Signed:	Date Signed:	Date Signed:

CNS377 2/93

Figure **4–5.** (*Continued*)

Care Plan Based on Nursing Diagnosis

Date	Nursing Diagnosis	Expected Outcomes	Target Date	Resol Date
	Ineffective Breathing Pattern related to _neuro-muscular impairment_	① Achieve optimal lung expansion with adequate ventilation.	LTO	
	as evidenced by _C-6 spinal cord injury, poor chest expansion_	✗ Identify causative factors and relate adaptive ways of coping with them.	Strength: Knows this well.	
		③ Remain free of signs and symptoms of hypoxia.	LTO	
	Commmon Etiologies			
	Neuromuscular Impairment Pain Musculoskeletal Impairment Inflammatory Process Anxiety	④ Relate relief of symptoms and comfort in breathing.	LTO	
	Decreased Lung Expansion Decreased Energy or Fatigue Infection Tracheo-Bronchial Obstruction Structural Damage	⑤ Demonstrates effective breathing techniques and use of assistive devices.	LTO	

F i g u r e **4–6.** Sample page from a nursing care plan that uses a separate page for each nursing diagnosis.

Nursing Interventions	Date IMP/DC	Nursing Orders	Date IMP/DC
1. Assess causative or contributing factors.	5/10	− Auscultate lungs q 4° + prn + chart q 8°.	5/10 RA
2. Reduce or eliminate causative or contributing factors, if possible.	5/10	− Monitor use of incentive spirometer (he tries to skip when he's tired).	5/10 RA
3. Assist patient in use of respiratory devices and techniques.	5/10	− Reinforce need for practicing quad cough.	5/10 RA
4. Provide for adequate rest periods between treatments.	5/10		
5. Promote comfort.	5/10	− Encourage family to help him to ↑ mobility and to turn from side to side.	5/10 RA
6. Provide emotional support.	5/10		
7. Maintain adequate ventilation.	5/10	− Document vital capacity q 8 hours on flow sheet.	5/10 RA
8. Assess for signs and symptoms of hypoxia.	5/10		
9. Initiate health teaching and referrals as indicated.	5/10	− Record daily teaching on discharge planning sheet.	5/10 RA

Figure 4–6. (Continued)

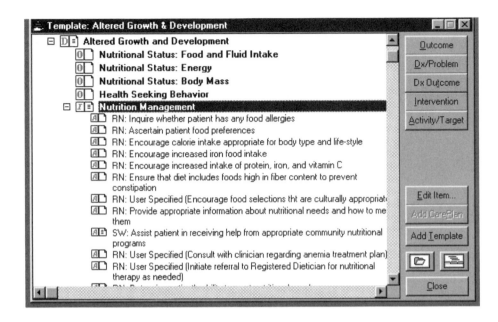

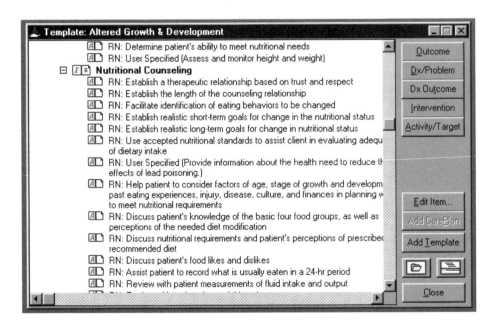

F i g u r e **4–7.** Two sample screens of a computerized care plan using NANDA, NIC, and NOC standardized language. Reproduced from CareManager software by permission of Ergo Partners, LC, *www.ergopartners.com.*

DISPLAY 4–6   Checklist to Evaluate the Plan of Care

1. Was the plan developed with the client (and, if appropriate, significant others and other involved health care providers)?

2. Have you addressed:
☐ Actual and potential problems that must be addressed to achieve the overall outcomes in a safe and timely way?
☐ Problems that require individualized, not routine, nursing interventions?

3. If you identified problems that aren't on the plan of care, have you made sure that they are addressed somewhere in the patient's record (eg, chest tube management might be addressed by physician's orders)?

4. Are the outcomes:
☐ Derived from the diagnoses or problems?
☐ Measureable?
☐ Mutually formulated with the patient and other key players?
☐ Realistic and attainable?
☐ Written according to the rules (patient-centered; measurable verbs; clear about who, what, when, how, and where)?

5. Do the nursing orders:
☐ Include interventions that focus on controlling the *underlying cause* or risk factors of the problem (or, if that's not possible, treating the *problem*)?
☐ Clearly direct interventions (addressing who, what, when, how, and how much)?
☐ Incorporate use of resources and strengths?
☐ Show the signature of the prescriber?

6. Does the plan:
☐ Reflect current policies and practice standards?
☐ Apply research and scientific principles?
☐ Address developmental, psychosocial, spiritual, cultural, and biologic needs?
☐ Include interventions for health promotion and teaching?
☐ Provide for continuity (eg, is it easily accessible, clear, and concise)?
☐ Aim to reduce costs while promoting convenience and comfort?

Box 4–1 Critical Thinking During Planning
Ten Key Questions*
1. What **major outcomes** (observable results) do we need to see?
2. What **problems, issues, or risk factors** must be addressed to achieve the major outcomes?
3. What are the **circumstances** (what is the context)?
4. What **knowledge** is required?
5. How much room is there for **error?**
6. How much **time** do we have?
7. What **resources** can help me/us?
8. Whose **perspectives** must be considered?
9. What's **influencing thinking?**
10. **What can be done** to prevent, control, or eliminate the problems or issues addressed in above in #2?

---

*Adapted from Alfaro-LeFevre (1999). *Critical thinking in nursing: A practical approach* (p. 45). Philadelphia: W. B. Saunders.

CRITICAL THINKING EXERCISE XIV

Determining Interventions and Recording Nursing Orders

To complete this session, read pages 142–157. Example responses can be found on page 247.

Part I.

1. What's the point of classifying interventions into direct and indirect interventions? (Three sentences or less.)

2. How do the words "see, do, teach, record" help you remember what you need to consider when determining interventions?

3. After you identify a problem, what two questions do you need to ask to determine interventions?

4. Explain how to weigh risks and benefits. (Five sentences or less.)

Part II.

For each problem and outcome listed here, list some appropriate nursing interventions that might achieve the outcome.

1. *Risk for Impaired Skin Integrity related to prescribed bed rest and loss of sensation in lower extremities.*
   Outcome with corresponding indicators: Maintains intact skin.
   Indicators: Absence of redness or irritation; management of risk factors.
   List appropriate nursing interventions:

2. *Risk for Ineffective Airway Clearance related to thoracic, incision pain.*
   Outcome: Demonstrates effective airway clearance.
   Indicators: Coughs effectively every 3 hours; lungs clear.

List appropriate nursing interventions:

3. *Constipation related to insufficient exercise and inadequate fluid and roughage in-take as evidenced by no bowel movement in 4 days.*
   Outcome: Reports or demonstrates no constipation.
   Indicators: Daily soft bowel movements; exercises 20 minutes every day; drinks minimum of 2000 mL daily; demonstrates adequate roughage intake.
List appropriate nursing interventions:

Part III.

For medical problems, a major independent responsibility of the nurse is to monitor for potential complications. For each of the following problems, identify potential complications and determine how and how often you plan to monitor for the problems. (You may need to use an additional resource, such as a medical–surgical textbook for this section.)

1. Intravenous infusion at 25 mL/h
   Potential complications:

   Plan for monitoring to detect potential complications:

2. Insulin-dependent diabetes
   Potential complications:

   Plan for monitoring to detect potential complications:

3. Foley catheter
   Potential complications:

Plan for monitoring to detect potential complications:

Try This on Your Own

Try weighing risks and benefits and making decisions about interventions. Consider the following interventions and decide whether you'd prescribe them and whether there was anything you could do to minimize the risks involved.

1. Your neighbor calls at 10 PM and tells you her 9-year-old has chickenpox and generally is irritable and uncomfortable. She asks you if you think it would be okay to give her Children's Tylenol®. What would you tell her? What would you have told her if it were *aspirin*? Be sure to look these drugs up before answering.

2. Mr. Ogden is weak from being on bed rest. He reports being depressed because he's become so dependent on others. He's now allowed to go to the bathroom on his own and requests that he be allowed to do his daily hygiene unsupervised in the bathroom. You are concerned that he might tire in the bathroom. Would you prescribe for him to be allowed to do his morning care alone in the bathroom? If so, what would you do to minimize the risks?

3. Your patient has a left chest tube and doesn't want to lie tilted to his left side because it's painful. Even though his right lung is compromised from previous disease process, he insists on being turned only to the right side. Would you allow him to turn only to his right side? If so, what would you do to minimize the risks?

Summary

Methods of developing and recording the plan of care continue to change as health care providers seek to be more efficient. Multidisciplinary approaches bring "the best of all worlds" to care planning because they bring the expertise and perspectives of various professionals together. As we continue to change, remember that no matter what care planning method you use to meet today's standards, the plan of care must be able to answer all the following questions:

- What are the problems that must be prevented, resolved, or improved by the time of discharge?
- What are the expected outcomes (results) of care?
- What are the interventions required to prevent, resolve, or control the problems?
- Where can we find statements that monitor progress (evaluation)?
- When indicated, the plan also must give special attention to teaching needs, safety precautions, and discharge planning.

Evaluate your knowledge of this chapter. Check to see if you can achieve the learning outcomes on page 122.

Bibliography: See pages 199–201.

Implementation

LEARNING OUTCOMES

After mastering the content in this chapter, you should be able to:

- Identify ways you can be more prepared for getting change-of-shift report the next time you're in the clinical setting.
- Explain the importance of assessing and reassessing performing nursing interventions.
- Discuss how you'll set daily priorities the next time you're in the clinical setting.
- Explain when and how to delegate an action to an unlicensed helper.
- Address your accountability in relation to delegating actions.
- Describe how to reduce the likelihood of harm from an intervention.
- Address your role in relation to case management and variances in care.
- Describe the characteristics of effective charting systems.
- Chart effectively following guidelines from the facility you'll go to for your next clinical assignment.
- Discuss how you'll give a factual, organized change-of-shift report the next time you're in the clinical setting.

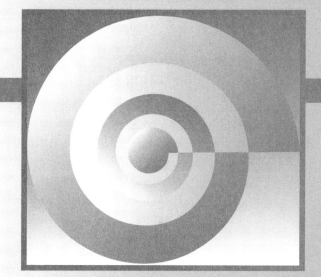

Standard I. *Assessment.* The nurse collects client health data.

Standard V. *Implementation.* The nurse implements interventions identified in the plan of care.*

Standard VI. *Evaluation.* The nurse evaluates the client's progress toward attainment of outcomes.*

Critical Thinking Exercises

■ **Critical Thinking Exercise XV:** Delegating, Case Management, Critical Paths, and Care Variances

■ **Critical Thinking Exercise XVI:** Principles of Effective Charting

What's in this chapter?

Whereas the last chapter addressed how to develop an initial comprehensive plan of care, this chapter focuses on the daily activities of *putting the plan into action*. It suggests steps for setting priorities at the beginning of the workday and answers the question, "When and how is it appropriate to delegate care to others?" It stresses the need to monitor responses to interventions by assessing and reassessing as you carry out the plan and provides guidelines for charting effectively (creating a record that clearly shows what happened, when it happened, where it happened, and how it happened).

*Excerpted from ANA Standards of Clinical Nursing Practice (ANA, 1998).

Implementation: Putting the Plan Into Action

Implementation, or *putting the plan into action,* includes:

- Preparing for report and getting report
- Setting daily priorities
- Assessing and reassessing
- Performing interventions and making necessary changes
- Charting
- Giving report
  Let's go through each of these activities step by step.

Preparing for Report and Getting Report

In the clinical setting, most often, you begin taking care of people after comprehensive planning has been done and *Implementation* already has begun—you get report from someone who's been implementing the plan in your absence. Being prepared and staying focused can be the key to getting a factual, relevant report that helps you get organized and set priorities early in the day.

Preparing for Report

Preparing for report—for example, learning about patient problems, looking up common treatments, reading charts, and getting to the unit early—can be the key to efficiency. Too often, there's little time for reading charts and looking up management of common problems during the course of the day. When you have time to prepare yourself for the day, you feel more confident, *are* more competent, and can begin giving care in a timely way.

Getting Report

Getting a factual, relevant report can be quite a challenge for several reasons: there often are interruptions and distractions as one shift ends and the other begins; there's so much information that it's hard to write quickly enough; and nurses giving report often are fatigued or they may know the patients so well that they forget to tell you the unique aspects of care that you may need to know.

Coming to report with a prepared worksheet helps you to stay focused and get the necessary facts. For example, look at Figure 5–1, which shows the worksheet I developed for myself when I was working part-time in an intensive care unit. I found that without the worksheet, my brain couldn't remember and organize all it had to know in the short amount of time I had. If you tailor a worksheet to direct you to gain the information you need in each particular setting, you will find that it helps you:

Name _Wm. French_____   Room: _145_____

Age _62_____   Med Dx: _Angina_

Dr. _O'Hara_____   Nsg Dx: _Activity Intolerance_

Mental Status: _ok_

Airway: _ok_

Lungs: _clear_

Oxygen: _at 2 l per cannula_

Heart rhythm: _reg - no pvc's_

GI:

GU:

Skin: _ok_

Activity Restrictions: _OOB to chair only_

Diet: _Reg. No Caf_

IV: _Hep lock @ hand_

Pain? _None since yesterday_

Relevant History

Hypertension

Special Concerns

- _For stress test tomorrow_
- _Wants to see priest for communion_

EKG: _ok_ Na _ok_ Cl _ok_ K _3.5_ CO_2 _ok_

VITAL SIGNS: _98⁴-72-22_ $\frac{140}{90}$ BLD SUGAR: _ok_

BLOOD GASES: _ok_ O_2 SATURATION: _ok_

F i g u r e **5–1.** Personal worksheet developed by the author when she was working in an intensive care unit. The worksheet was essential to getting organized and identifying information that was missed during report. For example, above, the two blanks next to "GI" and "GU" point to missing information in those categories.

- Get more information down quickly.
- Organize the information (even if the nurse gives you a disorganized report, you can quickly organize it by placing the data in the appropriate blanks).
- Identify missing information (blanks jog your memory about pertinent questions to ask).
- Keep personal notes during the day (pertinent data can go on the worksheet).
- Give a more organized report (you can be more organized and comprehensive by systematically covering all the categories on the sheet).

If you don't have a preprinted worksheet, develop one yourself and use it consistently. You'll be surprised how it will help you be more efficient.

Setting Daily Priorities

Setting priorities during *Implementation* requires applying the same principles of priority setting you learned in *Planning* (page 126). However, the steps for setting priorities on a daily basis are a little different because *Implementation* focuses more on *doing* than planning.

Below are suggested steps for setting daily priorities.

Steps for Setting Daily Priorities

Step 1. Make initial quick rounds on your patients, briefly checking the "big picture" of how they are doing (preferably, do this before you go to report or sit down to study the plan of care). **Rationale:** This helps you to identify problems requiring immediate attention and helps you to connect the actual patients with what you hear during report or read in patient records.

Step 2. Immediately after shift report, verify critical information such as intravenous (IV) infusions, operation of equipment, and so forth. **Rationale:** Verifying information you received during report prevents misunderstandings and helps you and the nurse who's leaving settle problems while both of you are available for clarification.

Step 3. Identify urgent problems (those posing an immediate threat to the patient (eg, chest pain or a disconnected IV line) and take appropriate action (eg, get help if needed). **Rationale:** Setting the wheels in motion to correct severe problems takes priority over taking time to analyze all the patient's problems.

Step 4. List your patients' major problems and ask the following questions:

- Which problems must be resolved today, and what happens if I wait until later?
- Which problems must I monitor today, and what could happen if I don't monitor them?
- To achieve the overall outcomes of care, which are the key problems or ones that I must resolve or manage today?
- Which of the patient's problems can I realistically work on today?

Rationale: You can only do so much in a day. Answering these questions helps you decide what *must* be done today.

Remember the following rule.

R U L E ▶

An essential part of setting daily priorities is asking the patient and family to identify their own biggest priorities for the day (eg, stating, "Tell me three main things you want to accomplish today."). **Rationale:** This helps you to avoid making assumptions about what's important to your patients. It also helps you to identify assumptions your patients may have made (sometimes their expectations are unrealistic) and helps set the tone for mutual goal setting.

Step 5. Determine the interventions that must be done to prevent, resolve, or manage the listed problems. List these interventions along with routine tasks such as baths and meals. **Rationale:** This helps you to get a big picture of the tasks of the day, which helps you to answer questions such as, "What must be done first?" and "How can I make the best use of my time?" For example, you may give a routine bath to promote hygiene and, at the same time, discuss problems with coping.

Step 6. Decide what things the patient or significant others can do on their own, what things to delegate to others, and what things you must do yourself (see *Key Points of Delegation* and *When Is It Safe to Delegate?* in Displays 5–1 and 5–2).

DISPLAY 5 – 1   Key Points of Delegation*

Delegation defined: Transferring to a competent individual the authority to perform a selected task in a selected situation while retaining accountability for results.

☐ **Remember the "five rights of delegation."**
  1. **The right task**—one that doesn't fall only under the scope of nursing's practice.
  2. **To the right person**—someone qualified and competent to do the job.
  3. **In the right situation**—see Display 5–2 (*When Is It Safe to Delegate?*).
  4. **With the right communication**—be clear and concise when describing the task, the goal, and what you want reported.
  5. **Performing the right evaluation**—as indicated, timely evaluation of the patient's response and worker's performance as the task is being done and after the task is completed.

☐ **Delegate with full knowledge of:**
  1. Your state practice act and applicable standards, policies, and procedures (eg, what you're allowed to delegate and to whom may vary from state to state and facility to facility).
  2. The worker's specific job description and competencies.
  3. (When delegating to patients or family caregivers) whether they have the required knowledge and skills.

*Summarized from Hansten, R. & Washburn, M. (2001, 1998).

DISPLAY 5-2   When Is It Safe to Delegate?

Delegate When:

☐ The patient is stable.
☐ The task is within the worker's job description and capabilities.
☐ The amount of RN time with the patient isn't significantly reduced.

Don't Delegate When:

☐ Complex assessment, thinking, and judgment are required.
☐ The outcome of the task is unpredictable.
☐ There's increased risk of harm (eg, taking blood from an artery can cause more severe complications than venipuncture).
☐ Problem solving and creativity are required.

Source: R. Alfaro-LeFevre workshop handouts © 2001.

Rationale: Encouraging the patient and family to be as independent as possible helps them take charge of their own care. Often, patients and families don't know what they are or aren't expected to do for themselves. Using less qualified workers appropriately allows you to spend more time accomplishing tasks that require the expertise of a registered nurse.

Step 7. Make a detailed personal worksheet for getting things done for the day and refer to it frequently. Be sure to consider the daily routine of the unit (eg, when meals are served). **Rationale:** You're likely to experience many distractions during the course of the day. Don't rely on memory. Although the daily routine of the unit shouldn't dictate your activities, it's vital to consider it when setting the schedule. For example, it's frustrating to both nurses and patients when meals arrive during baths or patients are called to physical therapy at inconvenient times.

Think About It

You're Accountable for Care You Delegate. *As the nurse, you're accountable for decisions made by unlicensed assistive personnel (UAP). For example, in one case, a nursing assistant caring for a young boy who was on a suicide watch told the nurse she was going on a break, leaving the child in the care of his mother. The mother left the room to go to the bathroom, leaving the child alone. The child slipped away. Although the child later was found unharmed, the nurse would have been accountable for any injury incurred. Pay attention to decisions made by UAP and be sure you know the training and qualifications of the UAP you supervise.*

Assessing and Reassessing: Monitoring Responses

Assessing patients before and after nursing interventions is a critical part of *Implementation*. To ensure patient safety, you must closely monitor responses to interventions to determine the appropriateness of the plan of care: How is the patient responding? Are you getting the expected results? If not, why not? As in the *Think About It* on page 143, a recipe for *disaster* is blindly putting a plan into action without monitoring patient responses.

Your time for direct patient care often is limited. Make it a habit to use every patient encounter as an opportunity to monitor physical and mental health status. For example, if you're helping someone bathe, assess skin status (by observing the entire body) and mental status (by using therapeutic communication techniques). Remember to assess with an open mind. It's very easy to be misled by others' opinions, as in the following example.

E X A M P L E

> **The Importance of Assessing With an Open Mind.** During report, Jodi, the evening nurse, was told, "Mrs. Thrift is a difficult patient—she won't ambulate." Later, when Jodi went in to give Mrs. Thrift her medications, she asked if there was something that was causing her to seem so tired. Mrs. Thrift responded by explaining that she hadn't slept well in weeks because she had just found out her daughter had breast cancer and was afraid her daughter might die. This was important information that hadn't been offered before. Jodi then was able to talk with Mrs. Thrift about her fears and concerns and offer a positive outlook by explaining that breast cancer, when detected early, has a good prognosis. By later that evening, Mrs. Thrift was ambulating and talking about how eager she was to get home to some normalcy.

Performing Nursing Interventions

Performing interventions involves getting prepared, performing the interventions, determining the response, and making necessary changes.

Preparation: Be Proactive—Promote Safety, Comfort, and Efficiency

Preparation can make the difference between risky, haphazard care that taxes both you and the person and efficient, safe care that promotes comfort and gets results. Before you perform an intervention, prepare to act: be sure you know what you're going to do, why you're going to do it, how you're going to do it, and how you'll reduce risks of harm.

Steps for Preparing to Act

1. Review the plan and be sure you know the rationale and principles behind the intervention. If you don't know the principles and rationale, you won't be able to adapt the procedure if necessary, and you may not even recognize if the intervention is no longer appropriate.
2. Decide whether you're qualified and competent to perform the interventions (if not, seek help).
3. Find out if the facility has procedures, protocols, guidelines, or standards that address how you should perform the interventions.

4. Assess the patient's *current status* and decide whether the interventions still are appropriate.

5. Predict possible outcomes: get a picture of what you're going to do, think about what might come up, what could go wrong, and what you'll do about it.
   • Weigh risks and benefits (page 146).
   • Identify ways to reduce risks of harm to the patient and yourself.
   • Determine how to promote comfort and reduce patient stress (eg, if someone is expected to sit for a long period of time, get a comfortable chair and offer distractions).

6. Obtain the necessary resources (eg, equipment, personnel) and make sure you planned enough time and an environment conducive to performing the interventions.

7. Involve the person and significant others. Explain what's to be done and why, and how long it will take; encourage them to voice questions, suggestions, or concerns.

R U L E ▶ Before performing any intervention, ask yourself, "Am I clear about what I'm going to do, how I'm going to do it, and why it's indicated for this specific person?"

Thinking Critically: What to Do if Things Go Wrong

Even when you're fully prepared, you may not get the desired response to your interventions. Let's look at what to do if you don't get the desired response, the problem shows no improvement, or the situation is aggravated by the interventions?

If you don't get the desired response, a red flag that says *something is wrong* should go up in your mind. Stop and ask some key questions:

1. Did I perform the interventions correctly?
2. Is the diagnosis correct, or has the problem or its cause changed? For example, suppose you were caring for someone with tachycardia, and the tachycardia didn't respond to cardiac medications. Your next question might be, "Could there be something else causing or contributing to the tachycardia? For example, is there anxiety, fever, or respiratory problem?"
3. Are there other interventions that would complement this intervention, increasing its effectiveness? For example, a backrub and talking with someone who's anxious is likely to enhance the effect of an antianxiety agent.
4. What could I be missing? Should I be getting a second opinion?

Remember the following rule:

V O I C E S

Compassion: No Substitute for Competence. "In superficial, short-term medical encounters, a smiling face and a gentle hand impress. In the long term, it's competence that you begin to value. Does this mean I found myself disinterested in compassion? Not at all. But I also found it didn't count for much unless it was bundled with competence."
—*Daniel Beckman, parent of an acutely ill child.*

(Beckman, D. [1993]. Andrew's not-so-excellent adventure. *Healthcare Forum J,* May/June, 90–96.)

RULE ▶
> Carry out all nursing actions with full understanding of the principles and rationales involved, *observing responses carefully.* If you don't get the desired response, start asking questions to find out what's wrong before continuing to act. When you find out what's wrong, make the necessary changes and record them on the plan of care as needed.

Case Management: Critical Paths and Care Variances

If you're using a critical path like the one on page 252 to guide your patient's care, it sets priorities for you on a day-by-day basis; that is, it does *unless you identify a variance in care.* A *variance in care* occurs when a patient hasn't achieved outcomes by the time frame noted on a critical path. For example, if the critical path states "by the second day after surgery, the patient will be out of bed in a chair three times a day," but your patient isn't well enough to be out of bed three times a day, you've identified a care variance.

What do you do if you identify a care variance? Care variances should trigger you to perform additional assessment to determine whether the delay is justified or whether actions need to be taken to improve the likelihood of achieving the outcome. Assessing for care variances by comparing your patient's *actual situation* to the critical path is crucial for safe and effective nursing care. The following rule and Table 5–1 emphasize the need for critical thinking when using critical paths.

RULE ▶
> When using critical paths, never assume your patient is ready to progress as planned: *look* for care variances. If you identify a care variance, consider whether you need to contact a case manager for additional assessment and treatment.

TABLE 5 – 1 Critical Paths Don't Replace Thinking	
Examples of Thinking Critically When Using a Critical Path	Examples of Not Thinking Critically When Using a Critical Path
"I'm familiar with this path. . . . I wonder how this particular patient is doing in relation to the predicted care for this problem."	*"I have a path for this patient, so this should be easy and straight-forward because I already know what problems are going to be."*
"It's going to take time to think through what's really going on with this patient, but I'd better make time."	*"There's no way I have time to go through everything I need to really understand this patient. I'd better just follow the path."*

Ethical/Legal Concerns

You're responsible, both legally and ethically, for protecting the client's right to privacy. Remember to keep patient comments and information to yourself and to limit access to patient records to those involved in the patient's care (students in an approved program also may have access for learning needs).

Ethically (and in some cases, legally), you're responsible for *emotional* outcomes of your interventions as well as *physical* outcomes. For example, in some states, it's against the law to tell people they have AIDS over the phone. You must tell them in person and provide counseling and support. Here's another example: Suppose your client is having a facial tumor removed, and you're planning to give him a pamphlet with graphic pictures of reconstructive surgery. As a prudent nurse, you must anticipate his response, stay with him, and provide support.

Think About It

Evidence-Based Practice Challenges Assumptions About Restraints. *Are your interventions based on evidence? Think about how you might apply the following information from a study on the use of restraints done by Rogers and Bocchino in 1999. They found that whereas many nurses assume that restraining confused patients protects them from injury and prevents complications, evidence points to the contrary. Their study shows that restrained patients are more likely to sustain serious injury when they fall, that they are hospitalized twice as long as those who aren't restrained, and that they are eight times more likely to die during hospitalization than nonrestrained patients. It also shows that restraints contribute to depression, anger, nosocomial (hospital-acquired) infection, pressure ulcers, and deconditioning, all of which leave patients in a worse condition than when they were admitted.*

CRITICAL THINKING EXERCISE XV

Delegating, Case Management, Critical Paths, and Care Variances

To complete this session, read pages 164–172. Example responses can be found on page 247.

1. Suppose one of the many tasks that had to be accomplished today was getting a 30-year-old woman who has had a routine cholecystectomy out of bed for the first time:

   a. Would you delegate this task?

   b. Why or why not?

2. Read "Think About It" on page 168.

    a. Why do you think the nurse is accountable for the child slipping away? (One to two sentences.)

    b. What could the nurse have done to decrease the likelihood of the child slipping away? (One to two sentences.)

3. Answer each letter below, using three to five sentences.

    a. How do you assess a patient for a care variance?

    b. What would you do if you identified a care variance and why?

    c. What can happen to the *patient* if you miss the fact that your patient is demonstrating a care variance?

    d. What can happen to *you* if you miss the fact that your patient is demonstrating a care variance?

Charting

After you give nursing care and evaluated responses, the next thing on your mind should be charting the assessments, interventions, and responses. Two reasons for this are:

1. You're likely to be more accurate and thorough if your memory is fresh.
2. Writing down what you've observed and done often jogs your memory about something *else* you need to assess or do. For example, you may be charting an abdominal assessment and realize that you forgot to check whether the nasogastric tube equipment is functioning properly.

Keep in mind that the purpose of your charting is to:

1. Communicate care to other health care professionals who need to be able to find out what you've done and how the person is doing.

2. Help identify patterns of responses and changes in status.

3. Provide a foundation for evaluation, research, and improvement of quality of care.

4. Create a legal document that later may be used in court to evaluate the type of care rendered. Your records can be your best friend or worst enemy. The best defense that you actually observed or did something is the fact that you made a note of it.

5. Supply validation for insurance purposes. The saying goes, "If it's not documented, they won't pay."

Different Ways of Charting

Because charting practices vary from one place to another, and because it seems like charting practices are changing almost as quickly as you can say the word *computer,* it's important to become familiar with some of the following ways of charting.

Source-oriented charting: Caregivers from each discipline (medicine, nursing, physical therapy) chart on separate sheets, writing narrative notes chronologically. For an example, see Figure 5–2 on page 181.

Focus charting®: Nurses use key words to organize charting (data, action, response), and the subject of the note isn't necessarily a problem (eg, may simply address a change in patient behavior). For an example, see Figure 5–3 on page 181.

Multidisciplinary charting: Caregivers from all disciplines write on the same record. For an example, see Figure 5–4 on page 182.

Flowsheet charting: These types of records cue you to chart specific information in specific spaces. If there's significant information to chart, you write in the allocated space; if there's no significant information to record, you place a check mark or dash in the space. Additional marks, such as an asterisk, also may be used to reflect when other pertinent information has been recorded somewhere else, such as on the medication record. For an example of flowsheet charting, see Figure 5–5 on page 183.

Charting by exception: Nurses refer to unit standards, policies, and protocols in the patient record, charting narrative notes only when the patient's data changes or care deviates from the norm. For an example, see Figure 5–6 on page 184.

Use of addendum sheets: Nurses' notes are supplemented by separate sheets for each type of situation (eg, discharge summary sheets, teaching sheets). For an example, see Figure 5–7 on page 185.

Computerized patient records (CPR), also called computerized medical records: Nurses chart directly onto computers. CPR aims to eliminate repetitive charting and increase data base access.

Some places also are moving toward having **online patient records,** which allows access to records from many different locations. For an example, see Figure 5–8 on page 186.

Think About It

Guard Your Passwords and Your Patients' Privacy. *When using computerized patient records, remember your role in preventing unauthorized access to patient records. To ensure patient confidentiality and protect yourself from malpractice, never share your password and log yourself off the computer whenever you leave the screen. Don't leave patient information displayed on the monitor where others can see it.*

No matter what type of charting method you use—whether you're using a handheld computer or handwriting your own notes—be sure that you're able to apply the following charting principles.

Principles of Effective Charting

1. Effective charting shows evidence of the following:
   - **Initial assessments and reassessments:** What did you observe when you first encountered the patient and at subsequent encounters, especially before and after interventions?
   - **Status of client problems:** What current signs and symptoms are present?
   - **Interventions and nursing care performed:** What did you do to meet the person's needs?
   - **The response or outcomes of care:** What results did you observe?
   - **Specific attention given to safety:** What did you do to ensure patient safety?
   - **The person's ability to manage care needs after discharge:** What did you observe in relation to the likelihood that the patient is able to manage his own care?
2. Effective charting systems should:
   - Be tailor-made to the types of problems frequently demonstrated by the patient population of the facility, to direct nurses to chart key aspects of patient care.
   - Reflect use of nursing process and be legally sound.
   - Discourage double documentation (charting the same thing in two different places) and irrelevant charting.
   - Increase the quality of nursing records while reducing the amount of time spent charting.
   - Be designed so crucial patient data (eg, assessments and interventions) are easily retrievable, thereby facilitating communication, evaluation, research, and quality improvement.

Learning to Chart Effectively

Learning to chart effectively requires knowledge, experience, and application of these principles of effective charting. As you improve your ability to assess people and discriminate between normal and abnormal findings, your charting will improve. It's also important to do two things:

1. **Practice using the specific type of charting you'll be using** before you go to the clinical setting.
2. **Read charts to learn from actual situations.** As you read the charts, ask yourself questions like "What are the diagnoses?," "Where's the evidence that the diagnoses exist?," "What are they doing to treat them?," and "How is this person responding?."

Although charting varies from place to place, there are some universal guidelines that apply to all charting. Take a few moments to review the guidelines beginning on page 76 in Chapter 2, which address how to chart the initial data base, then go on to read the following guidelines.

Guidelines: Charting During Implementation

- Chart as soon as possible after giving nursing care. If you can't get to the chart, jot down notes on a worksheet. Don't rely on memory.
- *Think* as you chart and after you chart, asking yourself questions like "Am I missing anything?"
- Follow each facility's charting policies and procedures. These are in place to ensure safe and effective care.
- Record important actions (eg, medication administration) immediately to be sure that others know the action has been completed.
- Record all variations from the norm (eg, abnormalities in respiration, circulation, mental status, or behavior) and any actions taken related to the abnormalities (eg, if you reported the abnormality or if you intervened in some way).
- Be precise. Your notes should give a description and timeline for sequence of events, answering the questions *what happened* and *when, how,* and *where it happened.*
- Focus on significant problems or events that communicate *what's different* about this person today. For example, don't record, "went to the bathroom unassisted," unless this is unusual.
- Stick to the facts. Avoid judgmental language.

E X A M P L E

> **Right:** Shouting, "Everyone had better stay away from me, or I'm likely to hit someone."
> **Wrong:** Angry and aggressive.

- Be specific. Don't use vague terms.

E X A M P L E

> **Right:** Abdominal dressing has an area of light pink drainage about 6 inches in diameter.
> **Wrong:** Noted moderate amount of drainage on abdominal dressing.

- Be concise, yet descriptive. You don't have to write complete sentences. Use adjectives and accepted abbreviations to give a good picture of activities and observations.

For example, *OOB to chair for a half hour—c/o slight dizziness on standing up but moved well.*

- Sign your name consistently using your first initial, last name, and credentials after each entry that you complete (eg, F. Nightingale, RN).
- When you forget to chart something, record it as soon as you can, marking it a late entry.

EXAMPLE

> 5/17 3:00 PM, Late entry: Stool was positive for blood at 10 AM this morning. Notified Dr. Eyler. R. Alfaro-LeFevre, RN.

- Record failure or refusal to follow prescribed regimen, as well as any actions you took. For example, *Refuses to go to physical therapy. Says it "doesn't do any good." Notified Dr. Frazier and Rochelle Hutton in physical therapy.*
- When charting narratively, use one of the following mnemonics to organize your charting.

Mnemonics Used for Charting

AIR-A (Assessment, Intervention, Response, Action). Chart the *assessment* data you observe, the *interventions* performed, the patient's *response* to interventions, and any *actions* you took based on the response.

DAR (Data Action Response). Chart the *data* you observe, the *action*s performed, and the *response* of the patient.

DIE (Data, Intervention, Evaluation). Chart the *data* you observe, the *interventions* performed, and your *evaluation* of the patient's response.

PIE (Problem, Interventions, Evaluation). Chart the status of the *problems,* the *interventions* performed, and the *evaluation* of the patient's response to the interventions.

SOAP, SOAPIE. See page 149.

CRITICAL THINKING EXERCISE XVI

Principles of Effective Charting

To complete this session, read pages 164–177. Example responses can be found on page 248.

1. List five functions that patient records serve.

2. Give two reasons why you should chart as soon as possible after giving nursing care.

3. Imagine a patient calls you into the room and tells you that she feels like she's choking on mucus but is afraid to cough because of abdominal incisional pain. You help her to get in a better position and then assist her to splint the incision with a pillow. She finally coughs up a gray mucus plug and thanks you for your help. You listen to her lungs, and they sound clear. You emphasize the importance of reporting incisional pain that interferes with breathing. Using the mnemonic DAR, AIR-A, or DIE, write a note that records this event.

4. What's wrong with the following two excerpts from nurses' notes?

  a. 5/8 Patient is difficult and uncooperative. R. Alfaro-LeFevre, RN.

  b. 5/8 Patient seems confused. R. Alfaro-LeFevre, RN.

5. Pretend you wrote the nurse's note below on the wrong chart. Correct it using the accepted method for correcting charting errors.

5/8 N/G tube draining light green drainage.

Giving the Change-of-Shift Report

Your change-of-shift reports should be accurate, factual, and organized. What you say and how you say it can make a big difference in the quality of care that your patient receives. The following guidelines are presented to help you establish good habits for giving report.

Guidelines: Giving Change-of-Shift Reports

- Use a written or printed guide to prompt you to be thorough and organized (eg, use a worksheet like the one on page 165 or a comprehensive flowsheet).
- Begin by giving general background information, including the following: name, age, attending and consulting physicians, date of admission, and current problems list (major medical, nursing, and multidisciplinary problems).

EXAMPLE

"Mrs. Ballard, in room 214 by the window, is a 35-year-old patient of Dr. Smith with a consultation to Dr. Jones. She was admitted on 5/25 with pneumonia. She is a diabetic. She had a tracheostomy on 5/26. Our main concern today has been keeping her airway clear and getting her to drink more fluids."

- Be specific. Avoid vague terms.

EXAMPLE

Right: "Mrs. Wu has had an increase in her respiratory rate to 32/min. Her heart rate is up to 122, and her temperature is 101°F."
Wrong: "Mrs. Wu seems to be having respiratory difficulty."
Right: "I gave Mrs. Wu 8 mg of morphine IM at 5:10 pm for incisional pain."
Wrong: "I gave Mrs. Wu a pain med for her pain."

- If you make an inference, back it up with evidence (eg, "I think she isn't happy with her doctor because she's made statements that she doesn't like his bedside manner.").
- Describe the presence of all invasive treatments (eg, IV lines, Foley catheters, nasogastric tubes).
- Stress abnormal findings (eg, rales in the lungs, abnormal vital signs) and variations from routine or the norm (eg, "This patient *won't* be medicated before surgery.")

Keeping the Plan up to Date

Although how to complete a comprehensive evaluation is addressed in the next chapter, it's important to remember that early on, during *Implementation*, you should be reflecting on how things are going, monitoring progress, and updating the plan as needed, Display 5–3 shows the type of questions you should be asking on a daily basis to make sure the plan of care is kept up to date. Display 5–4 lists questions to ask yourself to evaluate your workday.

VOICES

Patients' Well-Being Depends on Communicating and Relating. Nursing is incredibly relational. We are surrounded every day by many people. . . . we are invited into the most intimate moments of the lives of people who minutes before were strangers . . . we cannot truly care for people without knowing them, without knowing their values, fears, beliefs, relationships, and plans for their lives. So each day we are thrust deep into relational work that touches our own humanity in ways we often cannot anticipate. . . . Although we work hard physically and intellectually, it is often the emotional and relational aspects of nursing that are both the most rewarding and the most difficult, frightening and exhausting. . . . We need each other not just for support and understanding, but because the care requirements of patients are not limited to our shift or our day of assigned work. For us to do good work, to make a difference in the lives of our patients and their families, our work must be continuous, coordinated and well communicated—shift-to-shift and nurse-to-nurse.— Gladys Campbell, RN, MSN

(Campbell, G. [1997]. President's note. *AACN News, 14*[8], 2.)

DISPLAY 5 – 3   Determining if the Plan of Care Is up to Date

☐ Does your patient still exhibit the problems identified on the plan?
☐ Does your patient have problems that *aren't* addressed on the plan of care but may impede progress to outcome achievement?
☐ Are the expected outcomes still realistic?
☐ Are the interventions still relevant?

DISPLAY 5 – 4   Evaluating Your Workday

Ask yourself:
- How has the day gone in general?
- Have I completed everything I should have?
- Have I been organized and able to set priorities well?
- What factors are influencing how I set priorities and organize my day?
- How much time am I spending performing collaborative nursing interventions?
- How much time am I spending implementing independent nursing interventions?
- Could I be doing more? Am I trying to do too much?
- Have I been clear and specific when delegating actions and communicating with others?
- How would each of my patients evaluate me in relation to meeting their specific needs?
- What changes should I make tomorrow?

Summary

Implementation requires you to put the plan into action with an active, open mind—a mind that's constantly assessing and reassessing both patient responses and your own performance. Human responses are unpredictable. Monitor them carefully—be flexible and change approaches as needed on a day-to-day (even hour-to-hour) basis. With today's reduced length of stays and increased use of unlicensed helpers, your time with patients may be limited. Use every patient encounter as an opportunity to observe mental and physical status and to empower patients to care for themselves (through teaching, motivating, and so forth). Be sure you know how to delegate effectively (pages 167–168). Also, work to become competent in communicating patient care (charting and reporting), setting priorities, and developing positive relationships with patients, families, and peers.

Evaluate your knowledge of this chapter. Check to see if you can achieve the learning objectives on page 162.

Bibliography: See pages 199–201.

Date and Time	Problems and Diagnoses	Nursing Assessments and Comments
5/8/02 0800	#1 *Risk for Ineffective Airway Clearance related to thick secretions* #2 *Risk for Fluid Volume Deficit related to poor fluid intake*	Coughing up thick white mucus. He does this well, but needs to be reminded to work at it. Lungs have a few scattered rhonchi at both bases. Fluids encouraged, he does drink juices well. Apple juice on ice kept at bedside. _____ H. Laird, RN
1000		OOB to chair for 1/2 hour. States he feels very fatigued, but he is steady on his feet. Voided lge amount clear yellow urine. Allowed to rest before pulmonary function test. _____ H. Laird, RN
1100		To special studies via wheelchair for pulmonary function. _____ H. Laird, RN
1230		Returned via wheelchair. Assisted back to bed. Ate all of his lunch; said it was the first time he's been hungry. _____ H. Laird, RN

F i g u r e **5–2.** Example of source-oriented narrative nurse's notes.

Date	Focus	Progress Notes
5/8		
07:00	Wound care	D—States he's changed his mind about having wife do wound care at home. Says he wants to be self-sufficient and do own wound care. A—Encouraged him to view wound care video today. R—Requested to view video after AM care. R. Alfaro, RN

F i g u r e **5–3.** Example of focus charting, using DAR to stand for data, action, response.

2/5/02 11³⁰ Nsg : Walked the length of the hall x2.
Refuses to sit up in a chair & can't be
convinced. Discussed need to participate
in plan to the best of her ability. Says
she understands, but feels she is being
"pushed too hard". Will be allowed to rest
& try again this afternoon. H. Laird RN

2/5 4ᵖᵐ Nutrition: Pt. sleeping - no N/V per RN.
Currently NPO on TPN. Recommend 134%
calorie & 118% of current protein intake.
                                    E. Barnes RD

2/5/02 5⁰⁰pm Medicine: Re above note:
Will ↑ calorie & protein in TPN.
                                    John Kruk MD

F i g u r e **5–4.** Example of multidisciplinary charting.

© 1985
St. Luke's Hospital   NURSING/PHYSICIAN
Milwaukee, Wisconsin   ORDER FLOWSHEET
                           05-937555 Rev. 12/85

Date __6/14/02__   Karl Stitt

NRSG DX	NURSING/PHYSICIAN ORDER													
1	Neurologic assessment — include short term memory	08*	09*	1930*	2000*	2100*	2230*	01→	04→	06→				
1	Neurovascular assessment	08*	09*	1930*	2000*	2100*	2230*	01→	04→	06→				
1	Tolerance of ADL's	08	09✓											
1	Signs + Symptoms of Bldg	08✓	16✓											
*	NURSE INITIAL ▶ SIGNIFICANT FINDINGS ▼	LB	WS	WS	WS	WS	WS	JB	JB	JB	-			

NRSG DX#	TIME		INIT
1	0800	®arm still feels heavy, speech slow but pt states he feels he's improving every day. Needs minimal assistance c̄ ADL's. Is able to set up his own tray and do own bath with assistance when chair is placed in bathroom. Ambulated to nurses station with 1 person standby assist. ————	LB
1	1600	c/o mild blurred vision + ® hand numbness.	WS
1	1900	States he feels worse, like when he was first admitted. c/o ® hand feeling "like it's needed". Weak ® hand grasp, much diminished from ® arm. Has very slow slurred speech, difficulty forming words. Dr. Ferguson notified. Immediately came up to see pt. Orders written. Wife called by nurse. Notified of change in pt. status. ————	WS
1	2030	Speech improving. ®hand numbness decreasing ————	WS
1	2130	Unable to speak. Able to communicate through head nod + gestures. No ® arm grasp. Dr. Ferguson called. No new orders.	
1	2230	Able to speak, but talks slowly. Has difficulty forming words. c/o "funny feeling" on ® arm, but couldn't be more specific. States feeling went away in 5 min. Able to lift arm in full ROM. Strong ® hand grasp. ® hand grasp < ⊕. States ® hand numbness is decreasing. ————	WS

INIT LB	R.N. SIGNATURE Lorraine Buhler RN	INIT JB	R.N. SIGNATURE Joan Bishop RN	INIT	R.N. SIGNATURE
INIT WS	R.N. SIGNATURE Wenda Schuster RN	INIT JK	R.N. SIGNATURE Jackie Kruck RN	INIT	R.N. SIGNATURE

➡ See Reverse Side   NURSING/PHYSICIAN ORDER FLOW SHEET   Dist. White-Chart Yellow-Bedside

F i g u r e **5–5.** Example of flowsheet charting (From Burke, L. & Murphy, J. [1988]. *Charting by exception* [p. 123]. New York: John Wiley & Sons).

ASSESSMENT PARAMETERS

The following parameters will be considered a negative assessment. If the physical assessment is negative indicate with a "✔" followed by initials in the box after the particular assessment area. An asterisk (*) followed by initials in the box is to be used to chart the exceptions which require elaboration in the box to the right.

Head Assessment:

Fontanelles level; soft. Sutures approximated. No infections, lice, alopecia, scabies or crusting. No headache

Integumentary Assessment

Skin warm, dry and intact. Turgor elastic. No lesions, masses, lacerations, bruises or rashes. Mucous membranes moist and pink.

EENT Assessment

Vision clear with or without glasses. Responds to spoken voice. Tm's pearly; ext. canals clear, nares patent, moist, and no discharge. Mouth and throat without lesions, erythema or exudate, tonsils 1-2+. Neck supple. Trachea midline, able to make swallowing movements. No lymphadenopathy.

Respiratory Assessment   *See reverse side for respiratory rates

Resps quiet and regular. Rate within normal limits for age. No flaring or retractions. Breath sounds vesicular through both lung fields, bronchial over major airways with no adventitious sounds, no cough.

Cardiovascular Assessment   *See reverse side for heart rates

Regular apical pulse and rate within limits for age. No extra heart sounds. Peripheral pulses palpable bil. No edema. No cyanosis of circumoral areas or nail beds. Capillary refill brisk.

Gasrointestinal Assessment

Abdomen soft. Bowel sounds active all 4 quadrants. No pain with palpation. No abnormal movements. Tolerates prescribed diet without nausea & vomiting. Having BM's within normal pattern and consistency.

TEMPERATURE (one only) °C			PULSE	RESP	INIT	NURSE SIGNATURE	DATE	TIME
A	O	R	AP	R				
BLOOD PRESSURE ☐ MANUAL ☐ MONITOR ____ Cuff Size								
RECUMBENT BP	SITTING BP		STANDING BP					
RT	RT		RT					
LEFT	LEFT		LEFT					
WEIGHT			HEIGHT					
____ kg ☐ standing	Hc ____ cms		____ cms					
____ lbs ☐ infant scale chest	____ cms		____ ins					

F i g u r e **5–6.** Sample of pediatric nursing data base using normal assessment parameters and charting by exception (Courtesy Memorial Hospital, Easton, MD).

ANTICOAGULANT

Karl Stitt

KNOWLEDGE OR SKILL CRITERIA* TO BE MET BEFORE DISCHARGE BY THE ( ) PATIENT ( ) SPOUSE OR SIGNIFICANT OTHER:	TEACHING AND/OR REINFORCEMENT		MEETS CRITERIA
	(DATE/INITIALS)		(DATE/INITIALS)
1. Verbalizes basic Coumadin pharmacology (purpose, action, dosage)	6/4 JS		6/5 LB
2. Verbalizes possible major side effects.	6/4 JS		6/5 LB
3. Verbalizes time, date, and place of scheduled post-discharge Prothrombin Time tests and to check with M.D. for results.	6/4 JS		6/5 LB
4. Verbalizes importance of adherence to medication regimen and results of omission (thrombi, emboli, phlebitis).	6/6 JS		6/7 LB
5. Verbalizes precautionary measures to be taken while on Coumadin therapy:			
a. take only meds per M.D. order (no ASA meds)	6/5 LB		6/6 JS
b. aware of meds that alter Coumadin actions (BCPs, vitamins, hormones)	6/5 LB		6/6 JS
c. carry ID card or medic alert jewelry	6/6 KB		6/7 LB
d. prevent physical injury when possible (shave with electric shaver, do not go barefoot, etc.)	6/6 LB		6/7 LB
6. Verbalizes appropriate action if persistent bleeding occurs.	6/6 JS		6/7 LB
7. Verbalizes need to inform all M.D.s and dentists of anticoagulant therapy.	6/6 JS		6/7 LB

*SEE NURSE'S DISCHARGE NOTE FOR DOCUMENTATION ON TEACHING RE: ADL RESTRICTIONS, DIETARY CHANGES, MEDICATIONS, TREATMENTS, OR FOLLOW-UP MEDICAL CARE. 6/3 *Hard of hearing (both ears)* LB

SPECIAL LEARNING NEEDS:

TEACHING RESOURCES UTILIZED	DATE	INITIALS	TEACHING RESOURCES UTILIZED	DATE	INITIALS
Coumadin Medication Sheet (330-05)			*Anticoagulant teaching sheet.*	6/8	LB
MedicAlert Jewelry Information	6/6	JS			
ID Card for Anticoagulant Therapy	6/8	LB			

SIGNATURE	INITIALS	SIGNATURE	INITIALS	SIGNATURE	INITIALS
Lorraine Buhler RN	LB				
Glenda Schuster RN	JS				

ST. LUKE'S HOSPITAL, MILWAUKEE WI   PATIENT TEACHING RECORD   8/80; REV. 12/86, 5/87 X-12C

F i g u r e **5–7.** Sample addendum sheet for teaching (From Burke, L. & Murphy, J. [1988]. *Charting by exception* [p. 127]. New York: John Wiley & Sons).

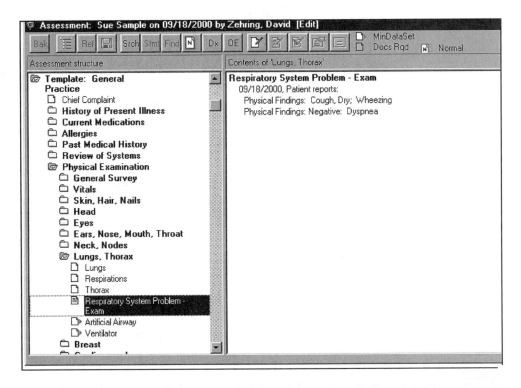

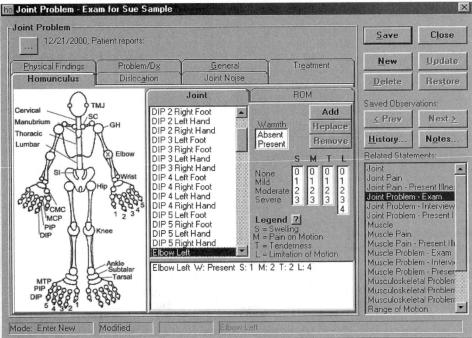

F i g u r e **5–8.** Two example screens of computerized documentation. Reproduced from CareManager software by permission of Ergo Partners, LC, *www.ergopartners.com.*

Evaluation

LEARNING OUTCOMES

After mastering the content in this chapter, you should be able to:

- Explain how to determine outcome achievement.
- Discuss how to decide whether to terminate, continue, or modify the plan of care.
- Describe the steps involved in a comprehensive evaluation of an individual plan of care.
- Explain how and why health care systems and organizations affect patient outcomes.
- Explain why it's important to perform all three types of evaluation studies—outcome, process, and structure—to improve care quality.
- Give four major responsibilities of staff nurses in relation to quality improvement (QI).

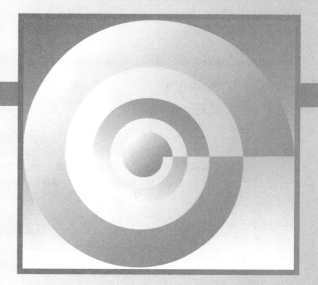

Standard V: Evaluation.
The nurse evaluates the client's progress toward attainment of outcomes.*

Critical Thinking Exercises

- ■ **Critical Thinking Exercise XVII:** Determining Outcome Achievement, Identifying Variables Affecting Achievement, and Deciding Whether to Continue, Modify, or Terminate the Plan

- ■ **Critical Thinking Exercise XVIII:** Quality Improvement

What's in this chapter?

Whereas the importance of *ongoing* early evaluation during *Implementation* was emphasized in Chapter 5, this chapter focuses on how to perform a *formal* evaluation of an individual plan of care; that is, how to decide whether to continue, modify, or terminate the plan and discharge the person. It also addresses the need to examine how health care delivery systems interact and impact on patient outcomes through QI studies aimed at correcting and improving care practices.

---

*Excerpted from ANA Standards of Clinical Nursing Practice (ANA, 1998).

Critical Evaluation: The Key to Excellence in Health Care Delivery

Critical evaluation—careful, deliberate, and detailed evaluation of various aspects of patient care—is the key to excellence in health care delivery. It can make the difference between care practices that are doomed to repeat errors and care practices that are safe, efficient, and constantly improving.

Most often, you'll be involved in evaluating an individual plan of care. However, you also may be asked to help in another type of evaluation—QI. QI studies aim to evaluate *groups of patients* or specific *aspects of care* to improve care quality for all (eg, "How can we achieve the same outcomes with less pain, in less time, and at a lower cost?").

Consumer Satisfaction: Maximizing Value

Evaluation provides the feedback needed to assess consumer satisfaction and maximize the value of health care delivery. To improve, we must consider both the needs and *wants* of consumers. We can't be satisfied with giving just "good" care—we must strive to give "the best" care possible. For example, consider how much improved nursing care can be if you work to manage the outcomes listed in Display 6–1.

Having addressed the importance of critical evaluation to improve care and maximize consumer satisfaction, let's look at what *Evaluation* entails in the context of an individual plan of care, then consider *Evaluation* in the context of QI.

DISPLAY 6 – 1   Improving Care and Maximizing Value

To improve care and maximize value, gathering, analyzing, and reporting data on the following health status outcomes is critical.
- ☐ **Quality of life:** Sense of well-being, presence of depression, success of pain management.
- ☐ **Functional status:** Ability to work, be independent, and do favorite activities.
- ☐ **Patient satisfaction:** Convenience, efficiency, and cost of care; sense that staff is attentive and sees each person as an individual.
- ☐ **Compliance measures:** Things done to help patients comply with treatment plan.
- ☐ **Impact of educational interventions:** Ability to manage own care after teaching has been done.

Evaluating an Individual Plan of Care

Evaluating an individual plan includes going through all the steps of the nursing process, as shown in the following diagram.

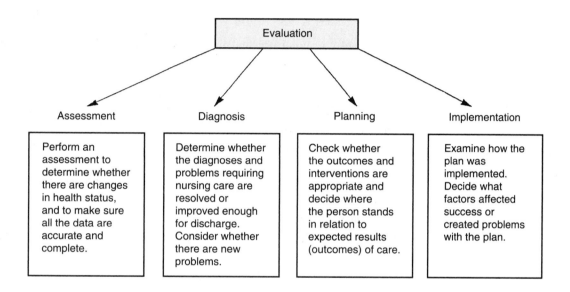

Once you complete these steps, you're ready to decide whether to continue, modify, or terminate the plan.

Determining Outcome Achievement

The following steps are suggested to evaluate outcome achievement.

Steps for Evaluating Outcome Achievement

1. Determine current health status and readiness to test for outcome achievement.
2. List the outcomes set forth in *Planning*.

E X A M P L E

"Will walk unassisted with crutches the length of the hall by 7/3."

3. Compare what the person is able to do in relation to the outcomes.

E X A M P L E

"Can walk unassisted the length of the hall but becomes unsteady toward the end of the hall."

4. Decide the extent of outcome achievement by asking the following questions:
   • Have the outcomes been completely met?
   • Have the outcomes been partially met?
   • Have the outcomes not at all been met?
5. Record your findings on the patient or client record (progress notes, plan of care).

Identifying Variables Affecting Outcome Achievement

Identifying the variables (factors) affecting outcome achievement requires analyzing information gained from assessing the patient and chart. You need to answer the following questions:

1. Were the outcomes and interventions realistic and appropriate for this individual?
2. Were the interventions consistently implemented as prescribed?
3. Were new problems or adverse responses detected early, and were appropriate changes made?
4. What's the person's opinion concerning outcome achievement and the plan of care?
5. What factors impeded progress?
6. What factors enhanced progress?
7. Do we need to search the literature for applicable research and practice articles? (This is especially important in complex situations.)

Deciding Whether to Continue, Modify, or Terminate the Plan

The final step is deciding whether to continue, modify, or terminate the plan.

• **Continue the plan** if the person hasn't achieved outcomes, but you haven't identified any factors that impeded or enhanced care and simply require more time. (Keep in mind that people failing to achieve desired outcomes in the expected time frame are demonstrating a *care variance*, which should be evaluated by a case manager.)

DISPLAY 6–2   Steps for Terminating the Plan of Care

1. Determine how health care will be managed at home (see Display 4–4, page 138, for the types of questions to ask for discharge).
2. Give verbal and written instructions for:
   ☐ Treatments, medications, activities, diet.
   ☐ What signs and symptoms to report.
   ☐ How to reach relevant community resources.
3. Ask the person to repeat (or show you) what has been learned (notes or instructions may be used to jog memory).
4. If the person (or caregiver) demonstrates knowledge of how to manage health care at home, terminate the plan according to facility policy.

- **Modify the plan** when outcomes haven't been achieved, when you identify new problems or risk factors, or when you identify ways to make care more effective.
- **Terminate the plan** if the person has achieved outcomes, has no new problems or risk factors, and demonstrates ability to care for herself. Display 6–2 gives steps for terminating the plan.

CRITICAL THINKING EXERCISE XVII

Determining Outcome Achievement, Identifying Variables Affecting Achievement, and Deciding Whether to Continue, Modify, or Terminate the Plan

To complete this session, read pages 190–193. Example responses can be found on page 248.

Part I.

Outcome Achievement. For each number below, compare the outcome criteria with the listed observable patient data. Circle "A" if the outcome has been *achieved*. Circle "P" if the outcome has only been *partially* met. Circle "N" if the outcome has *not* been met.

1. **Outcome:** Will demonstrate self-injection of insulin using aseptic technique.

   Observable Data: Able to give actual injection well, but I had to first point out she had contaminated the needle without noticing it.

   Answer: A P N

2. **Outcome:** Will demonstrate safe walking with crutches, including climbing and descending stairs.

   Observable Data: Demonstrates ability to use crutches for walking, climbing, and descending without problems.

   Answer: A P N

3. **Outcome:** Will relate the effect of increased exercise on insulin demand.

   Observable Data: States that insulin demand is not affected by increased exercise.

   Answer: A P N

4. **Outcome:** Will maintain skin free from signs of irritation.

   Observable Data: Skin is intact with some reddened areas noted on both elbows.

   Answer: A P N

5. **Outcome:** Will list the signs and symptoms of infection.

VOICES

Quality Improvement Ensures Patients Are Top Priority. The [QI] process is extremely important, because it not only contributes to the survival of healthcare institutions in a rapidly changing market, but also ensures that patients remain the primary focus of care delivery.—*Lyn Wooten, RN, MSN*

(Wooten, L. [2001]. Research corner: Focus is on continuous quality improvement process. *AACN News, 18*[1], 4.)

Observable Data: Lists pain, swelling, and drainage.

Answer: A P N

Part II.

How do you know whether to terminate, continue, or modify the plan?

Ongoing, Systematic Evaluation for Quality Improvement (QI)

The concept of QI is based on the philosophy that quality of health care always can be improved—what's considered acceptable quality today may be substandard tomorrow, especially if you consider modern advances such as diagnostic and treatment modalities, computers, and communication systems.

Almost every facility has a QI committee whose charge is to examine and improve care by doing three things:

1. **Staying up to date on research and practice articles** related to current care practices (eg, searching online each month for the latest pain management articles).
2. **Performing systematic and focused evaluation of patient records.** For example, consider the following case study, which shows how collecting and reviewing data about specific problems offers insight into how well care management practices are working and how they can be improved.
3. **Determining best practices and recommending improvement** based on evidence from clinical and research studies.

CASE STUDY

A QI nurse was studying data about how long patients stayed in the hospital for certain problems. He noted that patients who came to his hospital with pneumonia stayed 1 day longer than patients with the same diagnosis in most hospitals. He recognized this to be a problem: Why did it take patients in his hospital 1 day longer to get well enough to go home? After an in-depth study of the records of all patients who were admitted with pneumonia in the previous 2 years, he identified a simple but crucial delay in health care delivery: antibiotics weren't coming from the pharmacy in a timely fashion. On the whole, patients in his hospital started on antibiotics 12 to 24 hours after admission (compared to within 4 hours at other hospitals). Based on this information, new policies were made to ensure that antibiotics and other important medications were delivered to patient units immediately and were given within 4 hours of admission. The problem with length of stay was resolved.

Health Care Systems: Constantly Interacting and Affecting Outcomes

One of the most important things we know from years of QI studies is this: To identify strategies to correct or improve problems, you *must* look at how health care delivery systems are organized and how they all come together to affect patient outcomes. For instance, the case study just given shows a how a simple systems problem (the problem with drugs arriving late from the pharmacy) makes a major impact on outcomes for patients with pneumonia. Remember the following rule:

RULE ▶

> Patient outcomes—whether or not patients fare well—are greatly affected by how care delivery systems interact with one another. For example, patients are directly affected by whether the dietary, pharmacy, and nursing departments come together to give essential nourishment and treatments in a timely way. To prevent errors and improve efficiency, examine and reflect on how health care systems interact and impact on patient outcomes.

Think About It

Dietary and Housekeeping *Are* Your Job. *Don't allow yourself to fall into the "it's not my job" mentality. If there's a problem that's delaying or compromising patient care—whether it's insufficient linens, meal trays that are consistently late, or transport people who come ill equipped to take people for studies—it is your job to be sure that these problems are addressed. Avoid "Band-Aid solutions," ones that are quick fixes only (eg, borrowing linens all the time or consistently taking your time to call the dietary department about the same problem). Rather, report these types of problems to your supervisor so that department leaders can work together to address key issues.*

Three Types of Evaluation: Outcome, Process, and Structure

To ensure thorough monitoring of health care practices, QI studies should consider three types of evaluation:

Outcome Evaluation: Focuses on the *results,* or *outcomes* of care (eg, Were outcomes achieved? Are people satisfied with care?).

Process Evaluation: Focuses on *how the care was given* (eg, Were assessments and interventions performed consistently and in a timely way?).

Structure Evaluation: Focuses on the *setting* in which the care takes place (eg, Were the physical environment, staffing patterns, and organization communication practices adequate for efficient care management?).

Considering all three types of evaluation—outcome, process, and structure—provides a comprehensive examination of care management. Display 6–3 shows example questions for all three types of studies.

DISPLAY 6–3   Examples of Questions to Ask for Three Types
of QI Studies

- **Outcome Evaluation (focus on results):** How many of our patients undergoing emergency bowel surgery experience an infection severe enough to delay discharge?
- **Process Evaluation (focus on how care was given):** At what point was each of our patients undergoing emergency bowel surgery first given antibiotics?
- **Structure Evaluation (focus on setting):** In what setting were antibiotics given to each of our patients undergoing emergency bowel surgery (eg, emergency department, operating room, medical–surgical floor)?

Think About It

Use Three Approaches to Preventing Mistakes. *Although studies show that most mistakes result from basic flaws in the way the health system is organized, we all share accountability for ensuring patient safety:*
1. *Pay attention to things that you're doing that may create risk for errors.*
2. *Report systems that fail to adequately protect patients (eg, let the risk management department know if you think of a potential change in a policy or procedure that could reduce chances for human error).*
3. *Empower your patients by teaching them what to expect and letting them know that the main thing they can do to prevent mistakes is to become actively involved in managing their own care.*

Staff Nurses' Role

All staff nurses are accountable for participating in QI (most often for data collection and tracking outcomes). Although some of these QI studies may seem long and complicated, as the bedside nurse, you can make a valuable contribution to QI. Keep in mind the following:

- Be willing to get involved. As a nurse, you spend the most time with patients; if you see human problems or problems with hospital policies or procedures, report them to your supervising nurse. If you're asked to do extra documentation for the purpose of these studies, realize that the information gained from the records is essential to improving quality. Remember the following rule:

R U L E ▶

A large part of QI is focusing on your *own* personal improvement. Constantly reflect on how you can be more organized and prepared to meet your patients' needs. Be creative—think of ways you can overcome your limitations (eg, I developed the personal worksheet on page 165 to overcome my problem with getting organized during report; lots of nurses carry with them little notes and references that help them remember certain information).

- How you document is important. The records you create through ongoing documentation provide the basis for research that can benefit both health care consumers and nurses.
- QI studies may seem complicated and detailed, but they make your job more efficient and may make your (or your family's) next contact with the health care system more efficient.

Think About It

Holistic and Complementary Therapies Improve Quality. *Improving quality means considering all aspects of health care, including considering whether holistic and complementary therapies can improve results and reduce need for treatments such as medications. For example, music therapy has been used to help children with cerebral palsy improve balance, to help stroke survivors learn how to walk again, and to help women in labor feel less pain. Music therapy can make the difference between withdrawal and awareness, between isolation and interaction, between chronic pain and comfort—between demoralization and dignity. (From American Music Therapy Association. [2001]. [On-line]. Available: http://www.namt.com/quotes.html. Accessed January 20, 2001.)*

Summary

Critical evaluation—careful, deliberate, and detailed evaluation of various aspects of patient care—is the key to excellence in health care delivery. *Evaluation* in the context of nursing process usually refers to determining the effectiveness of an individual plan of care (ie, Did the patient achieve the outcomes in a timely manner?). Within the context of QI, *Evaluation* refers to ongoing studies of *groups of patients* to examine the effectiveness of care delivery practices. Comprehensive QI studies evaluate outcomes (results), process (how care was given), and structure (the setting in which care was given). Keep in mind that continuous improvement requires examining how health care delivery systems interact and impact on patient outcomes. You're responsible for improving your own ability to serve patients and for recognizing and reporting problems related to other departments (eg, dietary and pharmacy).

CRITICAL THINKING EXERCISE XVIII

Quality | *To complete this session, read pages 190–197. Example responses can be found on*
Improvement | *page 248.*

1. In five sentences (or phrases) or less, explain why QI studies are important.

2. Why is it important to consider outcome, process, and structure when performing QI studies?

3. Focusing on at least three different approaches to error prevention, write a personal plan for reducing risks of errors in your nursing practice.

Try This On Your Own

Visit *http://www.ahcpr.gov/,* **the home page of the Agency for Healthcare Research and Quality,** where you can find a wealth of clinical and consumer information from how to quit smoking and assess health plans (consumer information) to practice guidelines and information on outcomes and effectiveness (clinical information). Pick a few topics that interest you and see what you can learn.

Evaluate your knowledge of this chapter. Check to see if you can achieve the learning outcomes on page 188.
Bibliography: See pages 199–201.

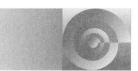

Bibliography

Alfaro-LeFevre, R. (2000a). Critical thinking is not usually rapid fire. *AACN News, 2,* 12.

Alfaro-LeFevre, R. (2000b). Don't worry! Be happy! Harmonize diversity through personality sensitivity. *Nursing Spectrum, 10* (16FL), 14–17. Available: *http://nsweb.nursingspectrum.com/ce/ce236.htm.*

Alfaro-LeFevre, R. (2000c). Improving your ability to think critically. [On-line]. Available: *http://nsweb. nursingspectrum.com/ce/ce168.htm.*

Alfaro-LeFevre, R. (1999a). *Critical thinking in nursing: A practical approach* (2nd ed.). Philadelphia: W.B. Saunders.

Alfaro-LeFevre, R. (1999b). *Instructor's manual for critical thinking in nursing: A practical approach.* Philadelphia: W.B. Saunders.

American Nurses Association. (1999). *Nursing quality indicators: Guide for implementation* (2nd ed.). Washington, DC: American Nurses Publishing.

American Nurses Association. (1998). *Standards of Clinical Practice* (2nd ed.). Washington, DC: American Nurses Publishing.

American Nurses Association. (1995). *Nursing: A social policy statement.* Kansas City, MO: Author.

American Nurses Association. (1994). *Registered professional nurses and unlicensed assistive personnel.* Washington, DC: American Nurses Publishing.

American Nurses Association. (1985). *Code of ethics for nurses with interpretive statements.* Washington, DC: American Nurses Publishing.

American Nursing Association's Code of Ethics Task Force. (2000). A new code of ethics for nurses. *American Journal of Nursing, 100*(7), 70–71.

Andrews, M., & Boyle, J. (1999). *Transcultural concepts in nursing care* (3rd ed.). Philadelphia: Lippincott Williams & Wilkins.

Aquilino, M., & Keenan, G. (2000). Having our say. *American Journal of Nursing, 100*(7), 33–38.

Benner, P. (2001). *From novice to expert.* Upper Saddle River, NJ: Prentice Hall.

Benner, P. (1982). Issues in competency-based testing. *Nursing Outlook, 30*(5), 303–309.

Berry, R. (1993a). Effective patient education, part 1: Teaching adults. *Nursing Spectrum* (PA Ed), *2*(23), 14–16.

Berry, R. (1993b). Effective patient education, part 2: Teaching children. *Nursing Spectrum* (PA Ed), *2*(24), 14–15.

Beyea, S. (Ed.). (2000). *The perioperative nursing data set.* Denver, CO: American Association of Perioperative Nurses.

Burfitt, S., Greiner, D., & Miers, L. (1993). Professional nurse caring as perceived by critically ill patients: A phenomenologic study. *American Journal of Critical Care, 2*(6), 489–549.

Burke, L., & Murphy, J. (1995). *Charting by exception: A cost-effective, quality approach.* Albany, NY: Delmar.

Canadian Nurses Association. (1987). *A definition of nursing practice: Standards for nursing practice* (Publication No. ISBNB 0-919 108-52-2). Ottawa, Canada: Author.

Carpenito, L. (2000a). *Handbook of nursing diagnosis* (8th ed.). Philadelphia: Lippincott Williams & Wilkins.

Carpenito, L. (2000b). *Nursing diagnosis: Application to clinical practice* (8th ed.). Philadelphia: Lippincott Williams & Wilkins.

Clark, C. (1999). *Integrating complementary health procedures into practice.* New York: Springer.

Coehn, E. (2000). *Nursing case management: From essentials to advanced practice application* (3rd ed.). St. Louis: Mosby.

Community Health Accreditation Program (CHAP). (1993). *Standards for excellence for home care organizations* (Publication No. 21-2327). New York: National League for Nurses and CHAP.

Covey, S. (1989). *The seven habits of highly effective people.* New York: Simon & Schuster.

Craft-Rosenberg, M., & Delaney, C. (1997). The keystone to a unified language. In M. Rentz & P. LeMone (Eds.), *Classification of nursing diagnosis: Proceedings of the Twelfth National Conference.* Glendale, CA: CINAHL.

Davidson, S., & Scott, R. (1999). Thinking critically about delegation. *American Journal of Nursing, 99*(6), 61–62.

DeCastillo, S. (1999). *Strategies, techniques, and approaches to thinking*. Philadelphia: W.B. Saunders.

DiVito-Thomas, P. (2000). Identifying critical thinking behaviors in clinical judgments. *Journal of Nursing Staff Development, 3*(16), 174–180.

Doble, R., Curley, M., Hession-Laband, E., Marino, B., & Shaw, S. (2000). The synergy model in practice. *Critical Care Nurse, 20*(3), 86–91.

Duchscher, J. (1999). Catching the wave: Understanding the concept of critical thinking. *Journal of Advanced Nursing, 29*(3), 577–583.

Edge, R., & Groves, J. (1999). *Ethics of health care: A guide for clinical practice*. Albany, NY: Delmar.

Fields, S. (1991). History-taking in the elderly: Obtaining useful information. *Geriatrics, 46*(8), 26–34.

Fielo, S. (2000). Screening: How to change world health. [On-line]. Available: *http://nsweb.nursingspectrum. com/ce/ce211.htm*. Accessed January 18, 2001.

Fischbach, F. (2000). *A manual of diagnostic tests*. Philadelphia: Lippincott Williams & Wilkins.

Fonteyn, M. (1999). *Thinking strategies for nursing*. Philadelphia: Lippincott Williams & Wilkins.

Foster, P. (1993). Helping students learn to make ethical decisions. *Holistic Nurse Practice, 7*(3), 28–35.

Good, V., & Schulman, C. (2000). Employee competency pathways. *Critical Care Nurse, 20*(3), 75–85.

Gordon, M. (1994). *Nursing diagnosis: Process and application* (3rd ed.). St. Louis, MO: Mosby-Year Book.

Grossman, S., & Valiga, T. (2000). *The new leadership challenge: Creating the future of nursing*. Philadelphia: F.A. Davis.

Gryfinski, J., & Lampe, S. (1990). Implementing focus charting: Process and critique. *Clinical Nurse Specialist, 4*(4), 201–205.

Hansten, R., & Washburn, M. (2001). Delegating to UAPs. [On-line]. Available: *http://www.nurseweek. com/ce/ce1680a.html*. Accessed February 7, 2001.

Hansten, R., & Washburn, M. (1999). Outcome-based care: An alternative to extensive redesign. *ADVISOR for Nurse Executives, 15*(2),12.

Hansten, R., & Washburn, M. (1998). *Clinical delegation skills: A handbook for professional practice* (2nd ed.). Gathersburg, MD: Aspen Publishers.

Hansten, R., Washburn, M., & Kenyon, V. (1999). *Home care nursing delegation skills: A handbook for practice*. Gathersburg, MD: Aspen Publishers.

Healthy People 2010 Objectives: Draft for public comment. [On-line]. Accessed from: *www.health.gov/healthy people*.

Hoffman, L., Wesmiller, S., Sciurba, F., Johnson, J., Ferson, P., Zullo, T., & Dauber, M. (1992). Nasal cannula and transtracheal oxygen delivery: A comparison of patient response after 6 months of each technique. *American Review of Respiratory Disease, 145*(4), 827–831.

Iyer, P., & Camp, N. (1999). *Nursing documentation: A nursing process approach* (3rd ed.). St. Louis, MO: Mosby-Year Book.

Johnson, M., Maas, M., & Moorehead, S. (2000). *Nursing outcomes classification* (2nd ed.). St. Louis, MO: Mosby.

Johnson, M., Bulechek, G., McCloskey Dochterman, J., Maas, M, & Moorehead S. (2001). *Nursing diagnoses, outcomes, and interventions: NANDA, NIC, NOC linkages*. St. Louis, MO: Mosby.

Johnstone, M. (1999). *Bioethics: A nursing perspective* (3rd ed.). Sydney, Australia: W.B. Saunders/Bailliere Tindall.

Joint Commission on Accreditation of Healthcare Organizations. (2000). *JCAHO and HCFA: Understanding the requirements for hospitals*. Oakbrook Terrace, IL: Author.

Jones, J.A. (1988). Clinical reasoning: Ethics, science, art. *Journal of Advanced Nursing, 13*(2), 185–192.

Krumberger, J. (1996). Culture: An inextricable component of care. *Critical Care Nurse, 16*(3), 118.

Lamond, D. , & Thompson, C. (2000). Intuition and analysis in decision making and choice. *Journal of Nursing Scholarship, 32*(3), 411–414.

Lampe, S. (1997). *Focus charting®: Documentation for patient-centered care* (7th ed.). Minneapolis, MN: Creative Nursing Management.

Lang, N. (Ed.). (1995). *Nursing data systems: The emerging framework*. Washington, DC: American Nursing Publishing.

Manion, J. (1998). *From management to leadership*. Chicago: American Hospital Publishers, Inc.

Manion, J. (1995). Understanding the seven stages of change. *American Journal of Nursing, 95*(4), 41–43.

Martin, K. (1999). The Omaha system: Past, present, and future. *On-Line Journal of Nursing Informatics*. Available: *http://cac.psu.edu/~dxm12/ojni.html*. Accessed August 1, 2000.

Martin, K., & Scheet, N. (1992). *The Omaha system: Applications for community health nursing*. Philadelphia: W.B. Saunders.

Mastal, M. (2000). Making the grade. *Nursing Spectrum, 10*(30FL), 8–9.

Maslow, A. (1970). *Motivation in personality.* New York: Harper & Row.

McCloskey, J., & Bulechek, G. (Eds.). (2000). *Nursing interventions classification (NIC): Iowa intervention project* (3rd ed.). St. Louis, MO: Mosby.

McIntosh, T. (1997). Empathy: Why patients recommend hospitals. *Healthcare Benchmarks, 4,* 39.

National Council of State Boards of Nursing (NCSBN). (1995, December). Delegation: Concepts and decision-making process. *Issues, December,* 1–4.

North American Nursing Diagnosis Association (NANDA). (2001). *Nursing diagnoses: Definitions and classification 2001–2002.* Philadelphia: Author.

Orem, D. (1980). *Nursing: Concepts of practice* (2nd ed.). New York: McGraw-Hill.

Ozbolt, J. (2001). Strategies for building nursing databases for effective nursing research. [On-line]. Available: *http://www.nih.gov/ninr/POR_Conf/ozbolt.pdf.* Accessed February 1, 2001.

Ozbolt, J.G. (1992). Strategies for building nursing databases for effectiveness research. In *Patient outcomes research: Examining the effectiveness of nursing practice* (NIH Publication No. 93-3411; pp. 210–218). Bethesda, MD: National Center for Nursing Research, National Institutes of Health.

Paul, R., & Binker, A. (Eds.). (1995). *Critical thinking: What every person needs to survive in a rapidly changing world.* Rohner Park, CA: Foundation for Critical Thinking and Moral Development.

Pesut, D., & Herman, J. (1999). *Clinical reasoning.* Albany, NY: Delmar Publishers.

Rehabilitation Nursing Foundation's Nursing Diagnosis Publications Task Force. (1995). *21 Rehabilitation nursing diagnoses.* Glenview, IL: Rehabilitation Nursing Foundation.

Rentz, M., & LeMone, P. (1997). *Classification of nursing diagnosis: Proceedings of the Twelfth National Conference.* Glendale, CA: CINAHL Information Systems.

Richardson, S. (2001). Making a spiritual assessment. *Nursing Spectrum, 11*(2FL), 12–15.

Rogers, P., & Bocchino, N. (1999). Is it possible? *American Journal of Nursing, 99*(10), 17.

Secretary's Commission on Achieving Necessary Skills. (1992). *Learning a living: A blueprint for high performance. A SCANS report for America 2000.* Washington, DC: U.S. Department of Labor.

Sheahan, S. (2000). Documentation of health risks and health promotion counseling by emergency department nurse practitioners and physicians. *Journal of Nursing Scholarship, 32*(3), 245–250.

Silver, J., & Winland-Brown, J. (2000). Power asymmetry and patient autonomy. *American Journal of Critical Care, 9*(5), 360–361.

Stevens, K. (2000). Mentoring on the cutting edge. *Reflections on Nursing Leadership, 26*(1), 31–32, 46.

Sugars, D., O'Neil, E., & Bader, J. (Eds.). (1991). *Healthy America practitioners for 2005: An agenda for action for U.S. health professional schools.* San Francisco, CA: The Pew Health Professions Commission.

Tanner, C. (1993). Thinking about critical thinking. *Journal of Nursing Education, 32*(9), 99–100.

Tanner, C. (1983). Research on clinical judgment. In W.L. Holzemer (Ed.), *Review of research in nursing education* (pp.1–32). Thorofare, NJ: Charles B. Slack.

Tanner, C., Benner, P., Chesla, C., & Gordon, D. (1993). The phenomenology of knowing the patient. *Image, 25*(4), 273–280.

Taylor, C., Lillis, C., & LeMone, P. (2001). *Fundamentals of nursing: The art and science of nursing care* (4th ed.). Philadelphia: Lippincott Williams & Wilkins.

Tompson, C., & Rebeschi, L. (1999). Critical thinking skills of baccalaureate nursing students at program entry and exit. *NLN Journal: Nursing and Health Care Perspectives, 20*(5), 248–254.

U.S. Department of Health and Human Services. (1996). *Healthy people 2000: Review 1995–1996.* Washington, DC: U.S. Government Printing Office.

U.S. Department of Health and Human Services, Public Health Service. (1990). *Healthy people 2000* (DHHS Publication No. [PHS] 91-50212). Washington, DC: Superintendent of Documents, U.S. Government Printing Office.

Valanis B. (1999). *Epidemiology in health care* (3rd ed). Stamford, CT: Appleton & Lange.

Webber, J., & Kelley, J. (1998). *Health assessment in nursing.* Philadelphia: Lippincott Williams & Wilkins.

Wells, S. (1996). Adding an "at home" path to your discharge plan. *American Journal of Nursing, 96*(10), 73–74.

Wilkinson, J. (2001). *Nursing process and critical thinking* (3rd ed.). Upper Saddle River, NJ: Prentice Hall.

Wolf, Z., Brennan, R., Ferchau, L., Magee, M., et al. (1997). Creating and implementing guidelines on caring for difficult patients: A research utilization project. *MEDSURG Nursing, 6*(3), 137–147.

Wolfe, Z., Serembus, J., Smetzer, J., Cohen, H., & Cohen, M. (2000). Responses of healthcare providers to medication errors. *Clinical Nurse Specialist: The Journal for Advanced Nursing Practice, 14*(6), 34–51.

Nursing Diagnoses

Organized alphabetically, this section is designed to provide you with easy access to basic information about commonly used diagnoses accepted for clinical testing by the North American Nursing Diagnosis Association (NANDA). This section is divided into three parts:

Part 1. Description of NANDA Taxonomy II domains and definitions of descriptors used in Taxonomy II. All of the diagnoses in parts 2 and 3 are listed using the new descriptors from Taxonomy II (see page 204)

Part 2. Alphabetical listing of all diagnoses accepted for testing as of 2001 (for listing according to Gordon's Functional Health Patterns, see inside back cover). Diagnoses listed with the symbol * after them aren't included in the quick reference section because they aren't yet well developed. For in-depth information on all of the diagnoses, I recommend that you read *Nursing Diagnosis: Definitions and Classifications 2001–2002* by NANDA and *Nursing Diagnosis: Clinical Application to Practice* by Lynda Carpenito.

Part 3. Quick Reference Guide (page 206). The definitions listed in this section are NANDA definitions unless otherwise stated, with minor adaptation in some cases for clarity. The information listed under the headings *Defining Characteristics, Related Factors, and Risk Factors* has been adapted from NANDA's *Nursing Diagnosis: Definitions and Classifications 2001–2002.*

Part 1.

NANDA Taxonomy II Domains[1]

Domain 1. Health Promotion: the awareness of well-being or normality of function and the strategies used to maintain control of and enhancement of that well-being or normality of function.

Domain 2. Nutrition: the activities of taking in, assimilating, and using nutrients for the purposes of tissue maintenance, tissue repair, and the production of energy.

Domain 3. Elimination: secretion and excretion of waste products from the body.

Domain 4. Activity/Rest: the productions, conservation, expenditures, or balance of energy resources.

Domain 5. Perception/Cognition: the human information processing system including attention, orientation, sensation, perception, cognition, and comprehension.

Domain 6. Self perception: awareness of the self.

Domain 7. Role Relationships: the positive and negative connections or associations between persons or groups of persons and the means by which those connections are demonstrated.

Domain 8. Sexuality: sexual identity, sexual function, and reproduction.

Domain 9. Coping/Stress Tolerance: contending with life events/life processes.

Domain 10. Life Principles: principles underlying conduct, thought, and behavior about acts, customs, or institutions viewed as being true or having intrinsic worth (eg, values and beliefs).

Domain 11. Safety/Protection: freedom from danger, physical injury, or immune system damage; preservation from loss; and protections of safety and security.

Domain 12. Comfort: sense of mental, physical, or social well-being or ease.

Domain 13. Growth/Development: age-appropriate

[1]Data from NANDA. (2001). pp. 221–232.

increases in physical dimensions, organ systems, and attainment of developmental milestones.

Taxonomy II NANDA Descriptors[2]

- *Ability:* Capacity to do or act
- *Anticipatory:* To realize beforehand, foresee
- *Balance:* State of equilibrium
- *Compromised:* To make vulnerable to threat
- *Decreased:* Lessened; lesser in size, amount or degree
- *Deficient:* Inadequate in amount, quality or degree; not sufficient; incomplete
- *Delayed:* To postpone, impede, and retard
- *Depleted:* Emptied wholly or in part, exhausted of
- *Disproportionate:* Not consistent with a standard
- *Disabling:* To make unable or unfit, to incapacitate
- *Disorganized:* To destroy the systematic arrangement
- *Disturbed:* Agitated or interrupted, interfered with
- *Dysfunctional:* Abnormal, incomplete functioning
- *Effective:* Producing the intended or expected effect
- *Excessive:* Characterized by an amount or quantity that is greater than necessary, desirable, or useful
- *Functional:* Normal complete functioning
- *Imbalanced:* State of disequilibrium
- *Impaired:* Made worse, weakened, damaged, reduced, deteriorated
- *Inability:* Incapacity to do or act
- *Increased:* Greater in size, amount or degree
- *Ineffective:* Not producing the desired effect
- *Interrupted:* To break the continuity or uniformity
- *Organized:* To form as into a systematic arrangement
- *Perceived:* To become aware of by means of the senses; assignment of meaning
- *Readiness for enhanced* (for use with wellness diagnoses): To make greater, to increase in quality, to attain the more desired

Part 2.

Alphabetical Listing of Diagnoses Accepted for Testing by NANDA

Note: Diagnoses are listed using revised descriptors from NANDA Taxonomy II (see above).

[2]From NANDA. (2001). p. 219.

Activity Intolerance
Activity Intolerance, Risk for
Adaptive Capacity: Intracranial, Decreased*
Adjustment, Impaired
Airway Clearance, Ineffective
Anxiety
Anxiety, Death*
Aspiration, Risk for
Autonomic Dysreflexia
Autonomic Dysreflexia, Risk for

Body Image, Disturbed
Body Temperature, Risk for Imbalanced
Bowel Incontinence
Breastfeeding, Effective*
Breastfeeding, Ineffective
Breastfeeding, Interrupted
Breathing Pattern, Ineffective

Cardiac Output, Decreased
Caregiver Role Strain
Caregiver Role Strain, Risk for
Communication, Impaired†
Communication, Impaired Verbal
Confusion, Acute
Confusion, Chronic
Constipation
Constipation, Colonic
Constipation, Perceived
Constipation, Risk for
Coping, Defensive
Coping, Family, Compromised
Coping, Family, Disabled
Coping, Family, Readiness for enhanced
Coping, Ineffective
Coping, Ineffective Community
Coping, Readiness for Enhanced Community

Decisional Conflict (Specify)
Denial, Ineffective
Dentition, Impaired
Development, Delayed, Risk for
Diarrhea
Disuse Syndrome, Risk for
Diversional Activity Deficit

Energy Field, Disturbed
Environmental Interpretation Syndrome, Impaired

*Diagnosis not included in Quick Reference section because it has little clinical usefulness or isn't well developed.

†Added by author; not on NANDA list as of 2001.

Failure to thrive, Adult
Falls, Risk for
Family Coping, Compromised
Family Coping, Disabled
Family Coping, Readiness for Enhanced
Family Process, Dysfunctional: Alcoholism
Family Processes, Interrupted
Fatigue
Fear
Fluid Volume, Deficient
Fluid Volume, Deficient, Risk for
Fluid Volume Excess
Fluid Volume, Imbalanced, Risk for

Gas Exchange, Impaired
Grieving[†]
Grieving, Anticipatory
Grieving, Dysfunctional
Growth, Risk for Disproportionate*
Growth and Development, Delayed

Health-Seeking Behaviors (Specify)
Health Maintenance, Ineffective
Home maintenance, Impaired
Hopelessness
Hyperthermia
Hypothermia

Infant Behavior, Disorganized
Infant Behavior, Disorganized, Risk for
Infant Behavior, Readiness for Enhanced
    Organized
Infant Feeding Pattern, Ineffective
Infection, Risk for
Injury, Risk for

Knowledge, Deficient (Specify)

Latex Allergy Response
Latex Allergy Response, Risk for
Loneliness, Risk for

Memory, Impaired
Mobility, Bed, Impaired*
Mobility, Impaired Physical

Nausea*
Noncompliance (Specify)
Nutrition, Imbalanced: Less than Body Requirements
Nutrition, Imbalanced: More than Body
    Requirements
Nutrition, Imbalanced: Risk for More than Body
    Requirements

Oral Mucous Membrane, Impaired

Pain, Acute
Pain, Chronic
Parental Role Conflict
Parent–Infant/Child Attachment, Risk for Impaired
Parenting, Impaired
Parenting, Risk for Impaired
Perioperative Positioning Injury, Risk for
Peripheral Neurovascular Dysfunction, Risk for
Personal identity, Disturbed
Poisoning, Risk for
Post-Trauma Response
Powerlessness
Powerlessness, Risk for*
Protection, Ineffective

Rape Trauma Syndrome[3]
Relocation Stress Syndrome
Relocation Stress Syndrome, Risk for
Role Performance, Ineffective

Self-Care Deficit, Bathing/Hygiene
Self-Care Deficit, Dressing/Grooming
Self-Care Deficit, Feeding
Self-Care Deficit, Toileting
Self-Esteem, Chronic Low
Self-Esteem Disturbance
Self-Esteem, Situational Low
Self-Esteem, Situational Low, Risk for
Self-Mutilation, Risk for
Sensory Perception, Disturbed (Specify: visual, auditory, kinesthetic, gustatory, tactile, olfactory)
Sexual Dysfunction
Sexuality Patterns, Ineffective
Skin Integrity, Impaired
Skin Integrity, Risk for Impaired
Sleep deprivation*
Sleep pattern, Disturbed
Social Interaction, Impaired
Social Isolation
Sorrow, Chronic*
Spiritual Distress
Spiritual Well-Being, Readiness for Enhanced
Suffocation, Risk for
Suicide, Risk for
Surgical Recovery, Delayed*
Swallowing, Impaired

---

[3]NANDA lists this as three different diagnoses (*Rape Trauma Syndrome, Rape Trauma Syndrome: Silent Reaction, Rape Trauma Syndrome: Compound Reaction*), all with the same definition.

Therapeutic Regimen, Ineffective Community
    Management of
Therapeutic Regimen, Ineffective Family
    Management of
Therapeutic Regimen, Effective Management of
Therapeutic Regimen, Ineffective Management of
Thermoregulation, Ineffective
Thought Processes, Impaired
Tissue Integrity, Impaired
Tissue Perfusion, Ineffective (Specify: renal,
    cerebral, cardiopulmonary, gastrointestinal,
    peripheral)
Transfer Ability, Impaired*
Trauma, Risk for

Unilateral Neglect
Urinary Elimination, Impaired
Urinary Incontinence, Functional
Urinary Incontinence, Reflex
Urinary Incontinence, Stress
Urinary Incontinence, Total
Urinary Incontinence, Urge
Urinary Incontinence, Urge, Risk For*
Urinary Retention

Ventilation, Impaired Spontaneous
Ventilatory Weaning Response, Dysfunctional
    (DVWR)
Violence, Other-directed, Risk for
Violence, Self-directed, Risk For

Walking, Impaired*
Wandering*
Wheelchair Mobility, Impaired

Part 3. Quick Reference Guide

Activity Intolerance

A state in which an individual has insufficient energy
to endure or complete required or desired daily
activities.

• Defining Characteristics

— *SUBJECTIVE DATA* (reported) —

Weakness or fatigue, exertional discomfort or dyspnea, reduced ability to perform desired activities.

— *OBJECTIVE DATA* (observed) —

Abnormal heart rate and blood pressure response to activity, electrocardiograph changes reflecting arrhythmias or ischemia.

• Related Factors

Deconditioned state (bed rest or immobility), generalized weakness, sedentary lifestyle, aging process, disease process (imbalance between oxygen supply and
demand, acute or chronic illness), medication side effects.

• Clinical Alert

Activity Intolerance often is related to compromised
respiratory, cardiac, or circulatory function.

• Compare With

*Activity Intolerance, Risk for; Disuse Syndrome, Risk
for; Fatigue.*

Activity Intolerance, Risk for

A state in which an individual is at risk for experiencing insufficient energy to endure or complete required
or desired daily activities.

• Risk Factors

See Related Factors for *Activity Intolerance.*

Adjustment, Impaired

The state in which a person is unable to modify his or
her lifestyle or behavior in a manner that promotes
adaptation to a change in health status.

• Defining Characteristics

— *SUBJECTIVE DATA* (reported) —

Nonacceptance of health status change; extended period of shock, disbelief, or anger regarding health status change; lack of future-oriented thinking.

— *OBJECTIVE DATA* (observed) —

Nonexistent or ineffective involvement in problem
solving or goal setting, lack of movement toward independence.

• Related Factors

Disability requiring change in lifestyle, inadequate
support systems, impaired cognition, sensory over-

load, assault to self-esteem, impaired locus of control, incomplete grieving.

• Compare With

Coping, Ineffective; Grieving, Dysfunctional.

Airway Clearance, Ineffective

Inability to clear secretions or obstructions from the respiratory tract to maintain a clear airway.

• Defining Characteristics
— *SUBJECTIVE DATA* (reported) —

Dyspnea.

— *OBJECTIVE DATA* (observed) —

Diminished breath sounds; orthopnea; adventitious breath sounds (rales, crackles, wheezes); ineffective or absent cough; sputum; cyanosis; difficulty vocalizing; changes in rate, rhythm, or depth of respirations; restlessness.

• Related Factors

Environmental: Smoking, smoke inhalation, secondhand smoke. *Obstructed airway:* Airway spasm, retained secretions, excessive mucus, artificial airway, foreign body in airway, exudates in alveoli. *Physiologic:* Neuromuscular impairment, bronchial wall hyperplasia, chronic obstructive lung disease, asthma, allergies.

• Compare With

Aspiration, Risk for; Breathing Pattern, Ineffective.

Anxiety

Uneasiness (mild or intense), the source of which is often nonspecific or unknown to the individual.

• Defining Characteristics
— *SUBJECTIVE DATA* (reported) —

Nervousness, tension; inability to relax, concentrate, or make decisions; lack of self-confidence; feelings of uncertainty, helplessness, or inadequacy; insomnia; somatic discomfort (eg, diarrhea, headache, chest discomfort); changes in eating habits.

— *OBJECTIVE DATA* (observed) —

Restlessness; increased perspiration, pulse rate, and blood pressure; pallor; tremors; extraneous movements; lack of initiative; self-deprecation; poor eye contact.

• Related Factors

Conscious or unconscious conflict about essential values or life goals; actual or perceived threat to self-concept, role function, security, or usual interaction patterns; situational or maturational crisis (eg, pregnancy, parenting); multiple stressors or demands; sleep deprivation; fear of pain, loneliness, physical or psychological harm; inability to cope with or control situations; loss(es).

• Clinical Alert

Sudden onset of anxiety, especially in the elderly, may be an early symptom of hypotension, hypoxemia, sepsis, or coronary disorders. Monitor vital signs carefully.

• Compare With

Fear.

Aspiration, Risk for

The state in which a person is at risk for entry of gastrointestinal (GI) or oropharyngeal secretions, or solids or fluids into the tracheobronchial passages.

• Risk Factors

Reduced level of consciousness; depressed cough and gag reflexes; impaired swallowing; presence of tracheostomy or endotracheal tube; incompetent lower esophageal sphincter; increased intragastric pressure; increased gastric residual; decreased GI motility; delayed gastric emptying; GI immaturity (infants); GI tubes; tube feedings; medication administration; situations hindering elevation of upper body; facial, oral, or neck surgery or trauma; wired jaws.

• Compare With

Airway Clearance, Ineffective; Suffocation, Risk for; Swallowing, Impaired.

Autonomic Dysreflexia

The state in which a person with a spinal cord injury at T7 or above experiences a life-threatening, uninhibited, sympathetic response of the nervous system to a noxious stimulus.

• Defining Characteristics
— *SUBJECTIVE DATA* (reported) —

Headache (a diffuse pain in different portions of the head and not confined to any nerve distribution area), chilling, paresthesia, blurred vision, chest pain, metallic taste, nasal congestion.

— *OBJECTIVE DATA* (observed) —

Individual with spinal cord injury at T7 or above with: paroxysmal hypertension (sudden periodic elevated blood pressure, systolic pressure over 140 mm Hg and diastolic above 90 mm Hg); bradycardia or tachycardia (pulse rate of less than 60 or over 100 beats per minute); diaphoresis or red splotches on skin (above the injury); pallor (below the injury); conjunctival congestion; Horner's syndrome (contraction of the pupil, partial ptosis of the eyelid, enophthalmos and sometimes loss of sweating over the affected side of the face); pilomotor reflex (gooseflesh formation when skin is cooled).

• Related Factors

Bladder or bowel distention (nonpatent catheter, bladder infection, constipation, impaction); spastic sphincter; acute abdomen, abdominal or thigh skin stimulation; lack of knowledge of prevention.

• Clinical Alert

This diagnosis requires *immediate* corrective measures (eg, raising the head of the bed, removing or correcting factors listed under Related Factors). If the condition doesn't respond promptly to initial treatment, emergency treatment with pharmacologic intervention is likely to be required.

Autonomic Dysreflexia, Risk for

See Related Factors for *Autonomic Dysreflexia*.

Body Image, Disturbed

A disruption in perception of body image.

• Defining Characteristics
— *SUBJECTIVE DATA* (reported) —

Unwanted change in appearance or lifestyle; fear of rejection or reaction by others or negative feelings about body; focus on past strength, function, or appearance; emphasis on remaining strengths, heightened achievement; preoccupation with change or loss; expansion of body boundary to incorporate environmental objects; personalization of part or loss by name; depersonalization of part or loss by impersonal pronouns; refusal to verify actual change.

— *OBJECTIVE DATA* (observed) —

Missing body part, change in structure or function, not looking at body part, not touching body part, hiding or overexposing body part (intentional or unintentional), trauma to nonfunctioning part, change in social involvement, change in ability to estimate spatial relationship of body to environment.

• Related Factors

Biophysical factors such as pregnancy, chronic disease, obesity, body changes related to adolescence or aging, loss of body part or function, effects of radiation or chemotherapy; cognitive or perceptual factors such as inaccurate interpretation of body or body parts; psychosocial, cultural, or spiritual factors.

Body Temperature, Risk for Imbalanced

The state in which a person is at risk for failure to maintain body temperature within normal range.

• Risk Factors

Extremes of age, extremes of weight, exposure to cold or hot environments, dehydration, inactivity or vigorous activity, medications causing vasoconstriction or vasodilation, impaired metabolic rate, sedation, inappropriate clothing for environmental temperature, illness or trauma affecting temperature regulation, infection.

• Compare With

Hyperthermia; Hypothermia; Thermoregulation, Ineffective.

Bowel Incontinence

A change in normal bowel habits characterized by involuntary passage of stool.

• Defining Characteristics
— *OBJECTIVE DATA* (observed) —

Involuntary passage of stool.

• Related Factors

Loss of sphincter control, neuromuscular disorder, inflammatory bowel disease, decreased level of consciousness, confusion, progressive dementia, depression, *Anxiety, Diarrhea.*

• Compare With

Diarrhea.

Breastfeeding, Ineffective

The state in which a mother and infant or child experience dissatisfaction or difficulty with the breastfeeding process.

• Defining Characteristics

— *SUBJECTIVE DATA* (reported) —

Unsatisfactory breastfeeding process, inadequate milk supply, persistence of sore nipples beyond first week of breastfeeding.

— *OBJECTIVE DATA* (observed) —

Mother: insufficient emptying of breast, no observable signs of oxytocin release (ie, let-down, or milk ejection, reflex), inadequate milk supply.
Infant: inability to latch onto breast; arching and crying at the breast; nonsustained suckling; insufficient opportunity for suckling; fussing, crying, and unresponsiveness to comfort measures within the first hour after feeding; weight loss, or failure to gain.

• Related Factors

Mother: frequent supplemental feedings with artificial nipple, lack of basic breastfeeding knowledge, history of breastfeeding difficulty or failure, interrupted breastfeeding, previous breast surgery, inverted or painful nipples, engorged breasts, maternal diet inadequate in nutrients or fluids, nonsupportive partner or family, maternal anxiety or ambivalence.
Infant: gestational age less than 34 weeks, structural anomaly, poor sucking reflex.

• Compare With

Breastfeeding, Interrupted; Infant Feeding Pattern, Ineffective.

Breastfeeding, Interrupted

A break in the continuity of the breastfeeding process as a result of inability or inadvisability to put baby to breast for feeding.

• Defining Characteristics

— *SUBJECTIVE DATA* (reported) —

Desire to maintain lactation and provide (or eventually provide) breast milk for infant's nutritional needs.

— *OBJECTIVE DATA* (observed) —

Infant doesn't receive milk from breast for some or all of feedings, mother–infant separation, lack of knowledge regarding expression and storage of breast milk.

• Related Factors

Maternal or infant illness, prematurity, maternal employment, contraindication to breastfeeding (eg, drugs, true breast milk jaundice), need to abruptly wean infant.

• Compare With

Breastfeeding, Ineffective; Infant Feeding Pattern, Ineffective.

Breathing Pattern, Ineffective

The state in which a person's inhalation or exhalation pattern does not promote adequate ventilation.

• Defining Characteristics

— *SUBJECTIVE DATA* (reported) —

Dyspnea, shortness of breath.

— *OBJECTIVE DATA* (observed) —

Changes in respiratory rate or depth of respirations; changes in pulse rate or rhythm; wheezing; fremitus; cough; nasal flaring; cyanosis; decreased diaphragmatic excursion; assumption of three-point position; use of accessory muscles; orthopnea; abnormal arterial blood gases; reduced vital capacity, forced-end expiratory volume, or oxygen saturation level; splinted or guarded respirations.

• Related Factors

Neuromuscular impairment, obstructive lung disease, restrictive lung disease, musculoskeletal impairment, decreased energy, *Fatigue, Anxiety, Acute pain,* medication side effects (respiratory depression).

• Clinical Alert

Report persistent *Ineffective Breathing Pattern* not responding to nurse-prescribed interventions immediately. This is especially important if confusion or severe anxiety is present because both of these are signs of hypoxemia.

• Compare With

Activity Intolerance; Airway Clearance, Ineffective.

Cardiac Output, Decreased

A state in which the heart is unable to pump blood with enough force to meet the body's metabolic demands.

• Defining Characteristics
— *SUBJECTIVE DATA* (reported) —
Fatigue, vertigo, dyspnea, orthopnea.

— *OBJECTIVE DATA* (observed) —
Low blood pressure; rapid heart rate; arrhythmias; angina; jugular vein distention; cyanosis of skin and mucous membranes; dependent edema; oliguria; decreased peripheral pulses; cold, clammy skin; rales; restlessness.

• Related Factors
To be developed.

• Author's Note
The defining characteristics of this problem represent a *collaborative problem* rather than a *nursing diagnosis.*

• Compare With
Activity Intolerance.

Caregiver Role Strain

The state in which a caregiver perceives difficulty in performing the family caregiver role.

• Defining Characteristics
— *SUBJECTIVE DATA* (reported) —
Inadequate resources; difficulty performing caregiving activities; concern regarding outcome for the care receiver; conflict with other role responsibilities; family conflict around issues of providing care; feelings of stress, nervousness, and depression.

— *OBJECTIVE DATA* (observed) —
Reduction in quality of care, increased family discord, long hours of caregiving without time off.

• Related Factors
Care receiver: severity of or prolongation of illness, unpredictable illness course, early discharge from skilled nursing facility, complexity or amount of care needed.
Caregiver: lack of preparation or experience, impaired physical or mental health, lack of respite or recreation, competing role commitments.
Other Factors: inadequate physical environment, family dysfunction.

Caregiver Role Strain, Risk for

The state in which a caregiver is at risk for perceiving difficulty in performing the family caregiver role.

• Risk Factors
See Related Factors for *Caregiver Role Strain.*

Communication, Impaired*

Decreased ability to send or receive messages (ie, has difficulty exchanging thoughts, ideas, or desires).

• Defining Characteristics
— *SUBJECTIVE DATA* (reported) —
Concern about being able to make self understood, or to understand directions, reluctance to speak, difficulty understanding or speaking dominant language.

— *OBJECTIVE DATA* (observed) —
Repetition of questions without apparent understanding of answers; inappropriate (or absent) speech or response; incongruence between verbal and nonverbal messages; stuttering, slurring, word-finding problems; weak or absent voice; confusion; use of sign language.

• Related Factors
Effects of cerebral impairment (expressive or receptive aphasia), hearing or auditory comprehension deficits, decreased ability to speak words, language barriers, lack of privacy, *Impaired Thought Processes.*

• Author's Note

Only *Impaired Verbal Communication* is on NANDA's list of diagnoses accepted for study. *Impaired Communication* has been included here because it includes a wider range of communication problems.

• Compare With

Communication, Impaired Verbal.

Communication, Impaired Verbal

A decreased or absent ability to speak, but the person can understand others.

• Defining Characteristics
— OBJECTIVE DATA (observed) —

Difficulty with dominant language, speech, or verbalization; does not or cannot speak.

• Related Factors

Physical barrier (tracheostomy, intubation), anatomic defect (cleft lip or palate), brain injury or disease causing expressive aphasia, psychological barriers (psychosis, fear), language barriers.

• Compare With

Communication, Impaired.

Community Coping, Ineffective

A pattern of community activities for adaptation and problem solving that is unsatisfactory for meeting the demands or needs of the community.

• Defining Characteristics
— SUBJECTIVE DATA (reported) —

Community does not meet its own expectations, expressed difficulty in meeting demands for change, expressed vulnerability, stressors perceived as excessive.

— OBJECTIVE DATA (observed) —

Deficits in community participation, deficits in communication methods, excessive community conflicts, high illness rates.

• Related Factors

Deficits in social support, inadequate resources for problem solving, powerlessness.

• Compare With

Community Coping, Readiness for Enhanced; Therapeutic Regimen, Ineffective Community Management of.

Community Coping, Readiness for Enhanced

A pattern of community activities for adaptation and problem solving that is satisfactory for meeting the demands or needs of the community but can be improved for management of current and future problems/stressors.

• Defining Characteristics
— SUBJECTIVE DATA (reported) —

Agreement that community is responsible for stress management.

— OBJECTIVE DATA (observed) —

Deficits in one or more characteristics that indicate effective coping, active planning by community for predicted stressors, active problem solving by community when faced with issues, positive communication among community members, positive communication between community aggregates and larger community, programs available for recreation and relaxation, resources sufficient for managing stressors.

• Related Factors

Social supports available, resources available for problem solving, community has a sense of power to manage stressors.

• Compare With

Community Coping, Ineffective; Therapeutic Regimen, Ineffective Community Management of.

Confusion, Acute

Abrupt onset of a cluster of global, transient changes and disturbances in attention, cognition, psychomotor activity, level of consciousness, and/or sleep–wake cycle.

• Defining Characteristics
— SUBJECTIVE DATA (reported) —

Hallucinations.

— *OBJECTIVE DATA* (observed) —

Fluctuation in cognition, fluctuation in sleep–wake cycle, fluctuation in level of consciousness, fluctuation in psychomotor activity, increased agitation or restlessness, misperceptions, lack of motivation to initiate and/or follow through with goal-directed or purposeful behavior.

• Related Factors

Age older than 60 years, dementia, alcohol abuse, drug abuse, delirium.

• Compare With

Confusion, Chronic; Environmental Interpretation Syndrome, Impaired; Sensory Perception, Disturbed; Thought Processes, Impaired.

Confusion, Chronic

Irreversible, long-standing, or progressive deterioration of intellect and personality characterized by decreased ability to interpret environmental stimuli, decreased capacity for intellectual thought processes and manifested by disturbances of memory, orientation, and behavior.

• Defining Characteristics

— *OBJECTIVE DATA* (observed) —

Clinical evidence of organic impairment, impaired interpretation/response to stimuli, progressive/long-standing cognitive impairment, no change in level of consciousness, impaired socialization, impaired memory (short term, long term), impaired personality.

• Related Factors

Alzheimer's disease, Korsakoff's psychosis, multi-infarct dementia, cerebral vascular accident, head injury.

• Compare With

Confusion, Acute; Environmental Interpretation Syndrome, Impaired; Sensory Perception, Disturbed; Thought Processes, Impaired.

Constipation

A state in which a person's bowel-elimination pattern is accompanied by difficult or incomplete passage of stool or passage of excessively hard stool.

• Defining Characteristics

— *SUBJECTIVE DATA* (reported) —

Feeling of rectal pressure or fullness, headache, abdominal pain, back pain, decreased appetite, nausea.

— *OBJECTIVE DATA* (observed) —

Decreased frequency of stools; hard, formed stools; straining at stool; palpable rectal mass.

• Related Factors

Bed rest, diet deficient in fluids or roughage, lack of exercise, lack of privacy, laxative dependence, painful defecation, pregnancy, side effects of medications, neuromuscular impairment.

• Clinical Alert

Untreated constipation can lead to fecal impaction and intestinal obstruction.

• Compare With

Constipation, Colonic; Constipation, Perceived; Constipation, Risk for.

Constipation, Colonic

The state in which a person's pattern of elimination is characterized by hard, dry stool that results from a delay in passage of food residue.

• Defining Characteristics

— *SUBJECTIVE DATA* (reported) —

Painful defecation, abdominal pain, rectal pressure, headache, decreased appetite.

— *OBJECTIVE DATA* (observed) —

Decreased frequency of stools; hard, dry stools; straining at stool; abdominal distention; palpable rectal mass; distended abdomen.

• Related Factors

Less than adequate fluid intake, less than adequate dietary intake, less than adequate fiber, less than adequate physical activity, immobility, lack of privacy, emotional disturbances, chronic use of laxatives and enemas, stress, change in daily routine.

• Compare With

Constipation; Constipation, Perceived.

Constipation, Perceived

The state in which a person makes a self-diagnosis of constipation when constipation does not exist and ensures a daily bowel movement through abuse of laxatives, enemas, and suppositories.

• Related Factors

Cultural or family health beliefs, faulty appraisal, impaired thought processes, obsessive–compulsive disorders.

• Defining Characteristics
— *SUBJECTIVE DATA* (reported) —

Expectation of a daily bowel movement with the resulting overuse of laxatives, enemas, and suppositories; expected passage of stool at same time every day.

• Compare With

Constipation; Constipation, Colonic.

Constipation, Risk for

A state in which a person is at risk for having a bowel-elimination pattern that's accompanied by difficult or incomplete passage of stool or passage of excessively hard stool.

• Risk Factors

Functional: Habitual denial/ignoring of urge to defecate, recent environmental changes, inadequate toileting (eg, timeliness, positioning for defecation, privacy), irregular defecation habits, insufficient physical activity, abdominal muscle weakness. *Psychological:* Emotional stress, mental confusion, depression. *Physiologic:* Insufficient fiber intake, dehydration, inadequate dentition or oral hygiene, poor eating habits, insufficient fluid intake, decreased motility of GI tract. *Pharmacologic:* Drugs that include constipation as a side effect (check drug regimen). *Mechanical:* Rectal abscess or ulcer, postsurgical obstruction, anal fissures, megacolon (Hirschsprung's disease), electrolyte imbalance, tumors, prostate enlargement, rectocele, rectal prolapse, neurologic impairment, hemorrhoids, obesity.

• Compare With

Constipation, Perceived; Constipation, Colonic.

Coping, Defensive

The state in which a person repeatedly projects falsely positive self-evaluation based on a self-protective pattern that defends against underlying perceived threats to positive self-regard.

• Defining Characteristics
— *OBJECTIVE DATA* (observed) —

Denial of obvious problems or weaknesses, rationalization, hypersensitivity to criticism, grandiosity, projection of blame or responsibility, superior attitude toward others, difficulty establishing or maintaining relationships, hostile laughter or ridicule of others, difficulty in reality testing perceptions, lack of follow-through or participation in treatment or therapy.

• Related Factors

Loss of job or ability to work, financial problems, marital problems, failure in school, legal problems, institutionalization, fear, aging.

• Compare With

Coping, Ineffective.

Coping, Ineffective

Impaired adaptive behaviors and problem-solving abilities in meeting demands and roles of life.

• Defining Characteristics
— *SUBJECTIVE DATA* (reported) —

Inability to cope or inability to ask for help.

— *OBJECTIVE DATA* (observed) —

Inability to meet role expectations or solve problems, impaired societal participation, destructive behavior toward self or others, inappropriate use of defense mechanism, change in usual communication patterns, manipulative behavior, high illness or accident rate.

• Related Factors

Situational or maturational crises, persistent stress, sensory overload, personal vulnerability, poor self-esteem, inadequate or unavailable support system, conflict with values or beliefs.

• Compare With

Adjustment, Impaired; Coping, Defensive; Denial, Ineffective.

Decisional Conflict (Specify)

Uncertainty about the course of action to be taken when choices involve risk, loss, or challenge to personal life values.

• Defining Characteristics
— *SUBJECTIVE DATA* (reported) —

Uncertainty about choices, concern about undesired consequences of actions being considered, vacillation between choices, delayed decision making, feeling of distress while attempting a decision, self-focusing, questioning of personal values and beliefs while attempting a decision.

— *OBJECTIVE DATA* (observed) —

Signs of distress or tension (eg, increased heart rate, increased muscle tension, restlessness, and so forth).

• Related Factors

Unclear personal values or beliefs, perceived threat to value system, lack of experience or interference with decision making, lack of relevant information, support system deficit, multiple or divergent sources of information.

• Compare With

Coping, Ineffective; Spiritual Distress.

Denial, Ineffective

The state of a conscious or unconscious attempt to disavow the knowledge or meaning of an event to reduce anxiety or fear to the detriment of health.

• Defining Characteristics
— *SUBJECTIVE DATA* (reported) —

Failure to perceive personal relevance of symptoms or danger, minimizing of symptoms, displacement of symptoms to other organs, displacement of fear or impact of the condition, inability to admit impact of disease on life pattern.

— *OBJECTIVE DATA* (observed) —

Lack of verbalization of fear of death or invalidism, delay in seeking (or refusal to accept) health care to the detriment of health, use of home remedies or self-medication to relieve symptoms, use of dismissive gestures or comments when speaking of distressing events, inappropriate affect.

• Related Factors

Illness or addiction accompanied by fear of death, separation, or loss of autonomy; *Anxiety*.

• Compare With

Adjustment, Impaired; Coping, Defensive; Coping, Ineffective.

Dentition, Impaired

Disruption in tooth development/eruption pattern or structural integrity of individual teeth.

• Defining Characteristics
— *SUBJECTIVE DATA* (reported) —

Toothache.

— *OBJECTIVE DATA* (observed) —

Excessive plaque, crown or root caries, halitosis, tooth enamel discoloration, loose teeth, excessive calculus, incomplete eruption for age (primary or permanent teeth), malocclusion or tooth misalignment, premature loss of primary teeth, worn down or abraded teeth, tooth fractures, missing teeth, erosion of enamel, asymmetric facial expression.

• Related Factors

Ineffective oral hygiene; sensitivity to heat or cold; self-care barriers; barriers to professional care; dietary habits; genetic predisposition; medication side effects; excessive fluoride intake; chronic vomiting or bulimia; tobacco; coffee, tea, or red wine intake; lack of knowledge regarding dental health; excessive abrasive cleaning agents use; bruxism (teeth grinding).

Development, Delayed, Risk for

At risk for delay of 25% or more in one or more of the areas of social or self-regulatory behavior, or skills of cognitive, language, or gross or fine motor nature.

• Risk Factors

Prenatal: Mother younger than 15 or older than 35 years, substance abuse, infections, genetic or endocrine disorders, unplanned or unwanted pregnancy, poor prenatal care, inadequate nutrition, illiteracy, poverty. *Individual:* Prematurity, seizures, congenital or genetic disorders, positive drug screening test, brain damage, vision impairment, hearing impairment or frequent otitis media, chronic illness, technology-dependent, failure to thrive, inadequate nutrition; foster or adopted child; lead poisoning; chemotherapy, radiation therapy, behavioral disorders, substance abuse. *Environmental:* poverty, violence, natural disaster. *Caregiver:* abuse, mental illness, mental retardation or learning disabilities.

Diarrhea

A state in which a person experiences a change in normal bowel habits characterized by the frequent passage of loose, fluid, unformed stools.

• Defining Characteristics
— *SUBJECTIVE DATA* (reported) —

Abdominal pain, cramping, urgency.

— *OBJECTIVE DATA* (observed) —

Loose liquid stools, increased frequency of stools, increased frequency of bowel sounds.

• Related Factors

Side effects of medications or radiation therapy, tube feedings, inflammatory or malabsorptive disorders, infectious processes, food intolerances, *Anxiety.*

• Compare With

Bowel Incontinence.

Disuse Syndrome, Risk for

A state in which a person is at risk for deterioration of body systems as the result of musculoskeletal inactivity.

• Risk Factors

Neuromuscular impairment (eg, paralysis, multiple sclerosis), musculoskeletal disorders, mechanical immobilization, prescribed immobilization, severe pain, altered level of consciousness, psychiatric disorders.

• Author's Note

This diagnosis is appropriate when interventions are aimed at promoting physiologic and psychosocial integrity and preventing complications of immobility.

• Compare With

Mobility, Impaired Physical.

Diversional Activity Deficit

Decreased stimulation from (or interest or engagement in) recreational or leisure activities.

• Defining Characteristics
— *SUBJECTIVE DATA* (reported) —

Boredom or disinterest.

— *OBJECTIVE DATA* (observed) —

Flat affect, restlessness, hostility.

• Related Factors

Lack of diversional activity (eg, chronic illness or disability, frequent lengthy treatments), sight or hearing loss, inability to participate in usual activities, retirement.

Energy Field, Disturbed

A state in which the flow of energy surrounding a person's being is disrupted, resulting in a disharmony of the body, mind, or spirit.

• Defining Characteristics
— *SUBJECTIVE DATA* (reported) —

Temperature change (warmth/coolness), visual changes (image/color), disruption of the field (vacant/hold/spike/bulge), movement (wave/spike/tingling/dense/flowing), sounds (tone/words).

• Related Factors

None listed.

Environmental Interpretation Syndrome, Impaired

Consistent lack of orientation to person, place, time, or circumstances for more than 3 to 6 months, requiring a protective environment.

• Defining Characteristics
— *OBJECTIVE DATA* (observed) —

Consistent disorientation in known and unknown environments, chronic confusional states, loss of occupation or social functioning from memory decline, inability to follow simple directions or instructions, inability to reason or concentrate, slow response to questions.

• Related Factors

Dementia (Alzheimer's disease, multi-infarct dementia, Pick's disease, AIDS dementia), Parkinson's disease, Huntington's disease, depression, alcoholism.

• Compare With

Confusion, Acute; Confusion, Chronic; Sensory Perception, Disturbed; Thought Processes, Impaired.

Failure to Thrive, Adult

Progressive physical and cognitive functional deterioration; ability to live with multisystem diseases, cope with ensuing problems, and manage care are remarkably diminished.

• Defining Characteristics

— SUBJECTIVE DATA (reported) —

No appetite or desire to eat, expression of feeling sad or low in spirits, expresses loss of pleasure in usually pleasurable activities, reports desire for death.

— OBJECTIVE DATA (observed) —

Doesn't eat when encouraged to do so; consumption of minimal or no food; weight loss; physical decline; frequent exacerbations of chronic health problems (eg, pneumonia, urinary tract infections); cognitive decline (eg, problems with responding appropriately to environmental stimuli, difficulty reasoning, decreased perception, decreased social skills, social withdrawal, behavioral changes with decreased participation in relationships); decreased participation in activities once enjoyed; difficulty performing simple self-care tasks; neglect of home environment or financial responsibilities; apathy; altered mood state;

• Related Factors

Depression, apathy, fatigue.

Falls, Risk for

Increased susceptibility to falling.

• Risk Factors

Adults: History of falls, wheelchair use, aged 65 or older, lives alone, lower limb prosthesis, use of assistive devices such as canes or walkers, illness (acute or chronic), impaired mobility, diminished mental status, medications (causing dizziness, drowsiness, fatigue, or weakness), alcohol use, nighttime sedative use, restraint use, unfamiliar surroundings, dimly lit room, throw rugs, poorly fitted shoes, no anti-slip material in bathroom. *Children:* Age younger than 2 years old, boys younger than 1 year of age, lack of automobile restraints, lack of gate on stairs, lack of window guard, bed located near window, unattended infant on bed or changing table/sofa, lack of supervision.

Family Coping, Compromised

The state in which usually supportive significant others provide insufficient, ineffective, or compromised support, comfort, assistance, or encouragement to someone with a health challenge.

• Defining Characteristics

— SUBJECTIVE DATA (reported) —

Concern about response of significant other(s), significant other(s) describes preoccupation with personal reaction or inadequate knowledge or understanding of health challenge.

— OBJECTIVE DATA (observed) —

Withdrawal or limited contact by significant other(s), inappropriate assistance or supportive behaviors, unrealistic expectations for abilities of challenged individual, overprotection of challenged individual.

• Related Factors

Inadequate or incorrect information or understanding by a primary support person, preoccupation with emotional conflicts and personal suffering, temporary family disorganization and role changes, concurrent situations or crises, inability of significant others to provide support with health challenge, prolonged disease or disability.

• Compare With

Family Coping, Disabled; Family Processes, Interrupted; Parental Role Conflict; Parenting, Impaired.

Family Coping, Disabled

The state in which a family demonstrates destructive behavior in response to an inability to manage internal or external stressors due to inadequate resources (eg, physical, psychological, cognitive, or behavioral) (Carpenito, 2000b).

• Defining Characteristics
— *SUBJECTIVE DATA* (reported) —

Distorted perception by significant others of client's health problem.

— *OBJECTIVE DATA* (observed) —

Neglectful care, prolonged over concern about family member(s) with health challenge, rejection, abandonment, adherence to usual routine without regard for needs of family member(s), assuming symptoms of client, neglect of self or other family members, decisions detrimental to economic or social well-being, agitation, aggression, dependence or helplessness of significant others.

• Related Factors

Family members: significant health challenge; chronically unexpressed feelings of guilt, anxiety, hostility, despair; inappropriate coping mechanisms; highly ambivalent relationships; arbitrary handling of resistance to treatment by caregivers; *Caregiver Role Strain.*

• Compare With

Caregiver Role Strain; Family Coping, Compromised; Family Processes, Interrupted; Parental Role Conflict; Parenting, Impaired.

Family Coping, Readiness for Enhanced

The state in which family members exhibit desire and readiness for enhanced growth related to ability to manage family member's health care challenges.

• Defining Characteristics
— *SUBJECTIVE DATA* (reported) —

Growing impact of crisis on personal values, priorities, goals, or relationships; interest in making contact with others in similar situation.

— *OBJECTIVE DATA* (observed) —

Movement toward health-promoting and enriching lifestyle, auditing and negotiating of treatment programs, choice of experiences that optimize wellness.

• Related Factors

Family experiencing significant health challenge to one or more of its members, another family member ready for self-actualization.

Family Process, Dysfunctional: Alcoholism

The state in which the psychosocial, spiritual, and physiologic functions of the family unit are chronically disorganized, leading to conflict, denial of problems, resistance to change, ineffective problem solving, and a series of self-perpetuating crises.

• Defining Characteristics
— *SUBJECTIVE DATA* (reported) —

Decreased self-esteem, worthlessness, anger/suppressed rage, frustration, powerlessness, anxiety/tension/distress, insecurity, repressed emotions, responsibility for alcoholic's behavior, lingering resentment, shame/embarrassment, guilt, hurt, unhappiness, emotional isolation/loneliness, vulnerability, mistrust, hopelessness, rejection.

— *OBJECTIVE DATA* (observed) —

Expression of anger inappropriately, difficulty with intimate relationships, loss of control of drinking, impaired communication, ineffective problem-solving skills, enabling to maintain drinking, inability to meet emotional needs of its members, manipulation, dependency, criticizing, blaming, alcohol abuse, broken promises, rationalization/denial of problems, refusal to get help/inability to accept and receive help appropriately, blaming, inadequate understanding or knowledge of alcoholism.

• Related Factors

Abuse of alcohol, family history of alcoholism, resistance to treatment, inadequate coping skills, genetic predisposition, addictive personality, lack of problem-solving skills, biochemical influences.

• Compare With

Family Coping, Compromised; Family Coping, Disabled; Family Processes, Interrupted; Coping, Ineffective Individual.

Family Processes, Interrupted

The state in which a family that normally functions effectively experiences dysfunction.

• Defining Characteristics

— SUBJECTIVE DATA (reported) —

Family unable to express or accept wide range of feelings, unable to express or accept feelings of members.

— OBJECTIVE DATA (observed) —

Family members: unable to meet physical, emotional, or spiritual needs; unable to relate to each other for mutual growth and maturation; unable to change or deal with traumatic experience constructively; unable to accept help; uninvolved in community activities; rigidity in functions and roles; absence of respect for individuality and autonomy of each other; failure to accomplish current or past developmental tasks; failure to send and receive clear messages; unhealthy decision-making processes; poor communication of family rules, rituals, symbols; perpetuation of family myths; inappropriate level and direction of energy; parents don't demonstrate respect for each other's views on child-rearing practices.

• Related Factors

Situation transition or crisis, developmental transition or crisis.

• Compare With

Family Coping, Compromised; Parental Role Conflict; Parenting, Impaired.

Fatigue

An overwhelming, sustained sense of exhaustion and decreased capacity for physical and mental work.

• Defining Characteristics

— SUBJECTIVE DATA (reported) —

Unremitting and overwhelming lack of energy; inability to maintain usual routines, need for additional energy to accomplish routine tasks; impaired ability to concentrate; decreased libido; disinterest in surroundings or introspection.

— OBJECTIVE DATA (observed) —

Emotionally labile or irritable, decreased performance, lethargy or listlessness, increase in physical complaints, accident-prone.

• Related Factors (Etiology)

Decreased or increased metabolic energy production, overwhelming psychological or emotional demands, increased energy requirements to perform activities of daily living, excessive social or role demands, states of discomfort, altered body chemistry (eg, medications, drug withdrawal, chemotherapy), anemia.

• Compare With

Activity Intolerance; Sleep Pattern, Disturbed; Self-Care Deficit.

Fear

A feeling of dread and is able to identify its sources.

• Defining Characteristics

— SUBJECTIVE DATA (reported) —

Apprehension, terror, or panic in response to an identifiable source; insomnia; dry mouth; appetite loss.

— OBJECTIVE DATA (observed) —

Aggression; irritability; vigilance; increased blood pressure, pulse, and respirations; increased perspiration, pallor, muscle tension; diarrhea, urinary frequency.

• Related Factors

Actual or perceived threat of pain, disability, disease, physical or psychological discomfort or harm, inability to control situations or cope effectively, loss (of objects, significant others, capabilities, role function, or independence); *Knowledge, Deficient.*

• Compare With

Anxiety.

Fluid Volume, Deficient

Decreased intravascular, extracellular, or intracellular fluid. This refers to dehydration, water loss alone without change in sodium.

• Defining Characteristics

— SUBJECTIVE DATA (reported) —

Dry mouth, thirst, weakness.

— OBJECTIVE DATA (observed) —

Sudden weight loss except with third spacing, dry skin and mucous membranes, decreased skin turgor, oliguria, concentrated urine, increased body temperature, rapid pulse, decreased pulse volume/pressure, output greater than intake, elevated hematocrit, changes in mental state, decreased blood pressure.

• Related Factors

Active fluid volume loss, failure of regulatory mechanisms.

• Clinical Alert

Report onset of confusion, hypotension, or arrhythmias (may indicate electrolyte imbalance or hypovolemia, which require immediate physician-prescribed interventions).

• Compare With

Fluid Volume, Deficient, Risk for.

Fluid Volume Deficient, Risk for

The state in which a person is at risk of experiencing vascular, interstitial, or intracellular dehydration.

• Risk Factors

See Related Factors for *Fluid Volume, Deficient.*

Fluid Volume Excess

Increased isotonic fluid retention.

• Defining Characteristics
— SUBJECTIVE DATA (reported) —

Anxiety, shortness of breath, orthopnea, ankle swelling, weight gain.

— OBJECTIVE DATA (observed) —

Restlessness; edema; taut, shiny skin; effusion; anasarca; weight gain; intake greater than output; S_3 heart sound; pulmonary congestion on chest radiograph; rales (crackles); change in respiratory pattern; change in mental status; decreased hemoglobin and hematocrit; blood pressure changes; central venous pressure changes; pulmonary artery pressure changes; jugular vein distention; positive hepatojugular reflex;

oliguria; specific gravity changes; azotemia; imbalanced electrolytes.

• Related Factors

Compromised regulatory mechanism, excess fluid or sodium intake.

Fluid Volume, Imbalanced, Risk for

A risk of decrease, increase, or rapid shift from one to the other of intravascular, interstitial, or intracellular fluid. This refers to the loss or excess of body fluids or replacement fluids.

• Risk Factors

See related factors for *Fluid Volume, Deficient* and *Fluid Volume Excess.*

Gas Exchange, Impaired

Excess or deficit in oxygenation or carbon dioxide elimination at the alveolar-capillary membrane.

• Defining Characteristics
— SUBJECTIVE DATA (reported) —

Dyspnea, apprehension, headache upon wakening, visual disturbances.

— OBJECTIVE DATA (observed) —

Confusion, somnolence, restlessness, irritability, tachypnea, hypercapnia, hypoxemia, rapid heart rate, abnormal arterial blood gasses or pH, abnormal skin color (cyanosis, pale, or dusky), diaphoresis, nasal flaring.

• Related Factors

Ventilation or perfusion imbalance, alveolar-capillary membrane changes.

• Clinical Alert

Identifying and treating *Risk for Ineffective Airway Clearance* or *Ineffective Breathing Pattern* is essential to preventing *Impaired Gas Exchange.*

• Compare With

Activity Intolerance; Airway Clearance, Ineffective; Breathing Pattern, Ineffective.

Grieving*

The state in which a person or group experiences a normal pattern of extreme feelings of loss and sadness in response to an actual or perceived loss (of an object, relationship, loved one, pet, capability, body part, body function, or job status).

• Defining Characteristics
— *SUBJECTIVE DATA* (reported) —

During the first year after a loss: sadness in response to loss; guilt; unresolved issues; anger; mood swings; difficulty expressing loss; inability to stop crying, concentrate, make decisions, or participate in meaningful activities or relationships.

— *OBJECTIVE DATA* (observed) —

During the first year after a loss: idealization of lost object or person; changes in eating habits, activity level, libido, sleep or dream patterns; reliving of past experiences; interference with life functions; regression; labile affect; decreased ability to concentrate or pursue tasks.

• Related Factors
Actual or perceived loss.

• Compare With
Coping, Ineffective; Grieving, Anticipatory; Grieving, Dysfunctional; Spiritual Distress.

Grieving, Anticipatory

The state in which a person or family experiences feelings of anxiety, fear, or sadness in response to a possible loss (of object, relationship, loved one, pet, capability, body part, body function, or job status).

• Defining Characteristics
— *SUBJECTIVE DATA* (reported) —

Distress at potential loss, guilt, anger, sorrow, denial of potential loss.

— *OBJECTIVE DATA* (observed) —

Change in eating habits, sleep patterns, activity level, libido, communication patterns.

• Related Factors
Anticipated loss.

• Compare With
Grieving; Grieving, Dysfunctional; Spiritual Distress.

Grieving, Dysfunctional

The state in which a person or group experiences prolonged and exaggerated feelings of loss and sadness in response to an actual or perceived loss (of an object, loved one, pet, capability, relationship, or body part).

• Defining Characteristics
— *SUBJECTIVE DATA* (reported) —

More than a year after a loss: inability to participate in meaningful activities or relationships because of symptoms associated with sadness over loss (see defining characteristics of *Grieving*).

— *OBJECTIVE DATA* (observed) —

More than a year after a loss: inability to participate in meaningful activities or relationships because of symptoms associated with sadness over loss (see defining characteristics of *Grieving*).

• Related Factors
Actual or perceived loss.

• Compare With
Coping, Ineffective; Grieving; Grieving, Anticipatory; Spiritual Distress.

Growth and Development, Delayed

The state in which a child's growth or development is below the norm for his or her age group.

• Defining Characteristics
— *OBJECTIVE DATA* (observed) —

Delay or difficulty in performing skills (motor, social, or expressive) typical of age group, altered physical growth, inability to perform self-care or self-control activities appropriate for age, regression in previously acquired skills, flat affect, listlessness, decreased responses.

• Related Factors
Inadequate caregiving (eg, indifference, neglect, abuse, inconsistent responsiveness, multiple caregivers), separation from significant others, environ-

mental and stimulation deficiencies, physical illness or disability, prescribed dependence.

Health Maintenance, Ineffective

Inability to manage and/seek help to maintain health.

• Defining Characteristics

— *SUBJECTIVE DATA* (reported) —

History of lack of health-seeking behavior.

— *OBJECTIVE DATA* (observed) —

Lack of knowledge regarding basic health practices, lack of adaptive behaviors to internal or external environmental changes, inability to take responsibility for meeting basic health practices in any or all functional patterns, failure to seek basic health information.

• Related Factors

Decreased communication skills (written, verbal, non-verbal), inability to make valid judgments, perceptual or cognitive impairment (complete or partial lack of gross or fine motor skills), developmental delay, ineffective coping skills, lack of resources, unavailable or inadequate support system, poor health habits.

• Compare With

Coping, Ineffective; Knowledge, Deficient; Therapeutic Regimen, Ineffective Management of

Health-Seeking Behaviors (Specify)

A state in which a person in stable health is actively seeking ways to change health habits or the environment to move toward a higher level of health.

• Defining Characteristics

— *SUBJECTIVE DATA* (reported) —

Desire to seek higher level of wellness or increase control of health practices, concern about the effect of current environmental conditions on health status.

— *OBJECTIVE DATA* (observed) —

Unfamiliarity with wellness community resources, behaviors not consistent with health promotion.

• Related Factors

Ability to meet basic health needs, achievement of age-appropriate illness prevention measures, good or excellent health, desire to enhance current health status or practices.

Home Maintenance, Impaired

The state in which a person or family is unable to maintain a safe, growth-promoting environment independently.

• Defining Characteristics

— *SUBJECTIVE DATA* (reported) —

Difficulty in maintaining home in a comfortable fashion, seeking of assistance with home maintenance, outstanding debts or financial crises, history of accidents.

— *OBJECTIVE DATA* (observed) —

Disorderly surroundings; unwashed or unavailable cooking equipment, clothes, or linen; accumulated dirt, food wastes, or unhygienic wastes; offensive odors; inappropriate household temperature; overtaxed family members (eg, exhausted, anxious); lack of necessary equipment or aids; presence of vermin or rodents; repeated hygienic disorders, infestations, or infections; hazards in the home.

• Related Factors

Individual or family member disease or injury; insufficient organization or planning; insufficient finances; unfamiliarity with available resources; impaired cognitive or emotional functioning; lack of knowledge, role models, or support systems; young children in home.

• Compare With

Injury, Risk for.

Hopelessness

A state in which a person sees limited or no alternatives or acceptable choices and is unable to mobilize energy on his or her own behalf.

• Defining Characteristics

— *SUBJECTIVE DATA* (reported) —

Inability to make choices, solve problems, or perform activity; apathy; indifference; decreased appetite.

— OBJECTIVE DATA (observed) —

Passive anger, flat affect, sighing, decreased response to stimuli, decreased verbalization, turning away from speaker, closing eyes or shrugging in response to speaker, decreased or increased sleep, lack of initiative, lack of involvement in care or passively allowing care.

• Related Factors

Prolonged activity restriction creating isolation, failing or deteriorating physiologic condition, long-term stress, abandonment, lost belief in transcendent values or God.

• Compare With

Powerlessness; Spiritual Distress.

Hyperthermia

A state in which body temperature is elevated above normal range.

• Defining Characteristics

— OBJECTIVE DATA (observed) —

Increased body temperature above normal range, flushed or warm skin, increased respiratory rate, tachycardia, malaise, irritability, seizures or convulsions.

• Related Factors

Heat exposure, vigorous activity, medications or anesthesia, inappropriate clothing, increased metabolic rate, illness or trauma, dehydration, decreased ability to perspire.

• Clinical Alert

Report temperature elevations associated with a shaking chill, hypotension, or confusion immediately (may indicate onset of septic shock). Also report frequent unexplained elevations, sustained elevations, or elevations accompanied by symptoms of infection.

• Compare With

Body Temperature, Risk for Imbalanced; Thermoregulation, Ineffective.

Hypothermia

The state in which a person's body temperature is reduced below 95°F.

• Defining Characteristics

— SUBJECTIVE DATA (reported) —

Sensation of feeling cold.

— OBJECTIVE DATA (observed) —

Body temperature below normal range, shivering, cool skin, pallor, confusion, slow capillary refill, tachycardia, cyanotic nail beds, hypertension, piloerection.

• Related Factors

Exposure to cold, inadequate clothing, evaporation of moisture from skin, illness or trauma, damage to hypothalamus, inability or decreased ability to shiver, medications causing vasodilation, alcohol consumption, malnutrition, decreased metabolic rate, inactivity, aging, neonatal period, prematurity.

• Compare With

Body Temperature, Risk for Imbalanced; Thermoregulation, Ineffective.

Infant Behavior, Disorganized

The state in which an infant experiences an alteration in integration and modulation of the physiologic and behavioral systems of functioning (ie, autonomic, motor, state, organizational, self-regulatory and attentional-interactional systems).

• Defining Characteristics

— OBJECTIVE DATA (observed) —

Change from baseline physiologic measures, tremors, startles, twitches, hyperextension of arms and legs, diffuse/unclear sleep, deficient self-regulatory behaviors, deficient response to visual/auditory stimuli, yawning, apnea.

• Related Factors

Pain, oral/motor problems, feeding intolerance, environmental overstimulation, lack of containment/boundaries, prematurity, invasive/painful procedures.

Infant Behavior, Disorganized, Risk for

The state in which an infant is at risk for alteration in integration and modulation of the physiologic and behavioral systems of functioning (ie, autonomic, motor, state, organizational, self-regulatory, and attentional-interactional systems).

• Risk Factors

See Related Factors for *Infant Behavior, Disorganized*.

Infant Behavior, Organized, Readiness for Enhanced

A state in which the pattern of modulation of the physiologic and behavioral systems of functioning of an infant (ie, autonomic, motor, state, organizational, self-regulatory, and attentional-interactional systems) is satisfactory but can be improved, resulting in higher levels of integration in response to environmental stimuli.

• Defining Characteristics
— *OBJECTIVE DATA* (observed) —

Stable physiologic measures, definite sleep–wake states, use of some self-regulatory behaviors, response to visual/auditory stimuli.

• Related Factors

Prematurity; *Pain, Acute*.

Infant Feeding Pattern, Ineffective

A state in which an infant demonstrates an impaired ability to suck or to coordinate the suck–swallow response.

• Defining Characteristics
— *OBJECTIVE DATA* (observed) —

Inability to initiate or sustain an effective suck; inability to coordinate sucking, swallowing, and breathing; coughing or choking with feeding.

• Related Factors

Prematurity, neurologic impairment or delay, oral hypersensitivity, prolonged NPO status, anatomic abnormality.

• Compare With

Aspiration, Risk for; Breastfeeding, Ineffective.

Infection, Risk for

The state in which a person is at increased risk for being invaded by pathogenic organisms.

• Risk Factors

Inadequate primary defenses (broken skin, traumatized tissue, decreased ciliary action, stasis of body fluids, change in pH of secretions, altered peristalsis); inadequate secondary defenses (decreased hemoglobin, leukopenia, suppressed inflammatory response); immunosuppression; inadequate acquired immunity; chronic disease; malnutrition; environmental hazards (work, travel); treatment-related hazards (invasive lines or procedures, surgery, medications); extremes of age; *Knowledge, Deficient (self-protection)*; high-risk behaviors (eg, unsafe sex, drug abuse).

• Compare With

Protection, Ineffective.

Injury, Risk for

The state in which a person is at risk for injury as a result of individual risk factors or environmental hazards.

• Risk Factors

Individual: extremes of age, deconditioned state, difficulty ambulating, lack of knowledge of hazards, impaired mental status, history of frequent falls, *Sensory Perception, Disturbed.*
Environmental: workplace hazards without adequate safety precautions (eg, hard-hats, protective goggles), steps in poor repair, poor lighting, lack of handrails or side rails, *Impaired Home maintenance.*

• Compare With

Aspiration, Risk for; Poisoning, Risk for; Suffocation, Risk for; Trauma, Risk for; Home maintenance, Impaired.

Knowledge, Deficient (Specify)

The state in which a person lacks the skills or information to successfully manage his or her own health care.

• Defining Characteristics
— *SUBJECTIVE DATA* (reported) —

Information seeking, dissatisfaction with ability to manage health care, incomplete or inaccurate information related to health care needs, difficulty performing skills.

— *OBJECTIVE DATA* (observed) —

Inaccurate demonstration of skill, behavior inconsistent with instruction, inappropriate or exaggerated behaviors (eg, hysteria, hostility, agitation, apathy).

• Related Factors

Cognitive limitation, lack of recall, lack of previous opportunity to learn, misinterpretation of information, lack of interest or motivation, unfamiliarity with information sources, inability to read or lack of access to written information, *Fear, Ineffective Denial.*

Latex Allergy Response

Allergic response to natural latex rubber products.

• Defining Characteristics

— *SUBJECTIVE DATA* (reported) —

Increasing complaint of total body warmth, GI symptoms (abdominal pain, nausea), general discomfort. History of latex allergy or any of the following objective data. Reluctance to attempt movement, pain with movement.

— *OBJECTIVE DATA* (observed) —

Type I Reactions: Immediate reactions (<1 hour) to latex proteins (can be life threatening); contact urticaria progressing to generalized symptoms; lip, tongue, uvula, and/or throat edema; shortness of breath; chest tightness; wheezing; bronchospasm leading to respiratory arrest; hypotension; syncope; cardiac arrest. May also include itching, redness, and swelling of the eyes, mouth, and face; tearing, itching, swelling, running, or congestion of the nose; generalized symptoms (flushing, generalized edema). *Type II Reactions:* Delayed onset of symptoms (eczema, irritation, redness, chapped or cracked skin, blister.)

• Related Factors

No immune mechanism response. See also risk factors for *Latex Allergy Response, Risk for.*

Latex Allergy Response, Risk for

At risk for allergic response to natural latex rubber.

• Risk Factors

Multiple surgical procedures, especially from infancy; allergy to bananas, avocados, tropical fruits, kiwi, chestnuts, poinsettia plants; history of allergies and asthma; daily latex exposure; frequent or continuous catheterization.

Loneliness, Risk for

A subjective state in which an individual is at risk for experiencing vague dysphoria.

• Risk Factors

Affectional deprivation, physical isolation, emotional/attentional deprivation, social isolation.

• Compare With

Relocation Stress Syndrome; Social Isolation.

Memory, Impaired

The state in which an individual experiences the inability to remember or recall bits of information or behavioral skills. Impaired memory may be attributed to pathophysiologic or situational causes that are either temporary or permanent.

• Defining Characteristics

— *SUBJECTIVE DATA* (reported) —

Reported experiences of forgetting, inability to recall recent or past events.

— *OBJECTIVE DATA* (observed) —

Observed experiences of forgetting, inability to determine if a behavior was performed, inability to learn or retain new skills or information, inability to perform a previously learned skill, inability to recall factual information.

• Related Factors

Acute or chronic hypoxia, anemia, decreased cardiac output, fluid and electrolyte imbalance, neurologic disturbances, excessive environmental disturbances.

• Compare With

Confusion, Chronic; Thought Processes, Impaired.

Mobility, Impaired Physical

A state in which a person experiences a limitation of ability for independent movement.

• Defining Characteristics

— SUBJECTIVE DATA (reported) —

Reluctance to attempt movement, pain with movement.

— OBJECTIVE DATA (observed) —

Inability to move purposefully (confinement to bed; problems with transfer, ambulation, limited range of motion; decreased muscle strength, control, or mass).

• Related Factors

Intolerance to activity or decreased strength and endurance, pain or discomfort, neuromuscular or musculoskeletal impairment, imposed restrictions of movement, medical protocol.

• Author's Note

This diagnosis is appropriate when interventions are aimed at increasing strength and endurance, restoring function, or preventing deterioration.

• Compare With

Activity Intolerance; Disuse Syndrome, Risk for; Self-Care Deficit.

Noncompliance (Specify)

The state in which a person expresses an informed decision not to adhere to a therapeutic recommendation, which may significantly compromise health status (see the following author's note).

• Defining Characteristics

— SUBJECTIVE DATA (reported) —

Decision not to adhere to therapeutic recommendation in spite of knowledge of possible consequences.

— OBJECTIVE DATA (observed) —

Behavior inconsistent with therapeutic recommendation, development of complications, exacerbation of symptoms, failure to make progress toward recovery, failure to keep or make appointments.

• Related Factors

Undesirable treatment side effects, previous unsuccessful experience with health regimens, lack of motivation and trust, spiritual/cultural values.

• Author's Note

This diagnosis is poorly developed. The right of an informed, responsible adult to choose not to comply with a therapeutic recommendation must be respected. More appropriate diagnoses to consider are listed below.

• Compare With

Coping, Ineffective; Denial, Ineffective; Family Coping, Disabled; Knowledge, Deficient; Therapeutic Regimen: Individual, Ineffective Management of; Spiritual Distress.

Nutrition, Imbalanced: Less Than Body Requirements

The state in which a person is experiencing an intake of nutrients insufficient to meet metabolic needs.

• Defining Characteristics

— SUBJECTIVE DATA (reported) —

Poor appetite; aversion to eating; lack of interest in food; impaired taste sensation; satiety immediately after ingesting small amount of food; abdominal pain with or without disease; abdominal cramping; frequent purging; perceived inability to ingest food; lack of information, misinformation; misconceptions regarding nutritional requirements.

— OBJECTIVE DATA (observed) —

Food intake calculated to be less than metabolic requirements; body weight 20% below ideal; decreased serum albumin, muscle mass or tone, subcutaneous fat; pale conjunctival and mucous membranes; excessive hair loss; weight inconsistent with perception of being fat.

• Related Factors

Poor appetite, stomatitis, dysphagia, poorly fitting dentures, fad dieting, poor food choices, inability to obtain or prepare food (eg, physical or financial limitations), eating disorders (eg, anorexia nervosa, bulimia), increased metabolic requirements (eg, burns, infection, cancer), absorption disorders (eg, Crohn's disease, cystic fibrosis), medication side effects.

• Compare With

Oral Mucous Membrane, Impaired; Self-Care Deficit, Feeding; Home maintenance, Impaired; Swallowing, Impaired; Infant Feeding Pattern, Ineffective.

Nutrition, Imbalanced: More than Body Requirements

The state in which a person is experiencing an intake of nutrients that exceeds metabolic needs.

• Defining Characteristics
— *SUBJECTIVE DATA* (reported) —

Eating in response to external cues such as time of day, social situation; eating in response to internal cues other than hunger (eg, *Anxiety*).

— *OBJECTIVE DATA* (observed) —

Excessive intake in relation to metabolic need; weight 20% over ideal for height and frame; triceps skin fold greater than 15 mm in men, 25 mm in women; percentage of body fat greater than that recommended based on age and sex; pairing food with other activities; concentrating food intake at end of day.

• Related Factors

Obesity in one or both parents; rapid transition across growth percentiles during infancy and childhood; use of solid food as major food source before 5 months of age; use of food as reward or comfort measure; frequent, closely spaced pregnancies; higher baseline weight at beginning of each pregnancy; inadequate exercise or activity patterns; poor dietary habits (eg, snacking, unbalanced meals, high-fat foods); lack of knowledge of nutritional value of food; dysfunctional eating patterns; disease (thyroid problems, diabetes); medication side effects (eg, steroids, birth control pills).

• Compare With

Imbalanced Nutrition: Risk for More than Body Requirements; Coping, Ineffective.

Nutrition, Imbalanced: Risk for More Than Body Requirements

The state in which a person is at risk of experiencing an intake of nutrients that exceeds metabolic needs.

• Risk Factors

See Related Factors for *Nutrition, Imbalanced: More than Body Requirements.*

Oral Mucous Membrane, Impaired

Disruptions in the tissue layers of the oral cavity.

• Defining Characteristics
— *SUBJECTIVE DATA* (reported) —

Oral pain or discomfort.

— *OBJECTIVE DATA* (observed) —

Coated tongue, stomatitis, lesions or ulcers, leukoplakia, edema, hyperemia, plaque, vesicles, hemorrhagic gingivitis, halitosis.

• Related Factors

Radiation to head or neck, oral surgery, periodontal disease, chemical irritants (eg, alcohol, tobacco, drugs), dehydration, ill-fitting dentures or braces, carious teeth, presence of endotracheal or nasogastric tube, NPO for more than 24 hours, ineffective oral hygiene, mouth breathing, malnutrition, infection, absent or decreased salivation, medication side effects (chemotherapy, immunosuppressants).

• Compare With

Tissue Integrity, Impaired.

Pain, Acute

A state in which a person experiences and reports the presence of severe discomfort or an uncomfortable sensation.

• Defining Characteristics
— *SUBJECTIVE DATA* (reported) —
Description of pain or discomfort.

— *OBJECTIVE DATA* (observed) —

Guarding or protective behavior; self-focusing; narrowed focus (altered time perception, withdrawal from social contact, impaired thought process); distraction behavior (moaning, crying, pacing, seeking out other people or activities, restlessness); facial mask of pain (eyes lack luster, beaten look, fixed or scattered movement, grimace); impaired muscle tone, autonomic responses (diaphoresis, blood pressure and pulse changes, pupillary dilation, changes in respiratory rate).

• Related Factors

Injuring agents (biologic, chemical, physical, psychological), problems with structure or function of organ or systems, drug tolerance.

• Clinical Alert

Report new onset of pain or unrelieved pain. Recognize that there are national guidelines for pain management available from the Department of Human Services.

• Compare With

Pain, Chronic.

Pain, Chronic

A state in which a person experiences pain that continues for more than 6 months in duration.

• Defining Characteristics

— *SUBJECTIVE DATA* (reported) —

Pain for more than 6 months; fear of re-injury; impaired ability to continue previous activities; poor appetite; changes in weight, behavior, or sleep patterns; depression; frustration; anger; *Hopelessness.*

— *OBJECTIVE DATA* (observed) —

Behavior changes, facial mask, guarded movement.

• Related Factors

Chronic physical or psychosocial disability, depression, problems with organ or system structure or function, drug tolerance.

• Clinical Alert

People with *Chronic Pain* may not demonstrate usual autonomic response associated with pain (increased pulse and blood pressure). They may also appear to be pain-free (eg, smiling, laughing); however, this is usually a result of efforts to overcome pain through distraction and should not be considered a sign that the person really isn't in pain.

• Compare With

Acute Pain.

Parental Role Conflict

The state in which a parent experiences role confusion and conflict in response to crisis.

• Defining Characteristics

— *SUBJECTIVE DATA* (reported) —

Concern or feeling of inadequacy or reluctance to provide for child's physical and emotional needs; concerns about changes in parental role or family functioning, communication, or health; actual or perceived loss of control over decisions related to child (or children).

— *OBJECTIVE DATA* (observed) —

Disruption in care routines; reluctance to participate in usual care activities, even with encouragement and support.

• Related Factors

Separation from child, invasive or restrictive modalities (eg, isolation, intubation), specialized care center policies, home care of a child with special needs (eg, apnea monitoring, postural drainage, hyperalimentation), change in marital status, interruptions of family life due to home-care regimen, *Caregiver Role Strain.*

• Compare With

Caregiver Role Strain; Family Coping, Disabled; Family Processes, Interrupted; Parenting, Impaired.

Parent–Infant/Child Attachment, Risk for Impaired

A state in which there is a risk for disruption of the interactive process between parent/significant other and infant that fosters the development of a protective and nurturing reciprocal relationship.

• Risk Factors

Inability of parents to meet the personal needs anxiety associated with the parent role, substance abuse, premature infant, ill infant/child who is unable to effectively initiate parental contact due to impaired behavioral organization, separation, physical barriers, lack of privacy.

• Compare With

Infant Behavior, Disorganized; Parental Role Conflict.

Parenting, Impaired

The state in which parent figure(s) experiences inability to create an environment that promotes the optimum growth and development of a child or children.

• Defining Characteristics
— *SUBJECTIVE DATA* (reported) —

Inability to control child, disappointment in gender or physical characteristics of child, resentment toward child, disgust at body functions of child, feeling of inadequacy.

— *OBJECTIVE DATA* (observed) —

Parental abandonment, child abuse or neglect, runaway child, absence of parental attachment, failure to make or keep appointments with health care providers, inattention to needs of child, inappropriate caregiving behaviors, inappropriate or inconsistent disciplinary measures, frequent accidents or illnesses, delay in growth and development of child (children).

• Related Factors

Parent figure(s): lack of (or ineffective) role model, physical and psychosocial abuse, lack of support from significant other, unmet social or emotional needs, multiple pregnancies, lack of knowledge, *Caregiver Role Strain.*
Parent figure(s) or child(ren): actual or perceived threat to physical or emotional survival, unrealistic expectations, introduction of new family member(s) (eg, birth, adoption), mental or physical illness, stress.
Child(ren): absent or inappropriate response.

• Compare With

Caregiver Role Strain; Family Coping, Disabled; Family Processes, Interrupted; Growth and Development, Delayed; Infant Behavior, Disorganized; Parental Role Conflict.

Parenting, Risk for Impaired

The state in which parent figure(s) is at risk for experiencing inability to create an environment that promotes optimum growth and development of a child or children.

• Risk Factors

See Related Factors of *Impaired Parenting.*

• Compare With

Caregiver Role Strain; Family Coping, Disabled; Family Processes, Interrupted; Growth and Development, Delayed; Infant Behavior, Disorganized; Parental Role Conflict.

Perioperative Positioning Injury, Risk for

A state in which the client is at risk for injury as a result of the environmental conditions found in the perioperative setting.

• Risk Factors

Disorientation, immobilization, muscle weakness, anesthesia, obesity, emaciation, edema.

Peripheral Neurovascular Dysfunction, Risk for

A state in which a person is at risk of experiencing a disruption in circulation, sensation, or motion of an extremity.

• Risk Factors

Fractures, trauma, burns, vascular obstruction, immobilization, orthopedic surgery, mechanical compression (eg, tourniquet, cast, brace, dressing, or restraint).

• Clinical Alert

Report deviations from baseline neurovascular assessment findings that don't respond to nurse-prescribed interventions immediately so that measures can be taken to prevent irreversible neuromuscular damage.

• Compare With

Tissue Perfusion, Ineffective (peripheral).

Personal Identity, Disturbed

Inability to distinguish between self and nonself.

• Author's Note

No defining characteristics or Related Factors listed by NANDA. This diagnosis was accepted for study in 1978 but hasn't been developed sufficiently to be clinically useful.

Poisoning, Risk for

The state in which a person is at risk of accidental exposure to (or ingestion of) drugs or dangerous substances in doses sufficient to cause toxicity.

• Risk Factors

Individual: reduced vision, occupational setting without adequate safeguards, lack of safety or drug education or precautions, cognitive or emotional difficulties, insufficient finances.
Environmental: large supplies of drugs in house; medicines or potential poisons (cleansers and so forth) stored in unlocked cabinets accessible to children or confused persons; availability of illicit drugs; flaking, peeling paint or plaster in presence of young children; chemical contamination of food and water; unprotected contact with heavy metals or chemicals; paint, lacquer, and other materials with volatile solvents in poorly ventilated areas or without effective protection; poisonous vegetation; atmospheric pollutants.

• Compare With

Home maintenance, Impaired.

Post-Trauma Response

A sustained, painful response to unexpected, extraordinary life event(s).

• Defining Characteristics
— *SUBJECTIVE DATA* (reported) —

Re-experience of the traumatic event that may be identified in cognitive, affective, or sensory motor activities (eg, flashbacks, intrusive thoughts, repetitive dreams or nightmares, excessive verbalization of the traumatic event, survival guilt or guilt about behavior required for survival). Psychic or emotional numbness (impaired interpretation of reality, confusion, dissociation, amnesia, vagueness about traumatic event).

— *OBJECTIVE DATA* (observed) —

Altered lifestyle: self-destructiveness, such as substance abuse, suicide attempt, or other acting-out behavior; difficulty with interpersonal relationships; phobia regarding trauma; poor impulse control; irritability and explosiveness; constricted affect.

• Related Factors

Disasters, wars, epidemics, rape, assault, torture, catastrophic illness, or accident.

• Compare With

Rape Trauma Syndrome.

Powerlessness

The state in which a person perceives a personal lack of control over certain events or situations that impact on outlook, goals, and lifestyle (Carpenito, 2000a).

• Defining Characteristics
— *SUBJECTIVE DATA* (reported) —

Lack of control or influence over a situation or outcome, continued illness or deterioration despite compliance with prescribed regimen, anger.

— *OBJECTIVE DATA* (observed) —

Irritability, aggression, violent behavior, lack of cooperation with planned care, unwillingness to seek information regarding health status.

• Related Factors

Illness-related regimen, inability to perform self-care, health care environment or routines, interpersonal interactions, previous lifestyle of maintaining or enjoying control.

• Compare With

Hopelessness.

Protection, Ineffective

A decrease in the ability to guard the self from internal or external threats such as illness or injury.

• Defining Characteristics
— *SUBJECTIVE DATA* (reported) —

Dyspnea, itching, fatigue, anorexia, frequent illnesses, insomnia, *Activity Intolerance.*

— *OBJECTIVE DATA* (observed) —

Deficient immunity, impaired healing, impaired clotting, maladaptive stress response, neurosensory alteration, chilling, perspiring, cough, restlessness, weakness, immobility, disorientation, pressure sores.

• Related Factors

Extremes of age; inadequate nutrition; alcohol abuse; abnormal blood profiles (leukopenia, thrombocytopenia, anemia, coagulation); drug therapies (antineoplastics, corticosteroids, immunosuppressants, anticoagulants, thrombolytics); treatments (surgery, radiation); diseases such as cancer, diabetes, and immune disorders.

• Compare With

Infection, Risk for; Injury, Risk for.

Rape Trauma Syndrome[3]

Actual or attempted sexual penetration (vaginal, anal, oral) against his or her will or consent, resulting in an acute phase of disorganization of lifestyle and a long-term process of reorganization.

• Defining Characteristics
— *SUBJECTIVE DATA* (reported) —

Emotional reactions (anger, fear, embarrassment, humiliation, self-blame, desire for revenge); GI symptoms (nausea, vomiting, anorexia); genitourinary discomfort (pain, tenderness); muscle tension; insomnia; nightmares; changes in sexual behavior, relationship with opposite sex, or lifestyle; *Anxiety; Fear.*

— *OBJECTIVE DATA* (observed) —

Changes in behavior, communication patterns, appearance, or lifestyle; reactivation of previous conditions (physical illness, psychiatric illness, alcohol or drug abuse). *Additional data for Silent Reaction:* lack of verbalization of the occurrence of rape.

• Related Factors

Attempted or actual sexual assault.

• Clinical Alert

Referral of this diagnosis to a professional qualified in rape counseling is likely to result in improved outcomes.

Relocation Stress Syndrome

Physiologic or psychosocial disturbances as a result of transfer from one environment to another.

• Defining Characteristics
— *SUBJECTIVE DATA* (reported) —

Apprehension, increased confusion (elderly population), depression, loneliness, concern about or unwillingness to transfer, increased verbalization of needs, insecurity, lack of trust, unfavorable comparison of post- to pre- transfer staff, anger, *Anxiety.*

— *OBJECTIVE DATA* (observed) —

Change in eating habits or weight, sleep disturbances, GI disturbances, dependency, restlessness, sad affect, vigilance, withdrawal.

• Related Factors

Past, concurrent, or recent losses; losses involved with decision to move; little or no preparation for the move; moderate to high degree of environmental change; history and types of previous transfers; feeling of powerlessness; lack of adequate support system; impaired psychosocial or physical health status; advanced age.

• Compare With

Loneliness; Powerlessness; Social Isolation.

Relocation Stress Syndrome, Risk For

State in which the person is at risk for physiologic or psychosocial disturbances as a result of transfer from one environment to another.

• Risk Factors

See related factors for *Relocation Stress Syndrome*

Role Performance, Ineffective

The state in which a person perceives a disruption in ability to perform usual roles.

• Defining Characteristics
— *SUBJECTIVE DATA* (reported) —

Change in self-perception of role, role conflict.

— *OBJECTIVE DATA* (observed) —

Change in others' perception of role.

• Related Factors

Change in capacity to resume role, lack of knowledge of role, change in usual patterns of responsibility.

• Compare With

Adjustment, Impaired; Parental Role Conflict; Sexuality Patterns, Ineffective; Home maintenance, Impaired.

Self-Care Deficit, Bathing/Hygiene[4]

A state in which a person experiences an impaired ability to perform or complete bathing or hygiene activities for oneself.

• Defining Characteristics
— *OBJECTIVE DATA* (observed) —

Inability to: wash body parts, obtain (or get to) water, regulate temperature or flow.

• Related Factors

Decreased mobility, strength, or endurance: pain, discomfort; perceptual, cognitive, neuromuscular, or musculoskeletal impairment; depression; *Anxiety* (severe); *Activity Intolerance.*

• Compare With

Activity Intolerance; Mobility, Impaired Physical.

Self-Care Deficit, Feeding[4]

A state in which a person experiences an impaired ability to perform or complete feeding activities for oneself.

• Defining Characteristics
— *OBJECTIVE DATA* (observed) —

Inability to bring food from a receptacle to the mouth.

• Related Factors

Decreased mobility, strength, or endurance; pain, discomfort; perceptual, cognitive neuromuscular, or musculoskeletal impairment; depression; *Anxiety* (severe); *Activity Intolerance.*

---

[4]Classify functional level by using the following code: (0) completely independent; (1) requires use of equipment or device; (2) requires help from another person for assistance, supervision, or teaching; (3) requires help from another person and equipment or device; (4) dependent, doesn't participate in activity.

• Compare With

Mobility, Impaired Physical; Activity Intolerance; Nutrition, Imbalanced: Less than Body Requirements.

Self-Care Deficit, Dressing/ Grooming[4]

A state in which a person experiences an impaired ability to perform or complete dressing and grooming activities for oneself.

• Defining Characteristics
— *OBJECTIVE DATA* (observed) —

Impaired ability to: put on or take off necessary items of clothing, obtain or replace articles of clothing, fasten clothing, maintain satisfactory appearance.

• Related Factors

Decreased mobility, strength, or endurance; pain, discomfort; perceptual, cognitive, neuromuscular, or musculoskeletal impairment; depression; *Anxiety* (severe); *Activity Intolerance.*

• Compare With

Activity Intolerance; Mobility, Impaired Physical.

Self-Care Deficit, Toileting[4]

Impaired ability to perform or complete toileting activities for oneself.

• Defining Characteristics
— *OBJECTIVE DATA* (observed) —

Inability to: get to toilet, sit on or rise from toilet, manipulate clothing for toileting, carry out toilet hygiene, flush toilet or empty commode.

• Related Factors

Decreased mobility, strength, or endurance; pain, discomfort; perceptual, cognitive, neuromuscular, or musculoskeletal impairment; depression; *Anxiety* (severe); *Activity Intolerance.*

• Compare With

Activity Intolerance; Mobility, Impaired Physical.

Self-Esteem, Chronic Low

Long-standing negative evaluation of self or personal capabilities.

• Defining Characteristics
— *SUBJECTIVE DATA* (reported) —

Long-standing or chronic symptoms of low self-esteem (see subjective data listed under defining characteristics of *Self-Esteem Disturbance*).

— *OBJECTIVE DATA* (observed) —

Long-standing or chronic signs of low self-esteem (see objective data listed under defining characteristics of *Self-Esteem Disturbance*).

• Related Factors

History of ineffective or abusive relationships; unrealistic expectations of child by parent, of parent by child, or of self; inadequate support; rejection or separation; inconsistent punishment; lack of stimulation; restriction of activity; inability to trust significant other.

• Compare With

Self-Esteem, Situational Low.

Self-Esteem Disturbance

Negative evaluation or feelings about self or about personal capabilities.

• Defining Characteristics
— *SUBJECTIVE DATA* (reported) —

Shame or guilt; inability to deal with events; rejection of positive feedback or exaggeration of negative feedback; hesitance to try new things or situations; lack of success in relationships, work, or other life events; difficulty making decisions.

— *OBJECTIVE DATA* (observed) —

Dependence on others' opinions; poor eye contact; nonassertive, passive, or indecisive behaviors; excessive seeking of reassurance; being overly conforming; self-negating verbalization; difficulty making decisions.

• Related Factors

Relationships characterized by abuse (verbal, sexual, physical), parental neglect, helplessness.

• Compare With

Adjustment, Impaired; Coping, Ineffective; Self-Esteem, Situational Low; Self-Esteem, Chronic Low.

Self-Esteem, Situational Low

The state in which a person who previously had a positive self-evaluation experiences negative self-evaluation or feelings in response to a loss or change.

• Defining Characteristics
— *SUBJECTIVE DATA* (reported) —

Episodic occurrence of symptoms of low self-esteem in response to a loss or change (see subjective data listed under defining characteristics of *Self-Esteem Disturbance*).

— *OBJECTIVE DATA* (observed) —

Episodic occurrence of signs of low self-esteem in response to a loss or change (see defining characteristics of *Self-Esteem Disturbance*).

• Related Factors

Unemployment, financial problems, divorce, legal difficulties, institutionalization, failure in school or work, hospitalization.

• Compare With

Adjustment, Impaired; Coping, Ineffective; Self-Esteem, Chronic Low; Self-Esteem Disturbance.

Self-Mutilation, Risk for

A state in which a person is at risk of performing an act upon the self to injure, not kill, which produces tissue damage and tension relief.

• Risk Factors

Borderline personality disorder (especially females 16 to 25 years of age); psychotic state (frequently males in young adulthood); emotionally disturbed or battered children; mentally retarded and autistic children; history of self-injury; history of physical, emotional, or sexual abuse; inability to cope with increased psychological or physiologic tension; feelings of depression, rejection, self-hatred, separation anxiety, guilt, and depersonalization; fluctuating emotions; command hallucinations; need for sensory stimuli; parental or emotional deprivation; dysfunctional family.

Sensory Perception, Disturbed (Specify: visual, auditory, kinesthetic, gustatory, tactile, olfactory)

A state in which a person experiences a change in the amount or pattern of incoming stimuli accompanied by a diminished, exaggerated, distorted, or impaired response to these stimuli.

• Defining Characteristics

— *SUBJECTIVE DATA* (reported) —

Hallucinations, *Fatigue, Anxiety.*

— *OBJECTIVE DATA* (observed) —

Disorientation to time, place, or person; measurable decreased sensory acuity; change in behavior or communication pattern; inability to solve problems; inappropriate responses; apathy; restlessness; irritability.

• Related Factors

Sensory organ deficits; impaired sensory reception, transmission, or integration; excessive or insufficient environmental stimuli; sleep deprivation; metabolic alterations (eg, fluid and electrolyte imbalance, acidosis, alkalosis); medication side effects; *Acute Pain;* stress.

• Compare With

Thought Processes, Impaired.

Sexual Dysfunction

A change in sexual function that is viewed as unsatisfying, unrewarding, or inadequate.

• Defining Characteristics

— *SUBJECTIVE DATA* (reported) —

Problem with sexual function, dissatisfaction with sex role, limitations imposed by disease or therapy, inability to achieve desired sexual satisfaction, seeking of confirmation of desirability, altered relationship with significant other, change of interest in self or others.

— *OBJECTIVE DATA* (observed) —

Frequent sex-related questions.

• Related Factors

Biopsychosocial alteration of sexuality, ineffectual or absent role models, physical or psychosocial abuse (eg, harmful relationships), vulnerability, values conflict, lack of privacy, lack of significant other, altered body structure or function (eg, pregnancy, recent childbirth, drugs, surgery, anomalies, disease process, trauma, radiation), misinformation or lack of knowledge.

• Compare With

Sexuality Patterns, Ineffective.

Sexuality Patterns, Ineffective

The state in which a person experiences, or is at risk for experiencing, a change in sexual patterns.

• Defining Characteristics

— *SUBJECTIVE DATA* (reported) —

Difficulties, limitations, or changes in sexual behaviors or activities.

— *OBJECTIVE DATA* (observed) —

Frequent sex-related questions.

• Related Factors

Knowledge or skill deficit about alternative responses to health-related transitions, altered body function or structure, illness or medical treatment, lack of privacy, lack of significant other, ineffective or absent role models, conflicts with sexual orientation or variant preferences, fear of pregnancy or of acquiring or transmitting a sexually transmitted disease, impaired relationship with a significant other.

• Compare With

Sexual Dysfunction.

Skin Integrity, Impaired

A state in which a person's skin is impaired.

• Defining Characteristics

— *SUBJECTIVE DATA* (reported) —

Itching, pain, numbness.

— *OBJECTIVE DATA* (observed) —

Nonblanchable erythema, denuded skin, destruction of epidermal and dermal skin layers.

• Related Factors

External factors: extremes of temperature, humidity, chemical substances, secretions or excretions, mechanical factors (shearing forces, pressure, restraints), trauma, radiation, immobilization.

Internal factors: imbalanced nutritional state (obesity, malnutrition), metabolic state, circulation, pigmentation or skin turgor; impaired sensation, skeletal prominence, developmental factors, immunologic deficits, medication side effects, edema, subcutaneous fat loss, decreased skin turgor.

• Compare With

Skin Integrity, Risk for Impaired; Tissue Integrity, Impaired.

Skin Integrity, Risk for Impaired

A state in which a person's skin is at risk of being impaired.

• Risk Factors

See Related Factors for *Impaired Skin Integrity.*

Sleep Pattern, Disturbed

Disruption of sleep time that causes discomfort or interferes with desired lifestyle.

• Defining Characteristics

— *SUBJECTIVE DATA* (reported) —

Difficulty falling asleep, awakening earlier or later than desired, interrupted sleep, not feeling well rested.

— *OBJECTIVE DATA* (observed) —

Changes in behavior and performance (eg, increased irritability, restlessness, disorientation, lethargy, listlessness), nystagmus, hand tremor, ptosis of eyelid, expressionless face, dark circles under eyes, frequent yawning, changes in posture, thick speech with mispronunciation and incorrect words.

• Related Factors

Internal sensory alterations: illness, psychological stress.
External sensory alterations: environmental changes, medication side effects, caregiving responsibilities.

• Compare With

Anxiety; Fatigue.

Social Interaction, Impaired

The state in which a person participates in an insufficient or excessive quantity, or ineffective quality, of social exchange.

• Defining Characteristics

— *SUBJECTIVE DATA* (reported) —

Discomfort in social situations; inability to receive or communicate a satisfying sense of belonging, caring, interest, or shared history.

— *OBJECTIVE DATA* (observed) —

Unsuccessful or dysfunctional social interaction behaviors, change in style or pattern of interaction.

• Related Factors

Knowledge or skill deficit about ways of enhancing mutuality, communication barriers, self-concept disturbance, absence of available significant others or peers, limited mobility, therapeutic isolation, sociocultural dissonance, environmental barriers, *Impaired Thought Processes.*

• Compare With

Communication, Impaired; Loneliness, Risk for; Social Isolation.

Social Isolation

The state in which a person experiences loneliness and perceives it as a negative or threatened state imposed by others.

• Defining Characteristics

— *SUBJECTIVE DATA* (reported) —

Lack of satisfying personal relationships or significant purpose in life, feelings of rejection or being different from others, inability to meet others' expectations, insecurity in public.

— *OBJECTIVE DATA* (observed) —

Absence of supportive significant other(s); sad, dull affect; communication deficits (eg, language barriers, withdrawal, poor eye contact); hostility in voice or behavior; preoccupation with own thoughts.

• Related Factors

Delay in accomplishing developmental tasks, immature interests, unusual physical appearance, chronic illness, impaired mental status, unacceptable social values or behavior, inadequate personal resources, absence of peers, inability to engage in satisfying personal relationships.

• Compare With

Communication, Impaired Verbal; Loneliness, Risk for; Social Interaction, Impaired.

Spiritual Distress

Distress of the human spirit, disruption in the life principle that pervades a person's entire being and integrates and transcends one's biologic and psychosocial nature.

• Defining Characteristics

— SUBJECTIVE DATA (reported) —

Concern with meaning of life, death, or belief systems; anger toward God; seeking to understand meaning of suffering, own existence, or moral or ethical implications of therapeutic regimen; inability to participate in usual religious practices; desire to talk with a chaplain or priest; anger toward religious representatives; nightmares, sleep disturbances.

— OBJECTIVE DATA (observed) —

Altered behavior or mood (eg, anger, crying, withdrawal, preoccupation, *Anxiety,* hostility, apathy, and so forth), use of gallows humor.

• Related Factors

Separation from religious or cultural ties, challenged belief and value system (eg, due to moral or ethical implications of therapy or intense suffering).

• Compare With

Spiritual Well-Being, Readiness for Enhanced.

Spiritual Well-Being, Readiness for Enhanced

Spiritual well-being is the process of an individual's developing/unfolding of mystery through harmonious interconnectedness that springs from inner strengths.

• Related Factors

(None listed.)

• Defining Characteristics

— SUBJECTIVE DATA (reported) —

A sense of awareness, self-consciousness, sacred source, unifying force, inner core, and transcendence; unfolding mystery; one's experience about life's purpose and meaning, mystery, uncertainty, and struggles; harmonious interconnectedness; relatedness, connectedness, harmony with self, others, higher power/God, and the environment.

• Compare With

Spiritual Distress.

Suffocation, Risk for

The state in which a person is at risk of suffocation (inadequate air available for inhalation).

• Risk Factors

Individual: reduced olfactory sensation or motor abilities, lack of safety education or precautions, cognitive or emotional difficulties, disease or injury process. *Environmental:* vehicle warming in closed garage, gas leaks, smoking in bed, use of fuel-burning heaters not vented to outside, clothesline. *Additional factors for children:* pillow or propped bottle placed in an infant's crib; playing with plastic bags or balloons, or inserting small objects into mouth or nose; discarded or unused refrigerators or freezers without removed doors; unsupervised bathing or swimming; pacifier hung around neck.

• Compare With

Aspiration, Risk for; Home Maintenance, Impaired.

Suicide, Risk for

At risk for self-inflicted life-threatening injury.

• Risk Factors

Behavioral: History of prior suicide attempt, impulsiveness, buying a gun, stockpiling medicines, making or changing a will, giving away possessions, sudden euphoric recovery from major depression, marked changes in behavior or attitude or school performance, threats of killing oneself, statements of desire to die or "end it all". *Situational:* Living alone, retired, relocation, institutionalization, economic instability, loss of autonomy or independence, presence of gun in the home, adolescents living in nontraditional settings (eg, juvenile detention center, prison, halfway house). *Psychological:* Family history of suicide, alcohol and substance use/abuse; psychiatric illness or disorder; history of childhood abuse; guilt; gay or lesbian youth. *Demographic:* Age (elderly, young adult males, adolescents); Race (Caucasian, Native American); Gender (male), widowed or divorced. *Physical:* chronic or terminal illness or pain. *Social:* Loss of important relationship, disrupted family life, grief, bereavement, poor support systems, loneliness, hopelessness, helplessness, social isolation, legal or disciplinary problem, cluster suicides.

• Clinical Alert

Specifically ask those at risk for suicide whether there is a risk for suicide. Get them to make a promise or contract not to attempt suicide within a specific time frame (eg, "Can you promise me that you will call me if you feel like you might harm yourself before I see you in the morning?").

Swallowing, Impaired

The state in which a person has decreased ability to voluntarily pass fluids or solids from the mouth to the stomach.

• Defining Characteristics
— *SUBJECTIVE DATA* (reported) —

Difficulty swallowing.

— *OBJECTIVE DATA* (observed) —

Observed evidence of difficulty in swallowing, stasis or pocketing of food in oral cavity, coughing or choking with swallowing attempts, drooling, evidence of aspiration.

• Related Factors

Neuromuscular impairment (eg, decreased or absent gag reflex, decreased strength or excursion of muscles involved in mastication or swallowing, perceptual impairment, facial paralysis, postcerebrovascular accident); congenital anomalies (cleft palate, tracheoesophageal fistula); mechanical obstruction (eg, edema, tracheostomy tube, tumor); limited awareness; reddened, irritated oropharyngeal cavity; weakness, *Fatigue.*

• Compare With

Aspiration, Risk for.

Therapeutic Regimen, Ineffective Community Management

A pattern of regulating and integrating into community processes programs for treatment of illness and the sequelae of illness that are unsatisfactory for meeting health-related goals.

• Risk Factors
— *OBJECTIVE DATA* (observed) —

Deficits in persons and programs to be accountable for illness care of aggregates, deficits in advocates for aggregates, deficits in community activities for secondary and tertiary prevention, illness symptoms above the norm expected for the number and type of population, number of health care resources are insufficient for the incidence or prevalence of illness(es), unavailable health care resources for illness care, unexpected acceleration of illness(es).

Therapeutic Regimen, Ineffective Family Management of

A pattern of regulating and integrating into family processes a program for treatment of illness and the sequelae of illness that is unsatisfactory for meeting specific goals.

• Defining Characteristics
— *SUBJECTIVE DATA* (reported) —

Desire to manage the treatment of illness and prevention of the sequelae, verbalized difficulty with regulation/integration of one or more effects or prevention of complication, verbalizes that family did not take action to reduce risk factors for progression of illness and sequelae.

— *OBJECTIVE DATA* (observed) —

Inappropriate family activities for meeting the goals of a treatment or prevention program, acceleration (expected or unexpected) of illness symptom of a family member, lack of attention to illness and its sequelae.

• Related Factors

Complexity of health care system, complexity of therapeutic regimen, decisional conflicts, economic difficulties, excessive demands made on individual or family, family conflicts.

Therapeutic Regimen, Effective Management of

A pattern of regulating and integrating into daily living a program for treatment of illness and its sequelae that is satisfactory for meeting specific health goals.

• Defining Characteristics
— *SUBJECTIVE DATA* (reported) —

Desire to manage the treatment of illness and prevention of sequelae, verbalized intent to reduce risk factors for progression of illness and sequelae.

— *OBJECTIVE DATA* (observed) —

Appropriate choices of daily activities for meeting the goals of a treatment or prevention program, illness symptoms are within a normal range of expectation.

• Related Factors

(None listed).

Management of Therapeutic Regimen, Ineffective

A state in which a person has a pattern of regulating and integrating into daily living a program for treatment of illness (and sequelae) that is unsatisfactory for meeting specific health goals.

• Defining Characteristics
— *SUBJECTIVE DATA* (reported) —

Desire to manage the illness and prevent sequelae; difficulty with regulation or integration of prescribed regimens for treatment of illness and its effects, or prevention of complications; report that no actions are being taken to include treatment regimens in daily routines or to reduce risk factors for progression of illness and sequelae.

— *OBJECTIVE DATA* (observed) —

Acceleration or lack of improvement of symptoms, choices of daily living ineffective for meeting the goals of treatment or prevention program.

• Related Factors

Complexity of health care system or therapeutic regimen, mistrust of regimen or health care personnel, in-

adequate assistive resources (eg, written schedule to follow regimen, devices to make following regimen easier), economic difficulties, excessive demands on individual or family, family conflict or patterns of health care inconsistent with therapeutic regimen, social support deficits.

• Compare With

Decisional Conflict; Health Maintenance, Ineffective; Home Maintenance, Impaired; Knowledge, Deficient; Powerlessness.

Thermoregulation, Ineffective (1986)

The state in which a person's temperature fluctuates between hypothermia and hyperthermia.

• Defining Characteristics
— *OBJECTIVE DATA* (observed) —

Fluctuations in body temperature above or below the normal range.

• Related Factors

Trauma, illness, immaturity, aging, fluctuating environmental temperature.

• Compare With

Body Temperature, Risk for Imbalanced.

Thought Processes, Impaired

Disruption in such mental activities as conscious thought, reality orientation, problem solving, judgment, and comprehension.

• Defining Characteristics
— *SUBJECTIVE DATA* (reported) —

Inaccurate interpretation of internal or external stimuli, hallucinations, delusions, phobias, obsessions, *Anxiety, Fear.*

— *OBJECTIVE DATA* (observed) —

Distractibility, cognitive dissonance, memory deficit, egocentricity, hyper- or hypovigilance, confusion, disorientation.

• Related Factors

Medications, substance abuse, electrolyte imbalance, depression, dementia, bipolar disorders, borderline personality, multiple demands or stressors, sleep deprivation, sensory bombardment.

• Compare With

Sensory Perception, Disturbed.

Tissue Integrity, Impaired

A state in which a person experiences damage to mucous membrane, corneal, integumentary, or subcutaneous tissue.

• Defining Characteristics

— *SUBJECTIVE DATA* (reported) —

Acute pain.

— *OBJECTIVE DATA* (observed) —

Damaged or destroyed tissue (corneal, mucous membrane, integumentary, or subcutaneous).

• Related Factors

Impaired circulation, nutritional deficit or excess, fluid deficit or excess, *Knowledge, Deficient,* impaired mobility, chemical irritants (body secretions or excretions, medications), temperature extremes, mechanical factors (pressure, shear, friction), radiation.

• Compare With

Oral Mucous Membrane, Impaired; Skin Integrity, Impaired.

Tissue Perfusion, Ineffective (Specify: renal, cerebral, cardiopulmonary, GI, peripheral)

A decrease in oxygen resulting in the failure to nourish tissues at the capillary level.

• Defining Characteristics

— *SUBJECTIVE DATA* (reported) —

Cardiopulmonary: chest pain, sense of impending doom, dyspnea. *Cerebral:* Confusion. *Gastrointestinal:* Abdominal pain or tenderness. *Peripheral:* Pain, claudication. *Renal:* history of kidney failure.

— *OBJECTIVE DATA* (observed) —

Cardiopulmonary: Abnormal respiratory rate, accessory muscle use, capillary refill greater than 3 seconds, abnormal blood gases, bronchospasms, arrhythmia, nasal flaring, chest retraction. *Cerebral:* Speech abnormalities, changes in pupillary reactions, extremity weakness or paralysis, impaired mental status, changes in motor response, behavioral changes, difficulty swallowing.
Gastrointestinal: Hypoactive or absent bowel sounds, nausea, abdominal distention. *Peripheral:* Pale skin color on elevation and color doesn't return on lowering of leg, slow healing of lesions, claudications, blood pressure changes in extremes, bruits, edema, positive Homans' sign, weak or absent pulses, skin discoloration, skin temperature changes, impaired sensations. *Renal:* Abnormal blood pressure, hematuria, oliguria or anuria, elevated BUN/creatinine ratio, diminished arterial pulsations.

• Related Factors

Hypovolemia, interruption of arterial or venous blood flow, hypervolemia, exchange problems, hypoventilation, impaired transport of oxygen across alveolar or capillary membrane, mismatch of ventilation with blood flow, decreased hemoglobin concentration, enzyme poisoning, impaired affinity of hemoglobin for oxygen.

• Clinical Alert

Report new onset of the above problems immediately to facilitate urgent medical evaluation.

• Compare With

Activity Intolerance; Cardiac Output, Decreased; Gas Exchange, Impaired; Peripheral Neurovascular Dysfunction, Risk for; Tissue Integrity, Impaired; Thought Processes, Impaired.

Trauma, Risk for

The state in which a person is at risk of injury to tissues (eg, wound, burn, fracture).

• Risk Factors

Individual: weakness; vision, balance, cognitive, or emotional difficulties; reduced temperature or tactile sensation; reduced hand–eye coordination, or large or small muscle coordination; lack of safety education or precautions; insufficient finances to purchase safety equipment or effect repairs; history of previous trauma. *Environmental:* slippery floors, stairs, or walkways (highly waxed, wet spots, icy or snowy spots); unanchored rugs or electrical wires; bathtub without hand grip or antislip equipment; unsteady ladders or chairs; unlighted rooms; unsturdy or absent stair rails; obstructed passageways; inappropriate call-for-aid mechanisms for immobile individuals; potential for igniting gas leaks; delayed lighting of gas burner or oven; experimenting with chemical or gasoline; unscreened fires or heaters; wearing plastic apron or flowing clothes around open flame; inadequately stored combustibles or corrosives (matches, oily rags, lye); overloaded fuse boxes; contact with rapidly moving machinery, industrial belts, or pulleys; sliding on coarse bed linen; struggling within restraints; faulty electrical plugs, frayed wires, or defective appliances; contact with acids or alkalis; playing with fireworks or gunpowder; contact with intense cold; overexposure to sun, sun lamps; cracked dishware or glasses; knives stored uncovered; guns or ammunition stored unlocked; large icicles hanging from roof; exposure to dangerous machinery; high-crime neighborhood and vulnerable clients; driving a mechanically unsafe vehicle, after partaking in alcohol or drugs, at excessive speeds, or without necessary visual or hearing aids; smoking in bed or near oxygen; overloaded electrical outlets; grease waste collected on stoves; thin or worn pot holders; misuse of bicycle or motorcycle helmets; unsafe road or road-crossing conditions; play or work near vehicle pathways (eg, driveways, lanes, railroad tracks).

Additional for children: unsafe storage of medications or potential poisons; inadequate stair gates; unsafe window protection; appliance cords or pot handles within reach; unsupervised bathing, swimming, or play; flammable toys or clothing; toys with sharp edges or small parts that can be removed; toys not approved for ages of children in home; balloons; availability of matches, candles, and cigarettes; inadequate car seats; absence of bicycle wheel guard or helmet for child riding on back; absence of adequate fences or gates in pool area; unfamiliar pets (dogs, cats).

• Compare With

Injury, Risk for.

Unilateral Neglect

The state in which a person is unaware of the hemiplegic side of his or her body, or unaware of objects, persons, or sounds on the hemiplegic side of the body.

• Defining Characteristics
— *OBJECTIVE DATA* (observed) —

Failure to see, hear, or feel stimuli on affected side; failure to purposefully use extremities on affected side; lack of awareness of positioning of extremities on affected side.

• Related Factors

Effects of stroke, brain tumor, or brain injury (hemianopsia, one-sided blindness, perceptual disturbances).

• Compare With

Sensory Perception, Disturbed (Visual); Self-Care Deficit.

Urinary Elimination, Impaired

A disturbance in urine elimination.

• Author's Note

Defining Characteristics and Related Factors aren't listed because this diagnosis is too nonspecific. See *Urinary Incontinence, Functional; Urinary Incontinence, Reflex; Urinary Incontinence, Stress; Urinary Incontinence, Total; Urinary Incontinence, Urge; Urinary Retention.*

Urinary Incontinence, Functional

Inability of a usually continent person to reach toilet in time to avoid unintentional voiding.

• Defining Characteristics
— *SUBJECTIVE DATA* (reported)—

Incontinence only in early morning, senses need to void, inability to reach commode in time, able to completely empty bladder.

— *OBJECTIVE DATA* (observed)—

Loss of urine before reaching toilet.

• Related Factors

Psychological factors, impaired vision, impaired cognition, neuromuscular limitations, altered environment, weakened supporting pelvic structures.

• Compare With

Urinary Elimination, Impaired; Urinary Incontinence, Reflex; Urinary Incontinence, Stress; Urinary Incontinence, Total; Urinary Incontinence, Urge.

Urinary Incontinence, Reflex

An involuntary loss of urine, occurring at somewhat predictable intervals when a specific bladder volume is reached.

• Related Factors

Tissue damage from radiation cystitis, inflammatory bladder conditions, or radical pelvic surgery; neurologic impairment above the level of sacral micturition center or pontine micturition center.

• Defining Characteristics
— *SUBJECTIVE DATA* (reported) —

No awareness of bladder filling; no urge to void, feelings of bladder fullness, or sensation of voiding; unable to cognitively initiate or inhibit voiding.

— *OBJECTIVE DATA* (observed) —

Involuntary urination at somewhat predictable intervals; predictable pattern of voiding; incomplete emptying with lesion above sacral micturition center.

• Compare With

Urinary Elimination, Impaired; Urinary Incontinence, Functional; Urinary Incontinence, Stress; Urinary Incontinence, Total; Urinary Incontinence, Urge.

Urinary Incontinence, Stress

A loss of urine of less than 50 mL occurring with increased abdominal pressure.

• Related Factors

Weak pelvic muscles or structural supports associated with age, surgery, or childbirth; high intra-abdominal pressure (eg, obesity, gravid uterus, coughing); incompetent bladder outlet; overdistention between voiding.

• Defining Characteristics
— *SUBJECTIVE DATA* (reported) —

Urinary urgency; urinary incontinence with coughing, sneezing.

— *OBJECTIVE DATA* (observed) —

Dribbling with increased abdominal pressure, urinary frequency (more often than every 2 hours).

• Compare With

Urinary Elimination, Impaired; Urinary Incontinence, Functional; Urinary Incontinence, Reflex; Urinary Incontinence, Total; Urinary Incontinence, Urge; Urinary Retention.

Urinary Incontinence, Total

A continuous and unpredictable loss of urine.

• Defining Characteristics
— *SUBJECTIVE DATA* (reported) —

Unawareness of bladder filling or incontinence, decreased sensation of perineal area.

— *OBJECTIVE DATA* (observed) —

Constant flow of urine at unpredictable times without urinary distention, incontinence not responding to treatment.

• Related Factors

Neuropathy preventing transmission of reflex indicating bladder fullness; neurologic dysfunction causing triggering of micturition at unpredictable times; independent contraction of detrusor reflex due to surgery, trauma, or disease affecting spinal cord nerves; anomaly (fistula).

• Compare With

Urinary Incontinence, Functional; Urinary Incontinence, Reflex; Urinary Incontinence, Stress; Urinary Incontinence, Urge.

Urinary Incontinence, Urge

Involuntary urine loss associated with a sudden, strong sensation of urgency.

• Related Factors

Decreased bladder capacity (eg, history of pelvic inflammatory disease, abdominal surgeries, indwelling urinary catheter), irritation of bladder stretch receptors causing spasm (eg, bladder infection), alcohol, caffeine, increased fluids, increased urine concentration, overdistention of bladder, enlarged prostate.

• Defining Characteristics

— *SUBJECTIVE DATA* (reported) —

Urgency, inability to reach bedpan or commode in time, frequent voiding.

— *OBJECTIVE DATA* (observed) —

Frequent urination, voiding immediately after urge to urinate.

Urinary Retention

Incomplete emptying of the bladder.

• Defining Characteristics

— *SUBJECTIVE DATA* (reported) —

Sensation of bladder fullness, dysuria.

— *OBJECTIVE DATA* (observed) —

Bladder distention; urine loss or voiding in small, frequent amounts; absence of urine output; dribbling; residual urine more than 100 mL.

• Related Factors

High urethral pressure caused by weak detrusor muscles, inhibition of reflex arc, strong sphincter, blockage, medication side effects.

• Compare With

Urinary Elimination, Impaired; Urinary Incontinence, Stress; Urinary Incontinence, Urge.

Ventilation, Impaired Spontaneous

A state in which the response pattern of decreased energy reserves results in a person's inability to maintain breathing adequate to support life.

• Defining Characteristics

— *SUBJECTIVE DATA* (reported) —

Dyspnea, apprehension.

— *OBJECTIVE DATA* (observed) —

Bradypnea, tachypnea, increased restlessness, decreased cooperation, increased use of accessory muscles, decreased tidal volume, increased heart rate, decreased Po_2, increased PCo_2, decreased oxygen saturation.

• Related Factors

Metabolic factors, respiratory muscle fatigue.

• Clinical Alert

These defining characteristics describe a degree of respiratory distress that is life threatening and requires immediate initiation of physician-prescribed interventions.

• Compare With

Ventilatory Weaning Response, Dysfunctional.

Ventilatory Weaning Response, Dysfunctional (DVWR)

The state in which someone cannot adjust to lowered levels of mechanical ventilator support, which interrupts and prolongs the weaning process.

• Defining Characteristics

— *SUBJECTIVE DATA* (reported) —

During weaning periods: increased need for oxygen, breathing discomfort, fatigue, warmth, increased concentration on breathing, apprehension.

— *OBJECTIVE DATA* (observed) —

During weaning periods: restlessness; increased blood pressure, heart rate, and respiratory rate; hypervigilance; lack of response to coaching; diaphoresis; wide-eyed look; decreased breath sounds; pallor, cyanosis; use of accessory muscles for respiration; agitation; deterioration in arterial blood gases or oxygen saturation; shallow, gasping breaths; paradoxical abdominal breathing; decreased consciousness level.

• Related Factors

Excessive airway secretions, sleep deprivation, inadequate nutrition, pain or discomfort, lack of trust in caregivers, insufficient information related to weaning process, perceived need for ventilator, prolonged ventilator dependence, previous unsuccessful weaning attempts, lack of motivation, nonsupportive environment, inappropriate pacing of weaning plan, *Fatigue, Anxiety, Fear.*

Violence, Self-Directed, Risk for

A state in which a person demonstrates behaviors that can be physically harmful either to the self or others.

• Related Factors

Antisocial character; history of aggressive acts; child or spouse abuse; organic brain syndrome; temporal lobe epilepsy; toxic reactions to medications, alcohol, illegal drugs; catatonic or manic excitement; panic states; hallucinations; rage reactions; suicidal behavior.

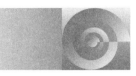

Example Responses to Critical Thinking Exercises

1. a. *Assessment* involves examining and interviewing the patient to determine health status. During *Diagnosis,* you analyze patient information and identify the problems requiring nursing or medical treatment. In *Planning,* the expected outcomes—goals of care—are determined, and the treatment plan is developed and recorded. In *Implementation,* you put the plan into action. Finally, In *Evaluation,* you evaluate whether the patient achieved the expected outcomes, and modify or terminate the plan as indicated. b. Paraphrase any of the benefits listed in Display 1–1. **2.** Use of nursing process is a requirement set forth by national practice standards (see Appendix A); it provides the basis for questions on state board exams; it promotes critical thinking in the clinical setting. **3.** The problems identified in *Diagnosis* are based on the information collected during *Assessment.* The outcomes identified during *Planning* are based on the problems determined in *Diagnosis.* The interventions used in *Implementation* are based on the outcomes identified during *Planning.* **4.** Post a copy of Display 1–6 at the nurses' station and lounge; have a conference on the importance of meeting patients' expectations; give patients short evaluation forms to evaluate satisfaction with their nursing care (nurses are more likely to pay attention to patient expectations if they are evaluated by them).

1. You can decide this by comparing yourself with Display 1–8. **3.** Compare your answer with Display 1–7. **4.** See Display 1–10.

Part I. 1. a. Tell me how you're feeling. b. How was your dinner? c. How do you feel about being here? d. Describe what you're feeling; tell me how you're feeling. **2.** a. So, you've been sick off and on for a month. What do you mean by *sick off and on*? b. You feel like nothing ever goes right for you. What's been happening? c. You have a pain in your side that comes and goes—can you explain more? d. You've had a funny feeling for a week. What do you mean by *funny?* **3.** a) C b) E c) S d) L e) O f) C g) S h) L i) O j) L k) E. **4.** d. How do you feel about feeding Susan? h. How would it be if your family visited? j. How do you feel about practicing more?

Part II. 1. a. You have a lot of ground-in dirt here. What's it from? b. I feel a lump on the back of your head. How did it happen? Does it hurt when I touch it? c. Your breathing is a little fast. How do you feel? d. Your eye seems inflamed. How does it feel? **2.** a. Show me where (and examine that area). Is there anything you think causes it? b. Show me where (and examine that area). Tell me more about how it feels. c. That's a common symptom of infection. Let's get a urine sample (and examine it). d. Where do you feel this bloating? Your stomach? Ankles? Where? (and examine the area).

CRITICAL THINKING EXERCISE IV

Part I. 1. 51 years old, no pain, feels better, feels relieved, denies being weary. **2.** Lab study results, talking slowly, frequent sighing, vital signs.
Part II. a. All the data listed under Part I, numbers 1 and 2. b. Physical condition seems to be improving. He is more comfortable. Seems weary/tired.
Part III. 1. Certainly valid: Lab studies, talking slowly, frequent sighing. Probably valid: 51 years old, no pain, feels better, vital signs. Possibly valid: Weary/tired. **2.** Compare age with birth date. Ask probing questions to clarify comfort state (*Are you sure you don't have any discomfort?*) Look for nonverbal signs of discomfort (eg, rubbing hand on chest). Spend quality time with him discussing how he feels physically and psychologically. Recheck vital signs.

CRITICAL THINKING EXERCISE V

1. You need to do both to facilitate recognition of both possible nursing problems and medical problems (see page 66). **2.** *Body systems:* Resp: 5, 6, 8, 10, 13, 14. Card: 6. Circ: 6, 15. GI: 9. Neuro: none specifically listed. GU: none listed, although you might have chosen to put 11 (childbirth) here. Skin: None listed. *Holistic nursing model:* (this organizes data according to Functional Health Patterns, but you may have chosen another model) Nutritional–Metabolic: 5, 6, 9, 10, 11, 13, 14, 15. Elimination: None listed. Activity-Exercise: 3, 8. Cognitive-perceptual: None listed. Sleep-rest: 8. Self-perception–self-concept: Role-relationship: 2, 3, 7. Sexual–reproductive: 1, 2. Coping-Stress: 10, 12. Value–belief: 4. **3.** You should think about how you can gain the missing information.

CRITICAL THINKING EXERCISE VI

1. a) N b) A c) N d) A e) A f) N g) A h) A i) N j) A.. **2.** Ask Mr. Moran to describe his daily activities. Ask him whether he has assistance with these routines. Ask what would make following the routines easier, how he could be more independent. Ask him to tell you any specific problems he sees in accomplishing daily routines. **3.** Ask Mr. Moran about his smoking history. If he's smoked, determine whether he still smokes. Ask Mr. Moran about his environment at home (air quality, such as humidity or dryness). Find out if he's ever been tested for allergies and whether contact with potential allergens has been avoided. Ask Mr. Moran to name three things that aggravate his breathing problems and three things that might help him do better.

CRITICAL THINKING EXERCISE VII

1. a. You may perform an action if you're qualified to do so (if you've demonstrated competency and have been given the authority). **b.** See Table 3–2. **2.** 1)q 2)f 3)b 4)a 5)g 6)c 7)k 8)m 9)l 10)o 11)d 12)j 13)e 14)f 15)n 16)h 17)i. **3. a.** 2,4,6 should have an "N". **b.** The following are nursing diagnoses: 2,3,5,6,9,11,12. **4.** Both models focus on treating health problems. The PPM model has a stronger focus on *early intervention* to prevent or manage potential complications.

CRITICAL THINKING EXERCISE VIII

1) b 2) a 3) c 4) e 5) g 6) h 7) f 8) d.

CRITICAL THINKING EXERCISE IX

Part I. 1. a. Problem: Urge incontinence. Cause: inability to hold large amounts of urine. Signs and symptoms: voiding immediately upon realization of need to void. b. Problem: Anticipatory Grieving. Cause: related to impending death of mother. Signs and symptoms: statements of extreme sadness over impending death. **2.** Because if they had signs and symptoms, they'd be *actual* diagnoses.

Part II. 1. *Ineffective Airway Clearance related to copious secretions as evidenced by inability to clear tracheostomy without suction.* **2.** *Imbalanced Nutrition: Less than Body Requirements related to poor appetite as evidenced by 15 lb below recommended weight.* **3.** *Powerlessness related to quadriplegia and rigorous physical therapy schedule as evidenced by report of depression and feelings of having no choices.*

Part III. 1. *Possible Ineffective Individual Coping.* **2.** *Risk for Fluid Volume Deficit related to fever.* **3.** *Risk for Ineffective Airway Clearance related to smoking history and recent general anesthesia.* **4.** *Possible Sexual Dysfunction.*

Part IV. A. 1, 4, 7, and **9** are correct. **B. 2.** May be legally incriminating. **3.** Addresses two problems in one diagnosis, isn't specific about where the pain is, isn't specific about what about the surgery is causing anxiety (eg, knowing too little? knowing too much?). **5.** Makes a value judgment that someone who's an atheist has *Spiritual Distress.* **6.** Doesn't focus on the *response* to the mastectomy or cancer. **8.** Renames a medical problem to make it sound like a nursing diagnosis. **10.** Neither the problem nor the related factors can be treated by nurse-prescribed interventions.

CRITICAL THINKING EXERCISE X

Part I. 1. PC: thrombus formation, phlebitis, extravasation, fluid overload related to IV. **2.** PC: brain swelling, bleeding, increased intracranial pressure related to concussion. **3.** PC: arrhythmias, hypotension, shock, congestive heart failure, pulmonary edema, re-infarction, embolus, cerebrovascular accident, cardiac arrest related to MI. **4.** PC: electrolyte imbalance, abdominal distention, bleeding, misplacement of the tube related to nasogastric tube.

Part II. You would ask a question like, *Looking at the big picture of this patient's situation, is it likely that he/she will be able to reach the desired outcomes in the expected timeframe using only nursing expertise for planning and management of care?* See *Identifying Problems Requiring Multidisciplinary Approaches* on page 119.

CRITICAL THINKING EXERCISE XI

Strengths: normal vital signs, moves all extremities with equal strength, strong peripheral pulses, abdomen soft, equal pupils. **Nursing Diagnoses:** *Risk for Injury related to dizziness: Risk for Impaired Patterns of Urinary Elimination related to inability to use the bed pan: Fear related to hospitalization as evidenced by statements of fear of hospitals and needles. Possible Impaired Family Processes.* **Potential Complications:** increased intracranial pressure, bleeding, phlebitis or extravasation at intravenous site.

CRITICAL   THINKING   EXERCISE   XII

1. Promote communication, direct care and documentation, provide a record that can be used for evaluation and research, provides insurance companies with a record of care requirements. **2.** Problems (eg, *Self-Care Deficit: Dressing*); outcomes (eg, dresses self without assistance by discharge); interventions (eg, have client practice buttoning clothing three times a day; evaluation/progress notes (eg, able to button and unbutton clothing with occasional help). **3.** Patient's perception of priorities, understanding of the whole picture of problems, patient's prognosis and overall health status, expected length of stay or contact, presence of clinical guidelines or critical paths related to specific situation. **4.** Severe dyspnea. Severe breathing problems are top priority unless the patient is hemorrhaging. **5.** Your state practice act, ANA standards, specialty organization standards (if you're in a specialty unit, like maternity), JCAHO standards, unique standards of the facility where you're working. **6.** Knowing the overall discharge outcomes helps you decide which problems need to be given a high priority in order to be ready for discharge in a timely fashion.

CRITICAL   THINKING   EXERCISE   XIII

Part I. 1. Outcomes are used to direct interventions, motivate patients and caregivers, and evaluate progress. **2.** Outcome, indicator, goal, objective. **3.** Outcome and indicator. **4. a.** Report the problem to whoever is responsible for achieving the outcome. **b.** Develop and initiate a plan of care to treat the problem. **5.** All nurses are responsible for detecting and reporting patients who may require case management (ie, patients who may require extra resources to achieve the expected outcomes in a timely manner).
Part II. 1. Measurable verbs help everyone to stay focused on observable data that will let you know how well the patient is progressing toward outcome achievement. For examples of measurable verbs, see page 134. **2.** Subject: Who is the person expected to achieve the goal? Verb: What actions must the person take to achieve the goal? Condition: Under what circumstances is the person to perform the actions? Performance Criteria: How well is the person to perform the actions? Target Time: By when is the person expected to be able to perform the actions? **3.** The following are incorrect. a. The verb isn't measurable. c. Nonspecific. How will we measure what is meant by "will improve"? f. No time frame listed; verb isn't measurable and observable. i. Verb isn't measurable. **4.** a. Will demonstrate healthy looking gums, without redness or irritation by Jan 15. b. Will not demonstrate signs and symptoms of Impaired Skin Integrity in the rectal area and area will be kept clean. c. Will be able to communicate basic needs through use of flash cards and through an interpreter when required.
Part III. a) C, P b) A c) C d) C, P
Part IV. a. View film on infant nutrition and formula feedings on 4/5. Describes the steps involved in sterilizing formula on 4/5. Demonstrate sterilizing baby formula on 4/6. b. Discuss with primary nurse on 2/2 how patient feels about going home. c. Attend group diabetic class on nutrition on 10/11. Discuss with primary nurse the relationship between blood sugar levels and eating certain foods on 10/11. Review printed diet restrictions on 10/11. d. Attend group diabetic class on insulin administration and monitoring of blood sugar level on 7/29. View teaching film on insulin administration and monitoring of blood sugar level on 7/29. Observe the nurse demonstrating the correct procedures for insulin administration and for testing blood sugar level on 7/30. Practice insulin self-administration based on morning blood sugar readings beginning 7/31.

CRITICAL THINKING EXERCISE XIV

Part I. 1. Classifying interventions into direct and indirect interventions allows you to examine nursing activities and time spent in direct contact with patients and activities and time spent performing activities on behalf of the patient, but away from the patient (eg, analyzing lab studies). **2.** See = What must be *assessed or observed* related to the intervention; do = what must be *done;* teach = what must be *taught or reinforced;* record = what must be *recorded* related to the intervention. **3.** What can be done about the cause(s) of this problem? What can be done to help this specific person achieve this specific outcome? **4.** See page 146.

Part II. 1. Monitor skin integrity, especially over bony prominences, with each position change. Post at bedside a schedule for turning every 2 hours, enlisting the client's maximum participation. Keep an air mattress on the bed. Ensure adequate vitamin C and protein intake. Keep sheets clean, dry, and unwrinkled. **2.** *Preoperatively:* Determine patient and family knowledge of coughing and deep breathing with incisional splinting. Teach as indicated and have patient return demonstration. *Postoperatively:* Monitor for incisional pain and medicate pm before pain is too intense. Teach the importance of asking for pain medication before pain is severe, changing positions, ambulating early, and coughing and deep breathing. Record pain level after medication is given. Record breath sounds q4h. Help client to cough and deep breath q2h the day of surgery and first postoperative day. **3.** Monitor daily bowel movements. Teach the relationship between exercise, diet, fluid intake, and bowel elimination. Develop a plan to increase roughage and fluid intake, and to increase exercise gradually (eg, using stairs instead of elevator).

Part III. 1. PC: Extravasation, phlebitis, thrombus formation, fluid overload, infection. Plan: Follow hospital policies or standards for care of IV therapy. Monitor vital signs q4h. Monitor IV site for signs and symptoms of infection, extravasation, phlebitis, thrombus q4h. Instruct patient to report discomfort or swelling at IV site. **2.** PC: Hypoglycemia/hyperglycemia. Plan: Follow hospital policies or standards for care of diabetics. Record daily caloric intake. Record blood sugars q4h. Instruct patient to report symptoms of dizziness or "feeling funny" in any way. **3.** PC: Infection, blockage of the catheter, bleeding. Plan: Follow hospital policies and standards for Foley catheter care. Monitor temperature q4–8h. Monitor urine color, odor, and amount. Record intake and output q8h. Monitor meatus for drainage or bleeding. Instruct patient to report catheter or bladder discomfort.

CRITICAL THINKING EXERCISE XV

1. a. No. b. Because it's the first time she's getting out of bed and you don't really know how she will respond. (See *When Should You Delegate*? on page 168). **2.** a. The nurse is accountable because she knew the UAP was leaving the child in the care of his mother, who may not have been aware of the possibility of her child sneaking out while she was in the bathroom. b. The nurse could have assigned another UAP to monitor the child or she could have clearly cautioned the mother not to leave her child unattended for any reason (rather, the mother should call if she needed to go to the bathroom or whatever). **3.** a. You perform a complete assessment and determine whether the patient is progressing as expected according to plan of care. For example, if the plan includes a critical path that states "chest tubes will be out by the second postoperative day," and the patient still has chest tubes, you've identified a variance in care. b. You should perform additional assessment to determine whether the delay is justified or whether actions need to be taken to improve the patient's likelihood of achieving the outcome. c. Additional assessments and interventions that may be required for the patient to progress may be omitted, resulting in harm to the patient or delays in recovery. d. If the patient is harmed, you may be accused of negligence. If there are delays in recovery, you may be accused of giving substandard care.

CRITICAL THINKING EXERCISE XVI

1. Patient records: 1. Communicate care to other health care professionals who need to be able to find out what you've done and how the patient's doing. 2. Help identify patterns of responses and changes in status. 3. Provide a foundation for evaluation, research, and improvement of the quality of care. 4. Create a legal document that may later be used in court to evaluate the type of care rendered. Your records can be your best friend or worst enemy—the best defense that you actually observed or did something is the fact that you made a note of it. 5. Supply validation for insurance purposes. The saying goes, "If it's not documented, they won't pay." **2.** You'll be more accurate when the information is fresh in your mind. Charting what you've done often jogs your mind to recognize when you've forgotten to do something *else* you should have done. **3. DAR:** D—States she feels like she's choking, but is afraid to cough because of incisional pain. A—Assisted to splint with pillow. R—Coughed up gray mucous plug. **DIE:** D—States she feels like she's choking, but is afraid to cough because of incisional pain. I—Assisted to splint incision with a pillow. E—Coughed up gray mucus plug. Lungs clear. **AIR-A:** A—States she feels like she's choking, but is afraid to cough because of incisional pain. I—Assisted to splint incision with a pillow. R—Coughed up gray mucus plug. Lungs clear. A—Emphasized importance of reporting pain that interferes with breathing. **4.** a. It's judgmental and has no supporting evidence. b. It has no supporting evidence—states opinion, not facts. **5.** You should have drawn a line through the note, then written the word *error,* followed by your initials.

CRITICAL THINKING EXERCISE XVII

Part I. 1) P 2) A 3) N. Insulin demand is affected by increased exercise. 4) P. 5) P. Fever and heat are also signs of infection.
Part II. Continue the plan if the patient hasn't achieved outcomes, but you haven't identified any factors that impeded or enhanced care. **Modify the plan** when outcomes haven't been achieved, and you've identified factors that enhanced or impeded care. **Terminate the plan** if the patient has achieved outcomes and demonstrates ability to care for himself.

CRITICAL THINKING EXERCISE XVIII

1. Information gained from these studies improves the quality and efficiency of patient care, and helps identify ways of improving nurses' job satisfaction. **2.** Considering all three types of evaluation—outcome (results), process (method), and structure (setting)—provides a comprehensive examination of care management. **3.** I'll follow policies and procedures carefully without skipping steps. I'll also pay attention to things that I'm doing that might make me prone to error and develop ways to prevent them (eg, ask people to wait when they want to talk to me and I'm pouring medications). I'll report things that make us all prone to error (eg, continually working with insufficient staff). I'll encourage my patients to take an active role in managing their health care.

Ethics Code and Practice Standards Related to Nursing Process

American Nurses Association Ethics Code[1]

As a nurse, you must:

- ✓ **Provide** services with respect for human dignity and the uniqueness of the client, unrestricted by considerations of social or economic status, personal attributes, or the nature of health problems.
- ✓ **Safeguard** the client's right to privacy by judiciously protecting information of a confidential nature; safeguard the client and public when health care and safety are affected by the incompetent, unethical, or illegal practice of any person.
- ✓ **Assume** responsibility and accountability for individual nursing judgments and actions.
- ✓ **Maintain** competence in nursing.
- ✓ **Exercise** informed judgment and use individual competence and qualifications as criteria in seeking consultation, accepting responsibilities, and delegating nursing activities to others.
- ✓ **Participate** in: (1) professional activities that contribute to the ongoing development of the profession's body of knowledge, (2) efforts to implement and improve standards of nursing, (3) efforts to establish and maintain conditions of employment conducive to high-quality nursing care, and (4) efforts to protect the public from misinformation and misrepresentation and to maintain the integrity of nursing.
- ✓ **Collaborate** with members of the health care professions and other citizens in promoting community and national efforts to meet the health needs of the public.

American Nurses Association (ANA) Practice Standards[2]

I **Assessment:** The nurse collects client health data.

II **Diagnosis:** The nurse analyzes assessment data in determining diagnoses.

III **Outcome Identification:** The nurse identifies expected outcomes individualized to the client.

IV **Planning:** The nurse develops a plan of care that prescribes interventions to attain expected outcomes.

V **Implementation:** The nurse implements the interventions identified in the plan of care.

VI **Evaluation:** The nurse evaluates the client's progress toward attainment of outcomes.

[1]Adapted from *Code for Nurses With Interpretive Statements* (ANA, 1985).
[2]From: American Nurses Association. (1998). *Standards of clinical practice* (2nd ed.). Washington, DC: American Nurses Publishing.

Canadian Nurses Association (CNA) Standard II[3]

Standard II. Nursing practice requires the effective use of the nursing process.

Nurses are required in any practice setting to do the following: (1) collection of data, (2) analysis of data, (3) planning of the intervention, (4) implementation of the intervention, and (5) evaluation.

---

[3]Summarized from *Canadian Nurses Association (CNA) Standards for Nursing Practice.* (1987). Prepared and revised by a Task Group to Develop a Definition of Nursing Practice and Standards for Nursing Practice. Ottawa: CNA.

B Example Critical Path/Care Map™*

*Adapted with permission from the Center for Case Management, South Natick, MA.

Brighton Medical Center Case CareMap™
Profile: Uncomplicated MI

Case Manager: _____   (Addressograph)

Patient Problem/ Nursing Diagnosis	DAY 1	DAY 2	DAY 3	DAY 4	DAY 5	DAY 6
Pain R/T ischemia	Pt. will verbalize pain or discomfort appropriately to RN	Pt. will be pain free	—	—	—	Pt. will be pain free at discharge
Activity intolerance R/T ischemia	Pt. will be able to tolerate BSC without chest pain Pt. can participate in "PT protocol" without chest pain	Pt. can participate in "PT protocol" without chest pain	—	—	—	Pt. will be discharged at anticipated activity tolerance as evidenced by B/P does not change by 20 torr and HR does not change by 20 BPM
Knowledge deficit R/T new MI	Pt. can state why admitted to hospital Pt. will understand the importance of notifying RN of chest pain	Pt. will demonstrate a readiness to learn Pt. will begin to read MI packet	Pt. will be able to state what an MI and angina are and risk factors & use of sublingual nitrates	Pt. demonstrates understanding of diet by making appropriate choices on menu Pt. can verbalize discharge needs	Pt. can verbalize community resources Pt. can take own pulse	Pt. can verbalize activity restrictions and rationale. Pt. can restate discharge instructions. Pt. will have completed all MI teaching packet goals
Anxiety R/T hospitalization	Pt. can verbalize fears and concerns related to hospitalization	—	Pt. displays appropriate coping skills	—	—	Pt. can identify appropriate resources and support systems
Potential for injury R/T bleeding (TPA)	Pt. will verbalize understanding of reasons to notify RN of signs of bleeding	—	—	—	—	Pt. can state rationale for risk factors of anticoagulation therapy

Critical Path					
Consults	Notify ER attending & family physician, Social Services, Quality Review, Case Manager	PT Dietary consultation	Social Services • home care referral	• Pharmacy consult (coumadin teaching)	
Tests	MCPs q 8° × 3 EKG, routine lab work/coag, CXR. O$_2$ sat	• ECG • MCP • 2 D echo • routine labs • O$_2$ sat	• ECG • schedule Holter monitor	Holter monitor	• coag. • routine labs • schedule stress test	• stress test
Treatments	I & O, weight, IV access, cardiac monitoring, B/P, V/S monitoring	• weight — Same as Day 1	D/C cardiac monitoring & transfer	IV access — Same as Day 3	IV access	D/C IV
Meds	• O$_2$ • Pa • Ntg • Reg meds • Lidocaine • MS • Sleeper Heparin • Tylenol • Beta blockers • Ca channel blockers and anxiety agent • Stool softener	Same • wean Lido • wean Ntg • O$_2$	Same wean Lido wean Ntg	Same Assess anticoag therapy (D/C heparin & consider ASA)		Discharge prescription with completed discharge form
Diet	Cardiac diet	—	—	—	—	
Activity	Bedrest with BSC ADL protocol	PT protocol —	—	—	— —	— —
Teaching	Orientation to unit & routine Dietary reading material	MI packet Progressive dietary teaching	—	Evaluate process & target problem areas • Coumadin teaching info bracelet	—	Discharge instruction review
Discharge Planning	Share CareMap if appropriate		Update to Social Service from QR transfer to general floor	As per Social Service	Consider outpatient needs	Discharge

C List of NIC Interventions and NOC Outcomes

Nursing Interventions Classification (NIC) Labels[1]

Abuse Protection Support
Abuse Protection Support: Child
Abuse Protection Support: Domestic Partner
Abuse Protection Support: Elder
Abuse Protection Support: Religious
Acid-Base Management
Acid-Base Management: Metabolic Acidosis
Acid-Base Management: Metabolic Alkalosis
Acid-Base Management: Respiratory Acidosis
Acid-Base Management: Respiratory Alkalosis
Acid-Base Monitoring
Active Listening
Activity Therapy
Acupressure
Admission Care
Airway Insertion and Stabilization
Airway Management
Airway Suctioning
Allergy Management
Amnioinfusion
Amputation Care
Analgesic Administration
Analgesic Administration: Intraspinal
Anaphylaxis Management
Anesthesia Administration
Anger Control Assistance
Animal-Assisted Therapy
Anticipatory Guidance
Anxiety Reduction
Area Restriction

Art Therapy
Artificial Airway Management
Aspiration Precautions
Assertiveness Training
Attachment Promotion
Autogenic Training
Autotransfusion

Bathing
Bed Rest Care
Bedside Laboratory Testing
Behavior Management
Behavior Management: Overactivity/Inattention
Behavior Management: Self-Harm
Behavior Management: Sexual
Behavior Modification
Behavior Modifications: Social Skills
Bibliotherapy
Biofeedback
Birthing
Bladder Irrigation
Bleeding Precautions
Bleeding Reduction
Bleeding Reduction: Antepartum Uterus
Bleeding Reduction: Gastrointestinal
Bleeding Reduction: Nasal
Bleeding Reduction: Postpartum Uterus
Bleeding Reduction: Wound
Blood Products Administration
Body Image Enhancement
Body Mechanics Promotion
Bottle Feeding

Bowel Incontinence Care
Bowel Incontinence Care: Encopresis
Bowel Irrigation
Bowel Management
Bowel Training
Breast Examination
Breastfeeding Assistance

Calming Technique
Cardiac Care
Cardiac Care: Acute
Cardiac Care: Rehabilitative
Cardiac Precautions
Caregiver Support
Case Management
Cast Care: Maintenance
Cast Care: Wet
Cerebral Edema Management
Cerebral Perfusion Promotion
Cesarean Section Care
Chemotherapy Management
Chest Physiotherapy
Childbirth Preparation
Circulatory Care: Arterial Insufficiency
Circulatory Care: Mechanical Assist Device
Circulatory Care: Venous Insufficiency
Circulatory Precautions
Code Management
Cognitive Restructuring
Cognitive Stimulation
Communicable Disease Management

[1]From McCloskey, J., Bulechek, G. (Eds.). (2000). *Nursing interventions classification (NIC): Iowa intervention project* (3rd ed.). St. Louis, MO: Mosby. Reprinted with permission.

Communication Enhancement: Hearing Deficit

Communication Enhancement: Speech Deficit

Communication Enhancement: Visual Deficit

Community Disaster Preparedness

Community Health Development

Complex Relationship Building

Conflict Mediation

Conscious Sedation

Constipation/Impaction Management

Consultation

Contact Lens Care

Controlled Substance Checking

Coping Enhancement

Cost Containment

Cough Enhancement

Counseling

Crisis Intervention

Critical Path Development

Culture Brokerage

Cutaneous Stimulation

Decision-Making Support

Delegation

Delirium Management

Delusion Management

Dementia Management

Developmental Care

Developmental Enhancement: Adolescent

Developmental Enhancement: Child

Diarrhea Management

Diet Staging

Discharge Planning

Distraction

Documentation

Dressing

Dying Care

Dysreflexia Management

Dysrhythmia Management

Ear Care

Eating Disorders Management

Electrolyte Management

Electrolyte Management: Hypercalcemia

Electrolyte Management: Hyperkalemia

Electrolyte Management: Hypermagnesemia

Electrolyte Management: Hypernatremia

Electrolyte Management: Hyperphosphatemia

Electrolyte Management: Hypocalcemia

Electrolyte Management: Hypokalemia

Electrolyte Management: Hypomagnesemia

Electrolyte Management: Hyponatremia

Electrolyte Management: Hypophosphatemia

Electrolyte Monitoring

Electronic Fetal Monitoring: Antepartum

Electronic Fetal Monitoring: Intrapartum

Elopement Precautions

Embolus Care: Peripheral

Embolus Care: Pulmonary

Embolus Precautions

Emergency Care

Emergency Cart Checking

Emotional Support

Endotracheal Extubation

Energy Management

Enteral Tube Feeding

Environmental Management

Environmental Management: Attachment Process

Environmental Management: Comfort

Environmental Management: Community

Environmental Management: Home Preparation

Environmental Management: Safety

Environmental Management: Violence Prevention

Environmental Management: Worker Safety

Environmental Risk Protection

Examination Assistance

Exercise Promotion

Exercise Promotion: Strength Training

Exercise Promotion: Stretching

Exercise Therapy: Ambulation

Exercise Therapy: Balance

Exercise Therapy: Joint Mobility

Exercise Therapy: Muscle Control

Eye Care

Fall Prevention

Family Integrity Promotion

Family Integrity Promotion: Childbearing Family

Family Involvement Promotion

Family Mobilization

Family Planning: Contraception

Family Planning: Infertility

Family Planning: Unplanned Pregnancy

Family Process Maintenance

Family Support

Family Therapy

Feeding

Fertility Preservation

Fever Treatment

Financial Resource Assistance

Fire-Setting Precautions

First Aid

Fiscal Resource Management

Flatulence Reduction

Fluid Management

Fluid/Electrolyte Management

Fluid Monitoring

Fluid Resuscitation

Foot Care

Forgiveness Facilitation

Gastrointestinal Intubation

Genetic Counseling

Grief Work Facilitation

Grief Work Facilitation: Perinatal Death

Guilt Work Facilitation

Hair Care

Hallucination Management

Health Care Information Exchange

Health Education

Health Policy Monitoring

Health Screening

Health System Guidance

Heat Exposure Treatment
Heat/Cold Application
Hemodialysis Therapy
Hemodynamic Regulation
Hemofiltration Therapy
Hemorrhage Control
High-Risk Pregnancy Care
Home Maintenance Assistance
Hope Instillation
Humor
Hyperglycemia Management
Hypervolemia Management
Hypnosis
Hypoglycemia Management
Hypothermia Treatment
Hypovolemia Management

Immunization/Vaccination
    Management
Impulse Control Training
Incident Reporting
Incision Site Care
Infant Care
Infection Control
Infection Control: Intraoperative
Infection Protection
Insurance Authorization
Intracranial Pressure (ICP)
    Monitoring
Intrapartal Care
Intrapartal Care: High-Risk
    Delivery
Intravenous (IV) Insertion
Intravenous (IV) Therapy
Invasive Hemodynamic
    Monitoring

Kangaroo Care

Labor Induction
Labor Suppression
Laboratory Data Interpretation
Lactation Counseling
Lactation Suppression
Laser Precautions
Latex Precautions
Learning Facilitation
Learning Readiness
    Enhancement
Leech Therapy
Limit Setting

Malignant Hyperthermia
    Precautions
Mechanical Ventilation
Mechanical Ventilatory Weaning
Medication Administration
Medication Administration: Ear
Medication Administration: Enteral
Medication Administration:
    Epidural
Medication Administration: Eye
Medication Administration:
    Inhalation
Medication Administration:
    Interpleural
Medication Administration:
    Intradermal
Medication Administration:
    Intramuscular (IM)
Medication Administration:
    Intraosseous
Medication Administration:
    Intravenous (IV)
Medication Administration: Oral
Medication Administration: Rectal
Medication Administration: Skin
Medication Administration:
    Subcutaneous
Medication Administration:
    Vaginal
Medication Administration:
    Ventricular Reservoir
Medication Management
Medication Prescribing
Meditation Facilitation
Memory Training
Milieu Therapy
Mood Management
Multidisciplinary Care
    Conference
Music Therapy
Mutual Goal Setting

Nail Care
Nausea Management
Neurologic Monitoring
Newborn Care
Newborn Monitoring
Nonnutritive Sucking
Normalization Promotion
Nutrition Management
Nutrition Therapy

Nutritional Counseling
Nutritional Monitoring

Oral Health Maintenance
Oral Health Promotion
Oral Health Restoration
Order Transcription
Organ Procurement
Ostomy Care
Oxygen Therapy

Pain Management
Parent Education: Adolescent
Parent Education: Childrearing
    Family
Parent Education: Infant
Parenting Promotion
Pass Facilitation
Patient Contracting
Patient-Controlled Analgesia
    (PCA) Assistance
Patient Rights Protection
Peer Review
Pelvic Muscle Exercise
Perineal Care
Peripheral Sensation Management
Peripherally Inserted Central (PIC)
    Catheter Care
Peritoneal Dialysis Therapy
Pessary Management
Phlebotomy: Arterial Blood
    Sample
Phlebotomy: Blood Unit
    Acquisition
Phlebotomy: Venous Blood
    Sample
Phototherapy: Neonate
Physical Restraint
Physician Support
Pneumatic Tourniquet Precautions
Positioning
Positioning: Intraoperative
Positioning: Neurologic
Positioning: Wheelchair
Postanesthesia Care
Postmortem Care
Postpartal Care
Preceptor: Employee
Preceptor: Student
Preconception Counseling
Pregnancy Termination Care

Prenatal Care
Preoperative Coordination
Preparatory Sensory Information
Presence
Pressure Management
Pressure Ulcer Care
Pressure Ulcer Prevention
Product Evaluation
Program Development
Progressive Muscle Relaxation
Prompted Voiding
Prosthesis Care
Pruritus Management

Quality Monitoring

Radiation Therapy Management
Rape-Trauma Treatment
Reality Orientation
Recreation Therapy
Rectal Prolapse Management
Referral
Religious Addiction Prevention
Religious Ritual Enhancement
Reminiscence Therapy
Reproductive Technology
   Management
Research Data Collection
Resiliency Promotion
Respiratory Monitoring
Respite Care
Resuscitation
Resuscitation: Fetus
Resuscitation: Neonate
Risk Identification
Risk Identification: Childbearing
   Family
Risk Identification: Genetic
Role Enhancement

Seclusion
Security Enhancement
Seizure Management
Seizure Precautions
Self-Awareness Enhancement
Self-Care Assistance
Self-Care Assistance:
   Bathing/Hygiene
Self-Care Assistance:
   Dressing/Grooming
Self-Care Assistance: Feeding

Self-Care Assistance: Toileting
Self-Esteem Enhancement
Self-Modification Assistance
Self-Responsibility Facilitation
Sexual Counseling
Shift Report
Shock Management
Shock Management: Cardiac
Shock Management: Vasogenic
Shock Management: Volume
Shock Prevention
Sibling Support
Simple Guided Imagery
Simple Massage
Simple Relaxation Therapy
Skin Care: Topical Treatments
Skin Surveillance
Sleep Enhancement
Smoking Cessation Assistance
Socialization Enhancement
Specimen Management
Spiritual Growth Facilitation
Spiritual Support
Splinting
Sports-Injury Prevention: Youth
Staff Development
Staff Supervision
Subarachnoid Hemorrhage
   Precautions
Substance Use Prevention
Substance Use Treatment
Substance Use Treatment: Alcohol
   Withdrawal
Substance Use Treatment: Drug
   Withdrawal
Substance Use Treatment:
   Overdose
Suicide Prevention
Supply Management
Support Group
Support System Enhancement
Surgical Assistance
Surgical Precautions
Surgical Preparation
Surveillance
Surveillance: Community
Surveillance: Late Pregnancy
Surveillance: Remote
   Electronic
Surveillance: Safety
Sustenance Support

Suturing
Swallowing Therapy

Teaching: Disease Process
Teaching: Group
Teaching: Individual
Teaching: Infant Nutrition
Teaching: Infant Safety
Teaching: Preoperative
Teaching: Prescribed
   Activity/Exercise
Teaching: Prescribed Diet
Teaching: Prescribed Medication
Teaching: Procedure/Treatment
Teaching: Psychomotor Skill
Teaching: Safe Sex
Teaching: Sexuality
Teaching: Toddler Nutrition
Teaching: Toddler Safety
Technology Management
Telephone Consultation
Telephone Follow-Up
Temperature Regulation
Temperature Regulation:
   Intraoperative
Therapeutic Play
Therapeutic Touch
Therapy Group
Total Parenteral Nutrition (TPN)
   Administration
Touch
Traction/Immobilization Care
Transcutaneous Electrical Nerve
   Stimulation (TENS)
Transport
Triage: Disaster
Triage: Emergency Center
Triage: Telephone
Truth Telling
Tube Care
Tube Care: Chest
Tube Care: Gastrointestinal
Tube Care: Umbilical Line
Tube Care: Urinary
Tube Care: Ventriculostomy/
   Lumbar Drain

Ultrasonography: Limited
   Obstetric
Unilateral Neglect Management
Urinary Bladder Training

Urinary Catheterization
Urinary Catheterization:
  Intermittent
Urinary Elimination Management
Urinary Habit Training
Urinary Incontinence Care
Urinary Incontinence Care: Enuresis
Urinary Retention Care

Values Clarification
Vehicle Safety Promotion
Venous Access Devices (VAD)
  Maintenance
Ventilation Assistance
Visitation Facilitation
Vital Signs Monitoring
Vomiting Management

Weight Gain Assistance
Weight Management
Weight Reduction Assistance
Wound Care
Wound Care: Closed Drainage
Wound Irrigation

Nursing Outcomes Classifications (NOC) Approved for Clinical Testing[2]

Abuse Cessation
Abuse Protection
Abuse Recovery: Emotional
Abuse Recovery: Financial
Abuse Recovery: Physical
Abuse Recovery: Sexual
Abusive Behavior Self-Control
Acceptance: Health Status
Activity Tolerance
Adherence Behavior
Aggression Control
Ambulation: Walking
Ambulation: Wheelchair
Anxiety Control
Aspiration Control
Asthma Control

Balance
Blood Glucose Control
Blood Transfusion Reaction
  Control
Body Image
Body Positioning: Self-Initiated
Bone Healing
Bowel Continence
Bowel Elimination
Breastfeeding Establishment:
  Infant
Breastfeeding Establishment:
  Maternal
Breastfeeding: Maintenance
Breastfeeding: Weaning

Cardiac Pump Effectiveness

Caregiver Adaptation to Patient
  Institutionalization
Caregiver Emotional Health
Caregiver Home Care Readiness
Caregiver Lifestyle Disruption
Caregiver-Patient Relationship
Caregiver Performance: Direct Care
Caregiver Performance: Indirect
  Care
Caregiver Physical Health
Caregiver Stressors
Caregiver Well-Being
Caregiving Endurance Potential
Child Adaptation to Hospitalization
Child Development: 2 Months
Child Development: 4 Months
Child Development: 6 Months
Child Development: 12 Months
Child Development: 2 Years
Child Development: 3 Years
Child Development: 4 Years
Child Development: 5 Years
Child Development: Middle
  Childhood (6–11 Years)
Child Development: Adolescence
  (12–17 Years)
Circulation Status
Coagulation Status
Cognitive Ability
Cognitive Orientation
Comfort Level
Communication Ability
Communication: Expressive
  Ability

Communication: Receptive Ability
Community Competence
Community Health Status
Community Health: Immunity
Community Risk Control: Chronic
  Disease
Community Risk Control:
  Communicable Disease
Community Risk Control: Lead
  Exposure
Compliance Behavior
Concentration
Coping

Decision Making
Depression Control
Depression Level
Dialysis Access Integrity
Dignified Dying
Distorted Thought Control

Electrolyte & Acid-Base Balance
Endurance
Energy Conservation

Family Coping
Family Environment: Internal
Family Functioning
Family Health Status
Family Integrity
Family Normalization
Family Participation in
  Professional Care
Fear Control

[2]From Johnson, M., Maas, M., et al. (Eds.). (2000). *Nursing outcomes classification* (2nd ed.). St. Louis, MO: Mosby. Reprinted with permission.

Fetal Status: Antepartum
Fetal Status: Intrapartum
Fluid Balance

Grief Resolution
Growth

Health Beliefs
Health Beliefs: Perceived Ability
  to Perform
Health Beliefs: Perceived Control
Health Beliefs: Perceived
  Resources
Health Beliefs: Perceived Threat
Health Orientation
Health Promoting Behavior
Health Seeking Behavior
Hearing Compensation Behavior
Hope
Hydration

Identity
Immobility Consequences:
  Physiological
Immobility Consequences: Psycho-
  Cognitive
Immune Hypersensitivity Control
Immune Status
Immunization Behavior
Impulse Control
Infection Status
Information Processing

Joint Movement: Active
Joint Movement: Passive

Knowledge: Breastfeeding
Knowledge: Child Safety
Knowledge: Conception Prevention
Knowledge: Diabetes Management
Knowledge: Diet
Knowledge: Disease Process
Knowledge: Energy Conservation
Knowledge: Fertility Promotion
Knowledge: Health Behaviors
Knowledge: Health Promotion
Knowledge: Health Resources
Knowledge: Illness Care
Knowledge: Infant Care
Knowledge: Infection Control

Knowledge: Labor & Delivery
Knowledge: Maternal-Child Health
Knowledge: Medication
Knowledge: Personal Safety
Knowledge: Postpartum
Knowledge: Preconception
Knowledge: Pregnancy
Knowledge: Prescribed Activity
Knowledge: Sexual Functioning
Knowledge: Substance Use Control
Knowledge: Treatment Procedure(s)
Knowledge: Treatment Regimen

Leisure Participation
Loneliness

Maternal Status: Antepartum
Maternal Status: Intrapartum
Maternal Status: Postpartum
Medication Response
Memory
Mobility Level
Mood Equilibrium
Muscle Function

Neglect Recovery
Neurological Status
Neurological Status: Autonomic
Neurological Status: Central Motor
  Control
Neurological Status:
  Consciousness
Neurological Status: Cranial
  Sensory/Motor Function
Neurological Status: Spinal
  Sensory/Motor Function
Newborn Adaptation
Nutritional Status
Nutritional Status: Biochemical
  Measures
Nutritional Status: Body Mass
Nutritional Status: Energy
Nutritional Status: Food & Fluid
  Intake
Nutritional Status: Nutrient Intake

Oral Health

Pain Control
Pain: Disruptive Effects

Pain Level
Pain: Psychological Response
Parent–Infant Attachment
Parenting
Parenting: Social Safety
Participation: Health Care
  Decisions
Physical Aging Status
Physical Fitness
Physical Maturation: Female
Physical Maturation: Male
Play Participation
Prenatal Health Behavior
Preterm Infant Organization
Psychomotor Energy
Psychosocial Adjustment: Life
  Change

Quality of Life

Respiratory Status: Airway
  Patency
Respiratory Status: Gas
  Exchange
Respiratory Status: Ventilation
Rest
Risk Control
Risk Control: Alcohol Use
Risk Control: Cancer
Risk Control: Cardiovascular
  Health
Risk Control: Drug Use
Risk Control: Hearing Impairment
Risk Control: Sexually Transmitted
  Diseases (STDs)
Risk Control: Tobacco Use
Risk Control: Unintended
  Pregnancy
Risk Control: Visual Impairment
Risk Detection
Role Performance

Safety Behavior: Fall Prevention
Safety Behavior: Home Physical
  Environment
Safety Behavior: Personal
Safety Status: Falls Occurrence
Safety Status: Physical Injury
Self-Care: Activities of Daily
  Living (ADL)

Self-Care: Bathing
Self-Care: Dressing
Self-Care: Eating
Self-Care: Grooming
Self-Care: Hygiene
Self-Care: Instrumental Activities
of Daily Living (IADL)
Self-Care: Non-Parenteral
Medication
Self-Care: Oral Hygiene
Self-Care: Parenteral Medication
Self-Care: Toileting
Self-Direction of Care
Self-Esteem
Self-Mutilation Restraint
Sensory Function: Cutaneous
Sensory Function: Hearing
Sensory Function: Proprioception
Sensory Function: Taste & Smell
Sensory Function: Vision
Sexual Functioning
Sexual Identity: Acceptance
Skeletal Function
Sleep

Social Interaction Skills
Social Involvement
Social Support
Spiritual Well-Being
Substance Addiction Consequences
Suffering Level
Suicide Self-Restraint
Swallowing Status
Swallowing Status: Esophageal
Phase
Swallowing Status: Oral Phase
Swallowing Status: Pharyngeal
Phase
Symptom Control
Symptom Severity
Symptom Severity: Perimenopause
Symptom Severity: Premenstrual
Syndrome (PMS)
Systemic Toxin Clearance: Dialysis

Thermoregulation
Thermoregulation: Neonate
Tissue Integrity: Skin & Mucous
Membranes

Tissue Perfusion: Abdominal
Organs
Tissue Perfusion: Cardiac
Tissue Perfusion: Cerebral
Tissue Perfusion: Peripheral
Tissue Perfusion: Pulmonary
Transfer Performance
Treatment Behavior: Illness or
Injury

Urinary Continence
Urinary Elimination

Vision Compensation
Behavior
Vital Signs Status

Weight Control
Well-Being
Will to Live
Wound Healing: Primary
Intention
Wound Healing: Secondary
Intention

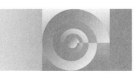# Glossary

Accountable. Being responsible and answerable for something.

Advanced practice nurse (APN). See Advanced practice registered nurse.

Advanced practice registered nurse (APRN). A nurse who, by virtue of credentials (completion of a masters program and certification) has a wide scope of authority to act (may include treating medical problems and prescribing medications).

Affective domain outcomes. Measurable goals that deal with changes in attitudes, feelings, or values.

Analyze. To examine and categorize pieces of information to determine where they might fit into the whole picture.

Anticipatory. Expected or foreseen.

Assessment. The first step of the nursing process, during which you gather and organize data (information) in preparation for the second step, Diagnosis.

Assessment tool. A printed form used to ensure key information is gathered and recorded during Assessment.

Authority. The power or right to act, prescribe, or make a final decision.

Baseline data. Information that describes the status of a problem before treatment begins.

Caring behavior. A way of acting that shows understanding and respect for others' ideals, values, feelings, needs, and desires.

CareMap™. See Critical pathway.

Case management. An approach to patient care that aims to improve patient outcomes and satisfaction while reducing overall cost and length or incidence of hospital stays.

Care partner. See Unlicensed assistive personnel (UAP).

Care variance. See Variance in care.

Client-centered outcome. A statement describing a measurable behavior of a client, family, or group that reflects the desired result of interventions (that the

problem, or problems, are prevented, resolved, or controlled).

Client goal. See Client-centered outcome.

Clinical pathway. See Critical pathway.

Collaborative problem. Potential complications of trauma, disease, or treatment (Carpenito, 1997b).

Cognitive domain outcomes. Measurable goals that deal with acquiring knowledge or intellectual skills.

Competence. The quality of having the necessary knowledge and skill to perform an action in a safe and appropriate manner.

Critical. Characterized by careful and exact evaluation and judgment.

Critical pathway. A standard plan that predicts the course of recovery and day-by-day care required to achieve outcomes for a specific health problem within a specific time frame.

Critical thinking. See Display 1–7 on page 23.

Cues. Pieces of information that prompt you to make a judgment.

Data. Pieces of information.

Data base assessment. Comprehensive data collected on initial contact with the patient to gain information about all aspects of the patient's health.

Data base form. See Assessment tool.

Deficient. Inadequate in amount, quality or degree; not sufficient; incomplete.

Defining characteristics. A cluster of cues (signs, symptoms, and risk [related] factors) often associated with a specific nursing diagnosis.

Depleted. Emptied wholly or in part; exhausted of.

Diagnostic error. When a health problem has been overlooked or incorrectly identified.

Direct care interventions. Actions performed through interaction with patients (eg, helping someone out of bed, teaching someone about diabetes).

Discharge goal. A client-centered outcome that describes what the patient will be able to do on discharge from a facility.

Definitive diagnosis. The most specific, most correct, diagnosis.

Definitive interventions. The most specific treatment required to prevent, resolve, or control a health problem.

Delegation. The transfer of responsibility for the performance of an activity while retaining accountability (ANA, 1993).

Diagnose. To make a judgment and identify a problem or strength based on evidence from an assessment.

Diagnosis. (1) The second step of the nursing process. (2) The *process* of analyzing data and putting related cues together to make judgments about health status. (3) The opinion or judgment that's drawn after the diagnostic process is completed.

Direct data. Information gained directly from the patient.

Diagnostic reasoning. A method of thinking that involves specific, deliberate use of critical thinking to reach conclusions about health status.

Diagnostic statement. A phrase that clearly describes a diagnosis; includes the problem name, etiology, and any evidence confirming the diagnosis.

Empathy. Understanding another's feelings or perceptions, but not sharing the same feelings or point of view (compare with Sympathy).

Etiology. Something known to cause a disease. The terms *risk factors* and *etiology* may be used interchangeably.

Expedite. To accomplish something quickly.

Focus assessment. Data collection that concentrates on gathering more information about a specific problem or condition.

Guidelines. See Display 4–1 on page 127.

Habits of inquiry. Thinking habits that enhance your ability to search for the truth (eg, following rules of logic).

Humanistic. See Caring behavior.

Indicator. Concrete, observable behaviors or states (eg, joint movement, absence of skin redness) that can be observed to determine outcome achievement.

Indirect care interventions. Actions performed away from the patient but on behalf of a patient or group of patients. These actions are aimed at management of the health care environment and interdisciplinary collaboration.

Indirect data. Information gained from sources other than the patient (eg, someone's wife).

Inference. How someone perceives or interprets a cue (eg, one person may perceive a person's silence as acceptance, whereas another may interpret it as defiance).

Intervention. Something done to maximize comfort and human functioning (eg, turning someone every 2 hours is an intervention to maintain skin integrity and assist lung function).

Intuition. Knowing something without having supporting evidence.

Judgment. An opinion that's made after analyzing and synthesizing information.

Life processes. Events or changes that occur during one's lifetime (eg, growing up, aging, maturing, becoming a parent, moving, separations, losses).

Long-term goal. An objective that's expected to be achieved over a relatively long time period, usually weeks or months.

Medical diagnosis. A problem requiring definitive diagnosis by a qualified physician or advanced practice nurse.

Medical domain. Activities and actions a physician is legally qualified to perform or prescribe.

Medical orders. Interventions ordered by a physician or advanced practice nurse to treat a medical problem.

Medical process. The method physicians use to expedite diagnosis and treatment of diseases or trauma. The medical process focuses mainly on problems with structure and function of organs or systems.

Multidisciplinary plan. A plan that's developed collaboratively by key members of the health care team (eg, nursing, physical therapy, medicine).

Need. A requirement that, if fulfilled, reduces stress and promotes a sense of adequacy and well-being.

Nurse extender. See Unlicensed assistive personnel (UAP).

Nursing assistant. See Unlicensed assistive personnel (UAP).

Nursing diagnosis. A clinical judgment about an individual, family, or community response to actual or potential health problems and life processes.

Nursing diagnoses provide the basis for selection of nursing interventions to achieve outcomes for which the nurse is accountable (NANDA, 1990). Nursing diagnoses often are called *human responses* because we, as nurses, focus on how people *are responding* to changes in health or life circumstances (eg, how they're responding to illness or to becoming a parent).

Nursing domain.   Activities and actions a nurse is legally qualified to perform or prescribe.

Nurse-prescribed intervention.   An action a nurse may legally order or initiate independently.

Nursing process.   A systematic, outcome-oriented method that nurses use to expedite diagnosis and treatment of actual and potential health problems.

Objective data.   Information that's measurable and observable (eg, blood pressure, pulse, diagnostic studies).

Outcome.   The result of prescribed interventions; usually refers to the *desired result* of interventions (ie, that the problem is prevented, resolved, or controlled) and includes a specific time frame for when the goal is expected to be achieved.

Outcome-based practice.   Health care practice that's focused on achieving desired results efficiently (ie, that patients achieve the expected results of care).

Palliative care.   Care that alleviates pain and suffering but doesn't cure.

Patient care technician.   See Unlicensed assistive personnel (UAP).

Physician-prescribed (or delegated) intervention.   An action ordered by a physician for a nurse or another health care professional to perform (Carpenito, 1997b).

Policies.   See Display 4–1 on page 127.

Primary care provider.   The health care professional designated to be in charge of managing the patient's major medical problems (may be a physician, advance practice nurse, or physician's assistant.

Proactive.   A way of thinking and behaving that accepts responsibility for one's actions and takes initiative to plan ahead to anticipate and prevent problems before they happen (comes from "act before").

Procedures.   See Display 4–1 on page 127.

Protocols.   See Display 4–1 on page 127.

Prognosis.   The predicted course or outcome of disease or trauma.

Psychomotor outcomes.   Measurable goals that deal with acquiring skills that require deliberate, specific muscle coordination to perform an activity (eg, walking with crutches).

Qualified.   Having the knowledge, skill, and authority to perform an action.

Quality care.   Cost-effective health care that increases the probability of achieving desired results and decreases the probability of undesired results.

Related factor.   Something known to be *associated with* a specific diagnosis. See Risk factor.

Risk factor.   Something known to cause or *contribute to* a specific problem (eg, *decreased vision* is a related factor of *Risk for Injury*).

Risk (potential) diagnosis.   A health problem that may develop if preventive actions aren't taken.

Sign.   Objective data that indicate an abnormality.

Subjective data.   Information the patient or client tells the nurse during Assessment (usually charted as "Patient states. . . .").

Short-term goal.   A client-centered outcome that's achieved as a stepping stone to reaching a long-term goal.

Standards.   See Display 4–1 on page 127.

Standard care plan.   See Display 4–1 on page 127.

Standard of care.   See Display 4–1 on page 127.

Standard of practice.   See Display 4–1 on page 127.

Standards of professional performance.   See Display 4–1 on page 127.

Sympathy.   Sharing the same feelings as another (compare with Empathy).

Symptom.   Subjective data that indicate an abnormality.

Syndrome diagnosis.   A cluster of nursing diagnoses often associated with a specific situation or event.

Uniform nursing language: A single system with a set of characters, conventions, and rules for conveying information about nursing practice; a system resulting from mapping terms among multiple nursing vocabulary.

Unlicensed assistive personnel (UAP).   Someone without a license to practice nursing who is hired to assist nurses in care delivery. These individuals may have a variety of job titles (eg, nursing assistant, nurse extender, care partner, patient care technician) and have varied job descriptions and capabilities.

Variance in care. When a patient hasn't achieved activities or outcomes by the time frame noted on a critical path. A variance in care triggers additional assessment to determine whether the delay is justified or whether actions need to be taken to improve the patient's likelihood of achieving the outcome. (Iyer, 1999).

Validation. The process of making sure the information you collect is factual and complete.

Wellness diagnosis. A clinical judgment about an individual, family, or community in transition from a specific level of wellness to a higher level of wellness (NANDA, 1990).

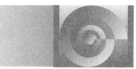

Index

Note: Page numbers followed by *f* indicate figures; page numbers followed by *t* indicate tables.